Transcultural
Health Care

Transcultural
Health Care

EDITORS:

George Henderson, Ph.D.
Martha Primeaux, R.N., M.S.N.

▲▼ Addison-Wesley Publishing Company
Medical/Nursing Division ● Menlo Park, California
Reading, Massachusetts ● London ● Amsterdam
Don Mills, Ontario ● Sydney

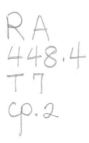
Sponsoring Editor: Pat Franklin
Production Coordinator: Madeleine Dreyfack
Production Editor: Nancy Sjoberg
Cover Designer: Judith Sager
Book Designer: Nancy Sjoberg

Library of Congress Cataloging in Publication Data

Main entry under title:
Transcultural health care.

    Includes index.
    1. Minorities—Medical care—United States.
2. Medical anthropology.   3. Medical anthropology—
United States.   4. Folk medicine—United States.
I. Henderson, George, 1932-   .   II. Primeaux,
Martha, 1930-   .   [DNLM: 1. Cross-cultural
comparison.   2. Health services.   3. Ethnic groups.
W 84.1 T771]
RA448.4.T7   362.1'0973   80-39991
ISBN 0-201-03237-6
ISBN 0-201-03452-2 (pbk.)

ABCDEFGHIJ-MA-83210

▲▼ Addison-Wesley Publishing Company
   Medical/Nursing Division
   2725 Sand Hill Road
   Menlo Park, California 94025

Preface

PURPOSE OF THIS BOOK

Basic human rights are violated every day in most American health care facilities. In a June '79 American Nurses' Association Commission on Human Rights hearing in Albuquerque, New Mexico, several health care professionals testified that the health care system discriminates against ethnic minority patients, nurses, and other health caregivers. Shirley A. Smuyak, Associate Dean for Research and Graduate Director of Nursing at Rutgers State University, cautioned, "At the minimum, we need to sensitize every health care professional to the cultural aspects of client care. At the other end—the large, complex social arena—we need to influence the government's expenditure of dollars to support theoretical studies of culture and the impact it has on health care."

Ample research findings support the assumption that to be optimally effective, every health care practitioner should have a minimal understanding of cultures other than her or his own. This book, intended for nurses and health practitioners, focuses primarily on Third World cultures; however, attention is also given to people of other backgrounds. In addition, considerable discussion centers on the subculture of poverty, which is the most pervasive negative characteristic of all cultures.

ORGANIZATION

This book is divided into three parts: Sociocultural Dimensions of Health Care, Folk Medicine, and Patient Care. The areas covered range from general and theoretical concerns to historical perspectives and finally to health care suggestions. Information is presented in a spiral arrangement, i.e. some topics discussed briefly in Part One are treated again, but in greater detail, in Parts Two and Three. We have found this format to be an educationally sound way of expanding on relevant issues and problems.

No two persons could attempt to write all the chapters in this book. Thus, rather than present a superficial treatment, we decided to draw on the expertise of several writers. More than ninety percent of the essays are written or co-authored by health care practitioners, and forty percent of the essays are original.

CONTENT

Each essay was judiciously written and selected to achieve four objectives: 1) to make our readers aware of cultural factors which impact positively or negatively on their behavior as well as that of their patients; 2) to explore multidisciplinary research on the premise that most Third World people receive inadequate health care; 3) to help our readers become more aware of their own beliefs, attitudes, and behaviors; and 4) to provide practical suggestions for more effective patient/client care.

Implicit throughout this text is the belief that *how* patient/client care is given is as important as *what* patient/client care is given. In human relations terms, the former is the *process* of helping, while the latter is the *content*. We know that there are effective, culturally aware caregivers scattered throughout the United States. Our concern is that they are too few in number. With these thoughts in mind we could have focused on the reprehensible *isms*—racism, sexism, and elitism. But while this approach would tell us what is wrong, it would not tell us what to do about it. For this reason, we place our major focus on strategies for change.

SPECIAL FEATURES

The introductory chapters at the beginning of each part are intended to be the threads holding the various essays together. However, each essay can also stand alone as a valuable compilation of information. Basic comprehensive data are provided in the end-of-part summaries. An obvious hazard to this approach is data overload. However, after much deliberation, we concluded that it is better to provide too much information than too little.

FINAL WORDS

If this book serves as an impetus for other books devoted to transcultural health care, our energy will have been well spent. If this book helps practitioners to provide more effective care, our dream will become a reality. But if neither of these goals is achieved, the intellectual growth we have attained will have made the effort worthwhile.

ACKNOWLEDGMENTS

We are grateful to the authors and publishers who granted us permissions to reprint their essays, and to Karin Weldin who critiqued them. Special thanks also go to Kris Gates, copy editor, and Nancy Sjoberg, production editor, who ensured quality editing and production of this manuscript. Finally, we thank Kristin Libbee for editorial assistance, and Susan Matthews and Leslie Gillies for typing portions of the manuscript.

George Henderson
Martha Primeaux
January 1981

List of Contributors

Murray Alpert, Ph.D., Professor and Director of Psychology, New York University School of Medicine, New York City

Teresa Campbell, M.S., Professor, Department of Nursing, California State College, San Francisco

Betty Chang, R.N., D.N.S., Assistant Professor, School of Nursing, University of California, Los Angeles

George M. Foster, Ph.D., Professor, Department of Anthropology, University of California, Berkeley

Mary L. Gottesfeld, M.S.S., Psychotherapist, New York City; Editor, *Clinical Social Work Journal*

Donn V. Hart, Ph.D., Professor, Department of Anthropology, Northern Illinois University, DeKalb

George Henderson, Ph.D., S. N. Goldman Professor of Human Relations and Chairperson, Department of Human Relations, Professor of Education and Associate Professor of Sociology, University of Oklahoma, Norman

Martin Kesselman, M.D., Professor of Clinical Psychiatry, Downstate Medical Center, Brooklyn; Director of Psychiatry, Kings County Hospital, Brooklyn

Luis R. Marcos, M.D., Med. Sc.D., Associate Professor of Psychiatry, New York University School of Medicine, New York City

Theresa Overfield, R.N., Ph.D., Associate Professor and Director of Research, College of Nursing, Brigham Young University, Salt Lake City

Martha Primeaux, R.N., M.S.N., Associate Professor and Assistant Dean, Director of Baccalaureate Program, College of Nursing, University of Oklahoma, Oklahoma City

Lora B. Roach, R.N., M.S.N., Assistant Professor, College of Nursing, University of Texas, Fort Worth

Ildaura Murrillo-Rohde, F.A.A.N., Ph.D., Professor and Associate Dean, School of Nursing, University of Washington, Seattle

Clarissa S. Scott, Ph.D., Instructor of Social Anthropology, Department of Psychiatry, University of Miami School of Medicine, Miami

Loudell F. Snow, Ph.D., Associate Professor, Department of Anthropology, Michigan State University, East Lansing

Raphella Sohier, R.N., M.S.N., Lecturer, College of Nursing, Wayne State University, Detroit

Donna Neal Thomas, B.S.N., M.S., Assistant Professor, College of Nursing, University of Oklahoma, Oklahoma City

Virgil J. Vogel, Ph.D., Professor, Department of Social Science, Truman College, City Colleges of Chicago, Chicago

Leonel Urcuyo, M.D., Assistant Professor of Clinical Psychiatry, New York University School of Medicine; Director of Child and Adolescent Psychiatry Service, Gouverner Hospital, New York City

Contents

A Self-Examination in Transcultural Issues

The purpose of this examination is to determine your grasp of selected transcultural issues. Most of the answers are found in the text. Answer each of the following questions by circling the letter before the best response. Correct answers to the questions and a transcultural awareness score are at the end of the examination. If you desire to repeat this test after you read the text, answer the questions on a separate sheet of paper. A pretest and posttest will give you a measure of your transcultural education.

1. Cardiovascular diseases and malignant neoplasms are the two leading causes of death for
   a. all ethnic groups.
   b. whites.
   c. Asian Americans.
   d. Hispanics.

2. Puerto Rico has a higher death rate from _____ than any other country that gathers such statistics.
   a. sickle cell
   b. hypertension
   c. tuberculosis
   d. malnutrition

3. _____ empirical evidence supports the assumption that race and/or ethnic group per se are related to the level of understanding between nurses and Third World patients.
   a. All
   b. No
   c. Most
   d. Little

4. Most Third World people have not assimilated into the American melting pot because of
   a. constitutional prohibition.
   b. communist sentiment.
   c. racism.
   d. all of the above.

5. Research findings conclude that
   a. there are more differences within ethnic groups than between them.
   b. there are more differences between ethnic groups than within them.
   c. few group differences are largely due to cultural conditions.

    d. few group differences are largely due to social conditions.

6. Pallor in the dark-skinned individual is observable by the absence of the underlying _____ tones that normally give the brown and black skin its "glow" or "living color."
   a. blue
   b. white
   c. red
   d. gray

7. The most difficult clinical sign to observe in the darkly pigmented individual is
   a. cyanosis.
   b. jaundice.
   c. erythema.
   d. petechiae.

8. Faith healing is practiced in which church?
   a. Church of Christ Scientist
   b. Seventh Day Adventist
   c. Eastern Orthodox
   d. Church of Jesus Christ of Latter-Day Saints
   e. None of the above
   f. All of the above

9. Among the Ojibwa, the _____ are the highest ranked medical practitioners.
   a. *midēwiwin*
   b. *wabenos*
   c. *jessakid*
   d. *chichicoya*

10. Both the Thai and Burmese believe that there are exactly _____ humoral ailments.
    a. 96
    b. 25

    c. 10
    d. 7

11. Which statement is true?
    a. Yang represents the female, negative force.
    b. Yang represents the female, positive force.
    c. Yin represents the female, negative force.
    d. Yin represents the female, positive force.

12. The traditional Chinese diet includes
    a. rare beef.
    b. soy sauce.
    c. milk.
    d. uncooked vegetables.

13. The belief that one's own group is superior is called
    a. self-actualization.
    b. racism.
    c. prejudice.
    d. ethnocentrism.

14. Which word does not belong in this list?
    a. Houngan
    b. Mambo
    c. Voodoo
    d. Obeah

15. The theoretical and philosophical foundation of Chinese medicine is
    a. the Taoist religion.
    b. existential philosophy.
    c. ayurvedic concepts.
    d. hippocratic concepts.

16. Among black Americans and Hispanics the most commonly cited reasons for witchcraft attacks are
    a. religion and fate.
    b. sexual jealousy and envy.
    c. pregnancy and menstruation.
    d. bad debts and unemployment.

17. Oils, incenses, and candles can be
    purchased in
    a. *pujos.*
    b. *poleos.*
    c. *evangelios.*
    d. *botanicas.*
18. Belief in the evil eye is known as
    a. *mal de ojo.*
    b. *mal de hija.*
    c. *mal de calleiro.*
    d. none of the above.
    e. all of the above.
19. Which is not a derogatory ethnic
    term?
    a. Hot dog
    b. Apple
    c. Oreo
    d. Banana
20. Which statement is true?
    a. Poor health is seldom an
       immediate cause of public
       dependency.
    b. Research to date reveals few
       similarities between cross-
       cultural and social class
       differences in health
       behavior.
    c. Susceptibility to pain is
       different and at vastly
       different levels for all
       humans.
    d. The people most in need of
       medical services are the ones
       who least often procure them.
21. Which statement is false?
    a. The upper classes get more
       preventive dental treatment.
    b. The lower classes are more
       often than the middle classes
       accepted in public outpatient
       clinics for psychotherapy.
    c. Most poor people distrust
       hospital personnel.
    d. All of the above are true.

22. _____ is a blessing
    from God.
    a. *Meidi*
    b. *Mitsva*
    c. *Shabbas*
    d. *Kosher*
23. People who speak different
    languages
    a. live in different worlds.
    b. live in different worlds with
       the same labels attached.
    c. see the world basically the
       same.
    d. pose little problem to psychia-
       trists trying to diagnose their
       illnesses.
24. From a traditional West African
    perspective, time
    a. does not have to be experi-
       enced to be real.
    b. is meaningful at the mathe-
       matical moment and not at
       the point of events.
    c. is reckoned according to its
       significant events.
    d. is not related to punctuality.
25. Which statement is not true of
    most black American families?
    a. They have their roots in
       West Africa.
    b. They include all relatives.
    c. Children born out of wedlock
       are stigmatized.
    d. Mothers tend to have the
       burden of socializing their
       children to live with the
       dangers of their environment.
    e. Low-income elders tend to
       be tolerated and respected.
26. In small group confrontation set-
    tings, traditional Asian Americans
    tend to
    a. be confrontive.
    b. be willing to discuss conflicts.

c.   withdraw.
d.   share inner feelings.
27. The _____ is a
     Mexican community.
     a.   *pochteca*
     b.   *barrio*
     c.   *jacol*
     d.   *calmecac*
28. *Hijos de crianza* are
     a.   foster children.
     b.   lovers.
     c.   musical instruments.
     d.   fond words of greeting.
29. Spiritualism and other forms of
     indigenous therapy are influential
     in the lives of
     a.   Puerto Ricans and black
          Americans but not Mexican
          Americans.
     b.   Mexican Americans and black
          Americans but not Puerto
          Ricans.
     c.   Puerto Ricans, Mexican
          Americans, and black
          Americans.
     d.   neither Puerto Ricans,
          Mexican Americans, or
          black Americans.
30. Most traditional Asian Americans
     a.   are not able to handle cultural
          conflicts.
     b.   are able to handle cultural
          conflicts and adequately
          resolve them.
     c.   are able to handle cultural
          conflicts but not able to
          adequately resolve them.
     d.   are not able to handle cultural
          conflicts but with proper
          guidance can cope.
31. Blacks were with the following
     explorers:
     a.   Cortez

     b.   Lucas Vasquez de Ayllon
     c.   Coronado
     d.   all of the above
     e.   none of the above
32. The vast majority of early
     Japanese immigrants (who
     came from southwestern
     Japan) were called
     a.   issei.
     b.   nisei.
     c.   sansei.
     d.   yonsei.
33. The traditional Hispanic
     American family pattern is
     a.   patriarchal-authoritarian.
     b.   patriarchal-laissez faire.
     c.   matriarchal-authoritarian.
     d.   matriarchal-laissez faire.
     e.   none of the above.
34. The Hopi-Tewa give the major
     responsibility of disciplining the
     child to
     a.   grandparents.
     b.   the father.
     c.   the oldest sibling.
     d.   mother's brother.
35. Pine Ridge Sioux begin toilet
     training a child
     a.   when he or she is weaned.
     b.   around 3 years of age.
     c.   when he or she can walk,
          talk, and understand the
          words.
     d.   when he or she gets tired of
          being untrained.
36. The only people in the United
     States banned from immigration
     by name and law in the nine-
     teenth century were
     a.   Chinese and Japanese.
     b.   Chinese and Mexicans.
     c.   Chinese and Africans.
     d.   Chinese and Italians.

37. Western-based culture as opposed to most other cultures
    a. does not distinguish between physical and mental illness.
    b. treats the whole person rather than concentrating only on the system involved.
    c. places the client's difficulties in the light of spiritual and religious values.
    d. distinguishes rather sharply between physical and mental illness.

38. Nonepileptic seizures are referred to as
    a. *bodega.*
    b. *ataque.*
    c. *colegio.*
    d. *dignidad.*

39. A traditional Asian family includes
    a. parents and unmarried children.
    b. parents, unmarried children, grandparents, and in-laws.
    c. parents, married children, and unmarried children.
    d. parents, married and unmarried children, grandparents, and in-laws.

40. Friendly inquisitiveness is considered _____ by traditional Native Americans.
    a. necessary
    b. nosiness
    c. helpful
    d. good manners

41. Unlike the traditional Western Anglo family, the traditional American Indian extended family is defined as
    a. mother, father, and children.
    b. three generations within a single household.
    c. several households representing significant relatives along vertical but not horizontal lines.
    d. several households representing significant relatives along vertical and horizontal lines.

42. The leading cause of death for nonwhites is
    a. hypertension.
    b. homicide.
    c. influenza.
    d. cancer.

43. Bahamian folk healers are called
    a. *espiritistas.*
    b. *obeah* men.
    c. *houngan* priests.
    d. *curanderos.*

44. According to black American folk medical beliefs, events made by God are called
    a. natural.
    b. unnatural.
    c. natural and unnatural.
    d. none of the above.

ANSWERS

1. a   2. c.   3. d   4. c   5. a   6. c   7. a   8. f   9. a
10. a   11. c   12. b   13. d   14. d   15. a   16. b   17. d   18. a
19. a   20. d   21. b   22. b   23. a   24. c   25. c   26. c   27. b
28. a   29. c   30. b   31. d   32. a   33. a   34. d   35. d   36. c
37. d   38. b   39. b   40. b   41. d   42. d   43. b   44. a

SCORE

40–44	Transculturally gifted
30–39	Transculturally above average
15–29	Transculturally average
10–14	Transculturally below average
Less than 10	Transculturally retarded

Introduction

Medical beliefs and practices can be measured in all cultures because human characteristics are universal. Furthermore, to the extent that medical beliefs and practices characterize subgroups of humanity, there are identifiable transcultural health beliefs and practices. For the sake of analysis, we shall presume that when a given ethnic group has to solve its health problems in a given environment, most of its members will develop patterns of behavior that can be conceptualized in the same way.

The essays in this book provide an analysis of the relationship between ethnicity, social class, and health care. Basic to this exploration are answers to several interrelated questions: What do people want from their medical system? What do they expect to get? What do they actually get from it? How effective is their system? When and under what conditions will they change to another system?

THEORETICAL PERSPECTIVE

Implicit in these questions is the assumption that sociocultural and religious variables are very important. As we focus on non-Western medical systems, we will juxtapose Western medicine, since it is considered the model of "modern" medicine. Peter Morley succinctly described the relationship between Western and non-Western medicine:

> Throughout the history of Western medicine, with a few exceptions, there has been a tendency to view traditional medical systems and beliefs from the vantage point of contemporary Western medical science, regarding them as not only "primitive," but archaic and largely irrelevant to both scientific medicine and the health of human populations. The emphasis has been on the quaint, but queer, customs and lore of the "savage." Imbued with the idea of progress, physicians, medical historians, and early anthropologists viewed "primitive" medicine as an early stage in evolutionary development. Traditional medicine, even as currently practiced in many non-Western societies, was therefore seen as a simple predecessor of complex modern scientific medicine.[1]

However, we shall not, as many writers have done, make the assumption that traditional medicine is based on prelogical beliefs. It would be relatively easy to define modern Western people as the *sine qua non* of scientific thought and other people as basically illiterate and unsophisticated, but this would be a gross distortion. In fact, both Western and non-Western medical systems are social rather than logical phenomena. Morley said it quite well:

> While modern industrial man submits to the scientifically-based *materia medica* of the allopathic physician, it does not necessarily follow that the former understands either the knowledge behind medical practice and its nosology, or the complexity of the treatment offered him by the latter.[2]

The crux of Western and non-Western medicine is that they are culturally determined; thus, it is a truism that the essence of medicine in Western and non-Western societies can be understood only as a social phenomenon. On close scrutiny, traditional and modern medical beliefs and practices are more interrelated than many scientists admit. Reflecting a power hierarchy, the traditional culture usually bends to make room for modern medical knowledge. Such unilateral change does have negative consequences. The belief that modern societies must reciprocate and make room for traditional medical systems is growing. There are good and bad practices in both systems.

Ethnoscience Approach

Our analysis includes the various ethnic groups' views of health and illness; thus, we have adopted an ethnoscience approach. Madeleine M. Leininger states that *"ethnoscience refers to the systematic study of the way of life of a designated cultural group with the purpose of obtaining an accurate account of the people's behavior and how they perceive and interpret their universe."*[3]

The ultimate goal of any ethnoscientific study is to describe the culturally relevant cognitive systems of a particular culture. This is done by collecting and analyzing data that have significant reliability and validity to the indigenous people being studied. Instead of telling indigenous people what they believe, we have selected chapters that let them tell us what they believe. This method of study is in step with Bronislaw Malinowski, who concluded that "the final goal, of which an Ethnographer should never lose sight . . . is, briefly, to grasp the native's point of view, his relation to life, to realize *his* vision and *his* world."[4]

The social class of the "curer" is an important health factor. A cursory study of world cultures reveals that variables such as education, income, residence, and religion of curers vary little with their patients in most traditional non-Western communities, but they vary greatly in most Western communities. Relatedly, the types of psychiatric disorders and the kind of treatment received by patients in modern Western communities tend to be a function of social class. This is less true in non-Western cultures. Despite conditions of homogeneity or heterogeneity, care should be taken when making generalizations about American "society."

In the etiology of mental disorders there are dramatic ethnic differences. Culture defines the situations that arouse certain anxieties and fears, and it also determines the degree to which responses are regarded as normal and abnormal. Although all psychoneurotic disorders occur in non-Western cultures, they differ from their Western counterparts in form and treatment. In addition to individual experiences that develop fears and anxieties, cultural beliefs cause members of societies to fear certain objects. For example, in some societies individuals worship snakes, whereas in others snakes are feared.

Physiological illness is similarly related to cultural conditioning. For example, studies of Western societies show that alcoholism is more prevalent among the Irish than among the Jews, and it is more prevalent among the French than the Italians. Low incidence of alcoholism among some ethnic groups is believed to be related to the restriction of the use of alcoholic beverages to religious ceremonies, special celebrations, and mealtimes. Even the pattern of alcoholism varies from one country to another. Alcoholism as a social problem is associated with cultural beliefs about the effects of alcohol; however, excessive drinking in all cultures brings about physiological changes in individuals. We shall be concerned primarily with methods of treating physiological and mental disorders in Third World people.

By now it should be clear that people who come from varying cultural backgrounds have varying health beliefs and practices. These backgrounds may be described from an *emic approach* or an *etic approach.* The emic approach focuses on the health system of a culture in its own terms, identifying both the cognitive units within the system and the classification of its subunits. This, then, is identifying the indigenous folk taxonomy. The etic approach seeks to discern medical system features that belong to more than one culture. Indeed, when viewing Third World cultures, we find more differences within than between them. It is mainly in the terms they use to classify health experiences that Third World cultures differ. The essays presented in this text compare and contrast indigenous taxonomy as well as ethnic group medical systems. The goal of this activity is to help care providers design plans that will meet Third World patients' needs.

Terminology

Much of our discussion focuses on racial and ethnic groups, especially Third World groups. It is important to note that the two terms—racial groups and ethnic groups—are not synonymous. On the one hand, race refers to a system by which humans are classified into subgroups according to specific physical and structural characteristics. These characteristics include skin pigmentation, stature, facial features, texture of body hair, and head form. The three commonly recognized racial types—Caucasoid, Mongoloid, and Negroid—greatly overlap each other. For this reason there are more similarities than differences between racial groups. On the other hand, ethnic groups refer to individuals who share a unique cultural and social heritage passed on from one generation to another. Additionally, race and ethnic groups should not be confused within a culture. Simply stated, culture is "the configuration of learned behavior and results of behavior whose components and elements are shared and transmitted by the members of a particular society."[5]

> Sometimes we tend to confuse race and ethnic groups within a culture. Great races do have different cultures. Ethnic groups within races differ in cultural content. But, people of the same racial origin and of the same ethnic groups differ in their cultural matrices. All browns, or blacks, or whites, or yellows, or reds, are not alike in the cultures in which they live and have their being. The understanding of the culture of another, or of groups other than our own, demands a knowledge of varied elements within a culture or the variety of cultural matrix.[6]

It is precisely this kind of understanding that we seek as we explore Third World medical beliefs and practices. This brings us to our final term, "Third World." We use it interchangeably with nonwhite men and women who are neither Western nor communist. The First World is comprised of capitalistic countries, the Second World is comprised of socialist countries, and the Third World is comprised of Africa, Asia, and South America. As people from these nations have settled in North America, they have maintained many of their cultural beliefs and behaviors. This, then, is the framework within which we present our analysis.

RELIGIOUS AND CULTURAL DIFFERENCES

The chapters focusing on patient care are at best introductions to the topic. Even so, these chapters vividly illustrate the importance of understanding religious and cultural differences. This awareness will help practitioners to realize that most behaviors exhibited by patients are neither capricious nor malicious. Rather, they are socially prescribed ways of dealing with pain and illness.

Religion

Although they have different historical backgrounds, each of the ethnic groups discussed in this book shares the perception that illness often is caused by supernatural force(s). A religious person often believes that being sick is God's punishment for some digression from His commandments. For this reason, religious leaders are very much a part of health care. In most instances, this means conferring with Roman Catholic priests or Protestant ministers associated with specific patients.

Too often, health professionals do not fully appreciate the impact of religious sects on health care. The importance of evangelistic groups is clear to social scientists who have studied them. Berton Kaplan's article, "The Structure of Adaptive Sentiments in a Lower-Class Religious Group in Appalachia," vividly describes the rituals of the Free Will Baptist Church.[7] Although his study was of the Free Will Baptist Church, Kaplan described behavior characterizing many other Christian denominations.

The premises of the evangelistic Christian sects—we are poor people but we have a mansion in heaven; thou shalt not be angry; give your love to Jesus; we belong to the fellowship of sufferers—can be construed as doctrines for being sick. Indeed, a deep pride in suffering can be instilled in the faithful. This is not to imply that there is a religious scheme to support illness. Instead, it implies that religious sentiments are functional for individuals seeking to cope with physical and mental illness.

The Roman Catholic Church is not unlike the Protestant churches. It acts as a bulwark of conservatism and presents obstacles in the path of medical progress and emancipation from folk practices. The Catholic church teaches obedience to its doctrines, to authority, and to one's parents. Acceptance of adversity is taught as a virtue that, like patience, will be rewarded in Heaven. Besides, it is God's Will.

A major difference between Catholic and Protestant religious expression of illness is that the former tends to be more restrained. Protestant evangelical sects are more like the Free Will Baptist Church of Appalachia:

> The free expression of feelings in rather uninhibited ways is a dominant sentiment in the group. Enter a revival and one witnesses yelling, wailing, crying, and the talking in tongues. During the sermon the audience participates in frequent yelling and prancing about. The songs are sung with the fullest possible emotional commitment, often with tears. After singing, the preacher and the congregation often break into what is called "talking in tongues," which is an expression of whatever comes to mind in a seemingly disorderly way with unique words, which are seen as presumably the Divine speaking through man.[8]

Expressions of pain are similarly uninhibited; however, beneath the yelling, wailing, and crying resides a fear of dying and death that is found in stoic patients, too.

But the health care picture is more complex than this. We must also recognize the function of the extended family. Whatever rituals an individual considers important, it is likely that they will be carried out in cooperation with members of his or her family.

Extended Family

Most hospital visitor regulations are designed for the nuclear family, which characterizes Anglos. We have tried to show that Third World cultures are mainly extended family units. The chapters only partially illustrate this point. Practitioners should be familiar with *compadrazgo,* or the *compadre* system, prevalent throughout Roman Catholic folk cultures in southern Europe, Latin America, and Puerto Rico. This is an artificial kinship system based on Catholic rituals. A godfather (*padrino*) and godmother (*madrina*) are chosen by a child's parents to sponsor the child's baptism through a special religious and social relationship. When the child is ill, it is not uncommon for his or her parents, siblings, grandparents, uncles, aunts, nieces, nephews, cousins, and godparents to show up at the bedside.

In Hispanic, Native American, and black cultures, relatives frequently consist of siblings and stepparents, who have no legal ties. Thus, the practice of determining relatives by checking family names can be both confusing and embarrassing. In most folk cultures grandparents are official or symbolic family leaders. Native American grandparents are both official and symbolic leaders. This arrangement may prove frustrating to practitioners who ask questions of parents but receive answers from grandparents. A similar condition exists in traditional Asian American families, where parents share esteem with grandparents, uncles, and aunts.

CURES AND FEARS

Margaret Clark provides an excellent summary of Mexican American health practices.[9] Although her observations are of barrio people, they also pertain to other ethnic groups. Faith is the most important element in folk cures. For example, it is not holy water itself that has curative power for Roman Catholic Hispanics; instead, faith in the water's curative power is the important factor. This also is true for home remedies—tonics, cough syrups, and laxatives—used by Third World people. It is not always necessary for physicians to prescribe additional medicine but to prescribe proper dosages of medicine an individual is already taking.

There are other debilitations when practitioners are not familiar with either ethnic group definitions of illness or indigenous cures. Among the poor in particular, being sick is a family phenomenon—all members of an individual's extended family are affected. Illness means loss of already scarce financial resources or the absence of someone to do household chores. For these reasons low-income adults are reluctant to accept the reality of their illness until kinship members confirm it and devise a plan to provide financial or household assistance.

In relation to how men deal with illness, the Hispanic concept of *macho* can be generalized to other ethnic groups. Black, Native American, and Asian American cultures dictate that men ignore or pretend to ignore pain until family members decide that they are sick. In summary, there are elaborate cultural norms surrounding illness. As noted earlier, in some ethnic groups, once an individual is given permission to be sick, he or she may moan and groan without the fear of peer censure.

The hospital epitomizes the alienation that Third World people experience in health care facilities. Cut off from his or her significant other persons (relatives and friends), a hospitalized patient of any group, but especially an ethnic minority person, feels frightened. The typical patient:

> . . . is dependent on a doctor and on the effectiveness or ineffectiveness of his treatment. He is dependent on others for visits, a cup of tea, his food and drink. Of course, it is true that in normal life we are also in a measure dependent on others, that we know the difficult feeling of having to wait on the decisions of others, but we also have great advantages denied to the sick: we arrange our own timetable, we can be productive in our work. Not so the patient; often he is not allowed to work, only to read a little, and he is certainly not the master of his time—his meals are at mealtimes, "lights out" is fixed, he is washed on time, etc. The sense of being passive which the need to lie in bed inactive readily breeds, soon spreads to the whole of his life.[10]

Under these conditions it is not surprising that the nurse quickly emerges as the patient's most significant other person in the hospital. More than anyone else, the nurse is present, and it is hoped, she or he cares about the patient. This caring is demonstrated in various behaviors.

PROFESSIONAL'S ROLE

Scattered throughout the text are explicit and implicit statements about the role of professionals in health care. Some of the skills involved in a professional role are listening, being empathic, recognizing the patient's as well as one's own self-interest and needs, being flexible, having a sense of timing, utilizing the patient's resources, and giving relevant information.

An effective practitioner listens in such a way that she or he is really able to hear what the patient (or client) is trying to say. This does not mean telling the patient what to say. Being empathic means identifying with the other person's point of view. Meaningful communication is impossible without empathy. An effective practitioner understands herself or himself and tries to gain similar understanding of the patient. Self-knowledge is a prerequisite to helping others. In the quest for self-knowledge, it is important to be flexible. Rarely is there one answer or a single interpretation for an event or situation. Furthermore, there will be instances in which patients may ask practitioners to give them answers when they really need help in finding their own answers.

Unless practitioners understand cultural norms and values, they may intervene at the wrong time, such as before the patient has had an opportunity to talk with relatives or a folk healer. The caregiver can help the patient to effectively blend orthodox and folk medical practices. This is best done with language that the patient understands. Help is help only when it is perceived as such. Clearly, this involves taking a nonjudgmental stance toward the patient and his or her culture. Little good can be accomplished if the practitioner tries to belittle religious beliefs and folk cultures.

Some readers may conclude that too little attention has been given to successful transcultural programs. One of the reasons for this omission is the relatively small number of successful programs. Since programs are devised by and comprised of people, it is our hope that the people who read this text will design and implement additional transcultural courses, institutes, and programs. On a smaller scale, we hope that individual attitudes, beliefs, and behavior will be favorably altered by this text. The hazard in our approach is that the data we present may serve to frighten or immobilize our readers. Perhaps the following observations will place our book within a meaningful behavioral context.

1. Care providers cannot solve patients' problems, but they may be able to help them solve their own problems.

2. Every patient's problem has more than one possible solution.

3. The easiest, least creative response to transcultural conflict is to pretend that it does not exist.

4. Every patient behaves according to unwritten ethnic group customs and traditions.

5. The most powerful factors in family decision making are precedent and cultural or religious norms.

6. Patient knowledge of scientific medicine is alienating, and every successful educational effort by practitioners tends to alienate patients from relatives and friends who do not have this knowledge.

7. Humor can help practitioners and patients over rough spots; we must be able to laugh at ourselves and with other people.

8. Previous transcultural experience is a valuable asset if it is used as a general guide. However, if viewed as offering the correct answer to every transcultural problem, experience (as well as the information in this book) will be a liability.

9. All care providers will make mistakes in transcultural interactions, but we should learn from our mistakes and not repeat them.

Questions for Each Chapter

If you answer the following questions after completing each chapter, transcultural health care will become a more meaningful concept.

1. Based on your experiences and previous reading, how accurate and relevant are the chapters?

2. What specific characteristics do ethnic groups have in common?

3. Which statements contradict beliefs that you hold? How do you reconcile these contradictions?

4. Cite examples of effective transcultural nursing methods or techniques that appear to be applicable to all ethnic groups. Which ones appear to have unique or limited value?

5. What unanswered questions do you have after reading each chapter? Where can you go to get answers to your questions?

References

1. Morley, P.; and Wallis, R., editors. 1978. *Culture and caring: Anthropological perspectives on traditional medical beliefs and practices.* Pittsburgh: University of Pittsburgh Press, pp. 5-6.

2. Morley, P.; and Wallis, R., editors. 1978. *Culture and caring: Anthropological perspectives on traditional medical beliefs and practices.* Pittsburgh: University of Pittsburgh Press, p. 15.

3. Leininger, M. 1970. *Nursing and anthropology: Two worlds to blend.* New York: John Wiley & Sons, Inc., p. 168.

4. Malinowski, B. 1922. *Argonauts of the Western Pacific.* London: George Routledge & Sons, p. 2.

5. Linton, R. 1945. *The cultural background of personality.* New York: Appleton-Century-Crofts, p. 32.

6. Moore, B. M. 1974. Cultural differences and counseling perspectives. *Tex. Personnel Guid. Assoc. J.* 3:41.

7. Kaplan, B. H. 1965. The structure of adaptive sentiments in a lower-class religious group in Appalachia. *J. Soc. Issues* 21:126-141.

8. Kaplan, B. H. 1965. The structure of adaptive sentiments in a lower-class religious group in Appalachia. *J. Soc. Issues* 21:134-135.

9. Clark, M. 1970. *Health in the Mexican-American culture: A community study.* Berkeley: University of California Press, Chapters 7 and 8.

10. Faber, H. 1971. *Pastoral care in the modern hospital.* Philadelphia: The Westminster Press, p. 22.

Transcultural
Health Care

PART I

Sociocultural
Dimensions

The chapters in Part I illustrate the importance of folkways, social class, religion, ethnic identity, and language. In short, they illustrate the importance of culture. *Folkways* are the normal, habitual ways ethnic groups do things. Some folkways, such as those pertaining to health care, are more closely adhered to than others. In social science jargon, folkways that must be followed because they are believed important to group survival are called *mores*. Certain health mores are practiced because it is believed that they are beneficial.

Wealth and income determine not only social class but also an individual's access to health care facilities. There is a cruel, vicious circle from which few poverty-stricken people can extricate themselves. Most low-income children attend inferior schools and, consequently, receive an inferior education. If they graduate from high school or a vocational school, most low-income persons who manage to get a job are disproportionately employed as unskilled and semiskilled laborers. Thus, low-income persons are likely to work in jobs hazardous to their health. At the end of the circle are inadequate health care systems that, if used, conflict with lower-class mores. All of our readings touch on social class variables.

Religion is a universal institution. Some religions, including Jewish sects, place considerable emphasis on the family. Health care professionals unaware of this emphasis are likely to engage in nonhelpful behavior. Raphella Sohier provides a sensitive view of the complexity that religious differences add to transcultural nursing. Equally complex is ethnic similarity. Practitioners frequently overlook the problem inherent in identifying too closely with their patients. Mary Gottesfeld calls our attention to the issue of countertransference.

Language is an integral aspect of culture. The arrogance of economically or politically dominant groups is seen in their failure to learn the languages of subordinate groups. The effect of denying interpreters to patients who speak English as a second language is the subject of research by Luis Marcos and associates. Although they may be difficult for some persons to read, the data generated by Marcos are crucial to bilingual-bicultural health care.

1

Health Care

George Henderson, Ph.D.
Martha Primeaux, R.N., M.S.N.

*Professor Henderson's interest in transcultural health care began in the early 1960s when he taught Introductory Sociology and Psychology in Detroit's Harper Hospital School of Nursing Program. For the past two years, he has taught coping skills to students enrolled in a health career preparatory program sponsored by the Oklahoma State Regents for Higher Education. As a consultant to the U. S. Commission on Civil Rights and the U. S. Department of Justice, Professor Henderson is involved in transcultural education issues on a national level. Several of his other books—*Understanding and Counseling Ethnic Minorities *(1979),* Introduction to American Education *(1978),* To Live in Freedom *(1972),* America's Other Children *(1971), and* Teachers Should Care *(1970)—also focus on Third World issues. He is Chairman of the Department of Human Relations, S. N. Goldman Professor of Human Relations, Professor of Education and Associate Professor of Sociology at the University of Oklahoma, Norman. At present, Professor Henderson is on leave and serving as a Distinguished Visiting Professor in the Department of Behavioral Sciences and Leadership at the U. S. Air Force Academy.*

Martha Primeaux is Assistant Professor in the Baccalaureate Program, University of Oklahoma College of Nursing, where she has been on the faculty since 1963. Her publications on American Indian health care have appeared in the Journal of Psychiatric Nursing, American Journal of

Nursing, *and* Current Practice in Gerontological Nursing. *She has conducted and participated in numerous workshops and symposia on American Indian health care as well as family planning and maternity/child nursing. Ms. Primeaux was one of the founders of the Indian Clinic of the Native American Center of the Oklahoma City Urban Indian Health Project. She is currently active in other health-related and nursing organizations and is on the advisory/editorial boards of* New Medicine *and* Family and Community Health.

THE NATION'S HEALTH

The phrase "a sound mind in a sound body" reflects an ideal that has remained constant from ancient to modern times, and medical research has brought us closer to this goal. Enormous improvements have been made in diagnostic procedures, surgical techniques, and both prophylactic and therapeutic medicine. Unfortunately, the delivery of health services has not kept pace with medical research. This is true despite unusually large government expenditures for health care delivery services. Particularly neglected are low-income communities, where a disproportionate number of Third World people reside.

Health care is the nation's third largest industry, employing more than 6 million persons, including 400,000 physicians, 150,000 dentists, 150,000 pharmacists, 980,000 registered nurses, 500,000 practical nurses, and 1 million nurse aides, orderlies, and attendants. In 1977 the nation's health bill came to $163 billion, 40% of which was tax dollars.[1]

Despite the fact that the United States currently spends more than $200 billion a year on health, large numbers of Americans suffer and die yearly from infirmities that modern medicine could prevent, mitigate, or cure if medical resources were unrestrictedly available. As Senator Edward Kennedy observed, "Smaller countries spend smaller amounts on health care than the United States, and they give more health care to their people. In many of these nations, fewer children die than in America, fewer women die in childbirth, and men and women live longer lives on the average."[2]

Neonatal mortality (the number of babies who die in their first year of life) and male and female longevity are two indices widely and frequently used to make international health comparisons. In a comparison of funds expended for health care and results produced, America does not fare well. America spends a slightly higher percentage of national income on health care than do Sweden and the United Kingdom. Even so, the infant mortality rate is lower in Sweden and England, and the life expectancy is higher.

The distinguished heart surgeon Dr. Michael DeBakey lamented that Russians lag behind Americans in the quality of medicine practiced, but Russia does a better job of taking care of the average citizen. In his words, "Well, I think care is more accessible in Russia in the sense that the whole population has accessibility to it.

It's accessible to everybody. In other words, they don't discriminate on the basis of finance in any way."[3] This is obviously not the case in America.

EFFECTS OF RACISM ON HEALTH CARE

Although all Americans might justifiably hope for better health care delivery systems, minority Americans have even more to wish for. As with many other services, minorities often receive the least and the last in health care. This difference in delivery of services may be attributed to the pervasiveness of racism in the United States.

Drawing on the findings of the National Advisory Commission on Civil Disorders (the Kerner Commission), Dr. John C. Norman wrote:

> America is, and has always been, a racist society. Bigotry permeates every level of every region of the country, North and South, business, labor, journalism, education, and medicine. The causes of racism are ignorance, apathy, poverty, and above all else a pervasive discrimination that has thwarted each and every citizen in all avenues of life.[4]

There are two kinds of racism: individual and institutional. *Individual racism* refers to the behavior of individuals that supports the belief of racial superiority of one or more groups over others. *Institutional racism* refers to the systematic oppression of people through institutional policies and practices. It is not uncommon for individuals chided for racist conditions to retort, "Don't blame me. I haven't done anything." Civil rights activists say that this is precisely the problem: they have done little, if anything, to understand or abate current conditions of racism. Through their ignorance and inaction, racism remains a destructive force in our nation's health care.

Nonwhites in particular are handicapped by poverty, discrimination, and sociopsychological barriers to health care. To most low-income nonwhite Americans, stories about cancer and drug research, birth control clinics, and government funding for research on vital areas of human medical treatment are akin to *Alice's Adventures in Wonderland*. Low-income Third World people receive the worst type of medical care. Nonwhite babies die at a rate 92% higher than for white babies, and nonwhite mothers die during childbirth at a rate four times that of white mothers.[5] In fact, the American nonwhite deaths at birth and during infancy are worse than the record of most of the world's urbanized nations. Clearly, the major issue for our Third World poor is not tax reform or welfare checks—it is survival.

Cardiovascular diseases and malignant neoplasms are the two leading causes of death for all ethnic groups, but they are higher for nonwhites than whites. The next three major causes of death for all groups in rank order are accidents, influenza and pneumonia, and homicide. Cancer is on the upswing in nonwhite communities. The mortality rate from cancer among nonwhites has increased more than 40% from 1954 to 1976. During this period, the death rate for nonwhites rose from 138 to

190 per 100,000 population, whereas the death rate for whites rose only 4% (from 149 to 155 per 100,000).[6]

Statistics compiled by the American Cancer Society show that there are striking racial differences in deaths from specific types of cancer. The mortality rate for cancers of the stomach, liver, esophagus, cervix, and uterus is higher for nonwhites than for whites. On the other hand, whites have a greater mortality from leukemia and cancers of the ovary, brain, and skin. Some researchers suspect that the higher cancer toll among nonwhites may stem from the fact that they tend to live in areas of high air pollution and are more likely than whites to be exposed to harmful chemicals on their jobs.

But cancer is not the only major medical problem for nonwhites. High blood pressure also afflicts a large number of them. Commonly known as hypertension, high blood pressure plays a direct role in the deaths of at least 100,000 men and women—both white and nonwhite—each year by placing severe strain on their hearts. The presence of high blood pressure is most severely felt in black communities. Some researchers estimate that at least one in seven black Americans has high blood pressure. Because black Americans get hypertension at a young age, it is more severe among black teenagers than white teenagers. Among black men 25 to 44 years of age, the death rate from hypertension-related heart disease is 15 times greater than among white men of the same age. Hypertension is 17 times greater among black women than it is among white women. Finally, hypertension kills more than 13,000 black Americans every year compared with sickle cell's death toll of 340. The nonwhite death rate for hypertension is 60 per 100,000, or more than twice the 27 per 100,000 rate for whites.[7]

The "Latin American" health problem has been intensified by large blocks of Spanish-speaking persons who have immigrated to the United States. A Colorado study determined that neonatal deaths were three times as high among Spanish-speaking groups as among Anglos (whites), reflecting less adequate conditions at and following delivery, a lack of prenatal care, and poor nutrition and deficient health care of the mother.[8]

Studies of Puerto Rico show that Puerto Ricans have a higher death rate from tuberculosis than any other country that gathers such statistics. Tuberculosis thrives in poor, overcrowded conditions, which are exactly the conditions in which many Puerto Ricans live, both in Puerto Rico and on the American mainland. These conditions are exacerbated by many Puerto Ricans being ignorant of sound health care and sanitation practices.[9]

Commenting on the health care of American Indians, Vine Deloria, Jr., said that although Indians of today are much better off than they were just a few years ago, they still have a long way to go to meet the standards of the more affluent Americans. Cultural conflict is still a problem, and the anomie and feelings of helplessness created by this conflict are still evident.[10]

Perhaps malnutrition, brought about in many different ways, is the most common problem among poor people—white and nonwhite. Malnutrition occurs when a person's food is inadequate either in terms of quantity or quality. Frequently, low-income living habits and environmental conditions result in a poor appetite, aversion to particular foods, or refusal to eat certain foods. It is not easy to tell whether a person is malnourished. Many malnourished people are fat due to their intake of large quantities of carbohydrates. Medical systems can be fully understood only by knowing a culture's food preferences.

Doris Y. Mosley identified six barriers to the delivery of health care to the poor:

1. Inability to pay, including the humiliation of "means tests," which establish medical indigence necessary to receive so-called free care.

2. Fragmentation of care—the depersonalization and confusion of referral to various medical specialty clinics. This is well illustrated by an example of an elderly indigent patient with 12 major diagnoses for which he was required to attend 10 clinics. He was too ill to do this, stopped attending any, and was labeled "uncooperative."

3. Operational features of providing the services, including travel, long waits, unattractive surroundings, and inconvenient hours. Also included are lack of communication, trust, and understanding between patients and health personnel and lack of time due to health personnel shortages. Understandably, hostility and isolation often result from these factors.

4. Low-income attitudes toward health care, resulting in differing perceptions of the health care system by patients and health personnel. This leads to misinterpretation of behavior and delay or nonutilization of services.

5. Racial discrimination in provision of services. Some hospitals previously closed to black people are still not utilized to maximum potential. Many still refuse to grant black physicians staff privileges.

6. Lack of facilities and manpower. Urban slums and ghettos as well as remote rural areas are unattractive to most professional health personnel and their families, who choose to live and practice in upper- and middle-class areas. Hospitals relocate in suburbs to escape deteriorating central city areas, and local politics often prevent establishment of areawide, centralized medical facilities.[11]

The preceding data are presented to facilitate an appreciation for the tremendous challenge facing health care professionals. Additional data can be found in other studies. This challenge cannot be met without understanding the concepts of culture, cultural diversity, and poverty.

IMPORTANCE OF CULTURE

No two cultures are precisely alike. As noted earlier, culture is the human-made part of the environment. The *material* components of culture are items human beings produce through creative thinking and technology. The *nonmaterial* components of culture consist of intangibles and symbolic abstractions. Because it is not biologically inherited, culture must be learned and transmitted to each successive generation. Optimum health is a cultural value shared by all health care professionals; however, not all patients share this value. Failure to understand this fact can result in defining patients who have values different than the care provider as "bad," "uncooperative," or "difficult."

The cultural context of a patient's (and nurse's) behavior refers to the implicit and explicit tendencies of subgroups to respond to stimuli according to their learned styles of coping. Each subgroup has its own unique ways of seeing, interpreting, and coping with its environment and the people in it. Nurses concerned with the why and what of a specific ethnic minority's health practices can get most of their answers by becoming familiar with the group's history, religion, kinship patterns, and social systems.

Cultural Diversity

America is a nation of great cultural diversity. Although all segments of our population share certain common elements in life patterns and basic beliefs, there are significant differences in subcultural attitudes, interests, goals, and dialects. Patients bring to medical settings cultural differences in perceptions of masculine and feminine roles, in rural and urban backgrounds, in ethnic groups, and in social classes.

Masculine and Feminine Roles. Until recently in our culture, men and women were expected to play different roles. One of the first lessons children learned from those around them was that their behavior must accord with that generally considered appropriate to their sex. A boy was not expected to take on feminine characteristics; a girl was handicapped if she were not feminine in dress, speech, and aspirations. "Good boys" and "good girls" were those who engaged in sex-appropriate behavior.[12] Gradually, sex stereotyping is disappearing—even in nursing.

Rural and Urban Backgrounds. Although they are not as striking as they used to be, differences in language, attitudes, and interests between rural and urban dwellers still exist. Some schools of nursing have orientation programs to acquaint students with patients who live in rural and urban areas.[13]

Ethnic Groups. Nearly every American can trace his or her ancestry back to some country across the seas. Each ethnic group has enriched our culture with its own particular types of music, food, customs, and dress. It usually takes two or more generations for the members of a new ethnic group to become sufficiently absorbed into the life of the community that they lose their separate identity. Some ethnic groups—mainly those of color—never achieve assimilation. The assimilation of the more recent immigrant groups seems to be unlikely; most of them are of the lower socioeconomic classes, and they tend to maintain their traditional beliefs, attitudes, and behaviors.[14]

Social Classes. The United States has rather clearly defined social classes. The social class to which the parents belong determines to a great extent a child's educational and occupational attainments. Numerous studies have documented how difficult it is for an individual to advance from one social class to another on the basis of ability and effort. Although 52% of 1977 white high school graduates had clerical jobs, only 30% of nonwhite graduates held such jobs. Furthermore, 25% of the nonwhites were employed in service occupations, but only 12% of whites were.[15] Black Americans, Hispanics, and American Indians are disproportionately represented in the lower socioeconomic classes.

POVERTY

Poverty is characterized by conditions of not enough—not enough money, food, clothes, adequate housing, prestige, or hope. Generally, when affluent people go without soap, hot water, light, food, medicine, and recreation, it is because they elect to do so. When poverty-stricken people go without these things, it is because they have no choice. Therein lies the major difference between the poor and the affluent. The former are controlled by the economic system, and the latter control it.[16]

Poverty has a familiar smell—a smell of rotting garbage and sour foods. It is the smell of children's urine and unwashed bodies. Above all else, it is the smell of people wasting away physically, socially, and psychologically. Urban poverty is much more visible than rural poverty. Dilapidated buildings, garbage-strewn alleys, and rats are the dominant characteristics of urban slums. These conditions blur the memory of clean, well-kept buildings that also characterize many urban poor neighborhoods. Although it is difficult to change the negative image of the urban slum, it is almost impossible to erase the idyllic picture of rural poverty frequently called "quaint," "picturesque," or "Americana." Nearly 40% of rural Americans are poverty stricken.

Migrant workers illustrate the plight of the poor. Hispanics comprise approximately 70% of the more than 500,000 migrant workers, each of whom earns less than $3000 per year. Life for the migrant is seasonal: a day here, a week there.[17] For example, migrants pick citrus fruits in California and Florida, beans and tomatoes in Texas, cherries and blueberries in Michigan, sugar beets in Kansas, cucumbers in South Carolina, and potatoes in Idaho and Maine.

Most migrants sleep in dilapidated structures that lack adequate heat, refrigeration, and sanitation facilities. They play on garbage-strewn grounds and drink polluted water. Communities in which migrants work tend to lack minimally adequate medical care and health services. Most migrant workers and their families are infected with intestinal parasites and have chronic skin infections and dental problems. Many have chronically infected ears that can result in partial deafness.

Because in America the norm is affluence, to be poor in America is to be among the most economically deprived persons in the world. All health care persons should understand this phenomenon. Telling an economically poor patient how well off he or she is compared with the poor in Latin America or Africa will have little positive effect.

The comparisons that reveal an ugly health picture for the poor in the United States were succinctly captured in the following statement by Richard D. Lyons:

> No finer medical treatment in the world may be found than what is now available at the Mayo Clinic in Minnesota, Johns Hopkins Hospital in Maryland, Methodist Hospital in Texas, Columbia-Presbyterian Medical Center in New York, or Stanford University Hospital in California. Yet only a few miles from these great humanitarian institutions, large segments of the nation's population receive hit-or-miss health care, with infrequent visits to doctors or public health nurses and virtually no dental treatment. The poor customarily enter a hospital only when they are very ill, often beyond help.[18]

The foregoing summary of statistics and practices characterizes the state of the nation's health and substantiates the assessment of experts that the United States has reached a crisis situation in health care. This situation can be summarized in the ideographs of the Chinese language, in which "two characters are used to write the single word 'crisis'—one is the character for 'danger' and the other is the character for 'opportunity.' "[19] One of the first requisites for a solution is improved nursing education.

NURSE'S ROLE

The nurse is a central figure in health care. Historically, the profession of nursing partly arose out of the practice of wealthy persons hiring servant girls to care for their sick and to perform tasks that illness prevented them from accomplishing. Many nurses feel that little has changed from those early attitudes regarding the status of nursing. Identified with the history of the female, especially mother-surrogate and healer roles, it has been difficult for nurses to shake the inferior status attached to women generally. Inadequate patient care is sometimes a result of the nurse's role conflict and low status rather than understaffing and ethnic or social class attitudes.

Much of the early day nurse training was accomplished by an apprenticeship that emphasized obedience to authority. A part of the current strain and unrest within the nursing profession derives from physicians and administrators who expect automatic and unquestioning response to their directives and orders. The more effective physicians and health administrators provide opportunities for nurses to exercise professional judgment. Most nurses seem to prefer situations where they can function more or less on their own, responding directly to patients' needs and deciding when intervention by a physician is appropriate.

How nurses administer a health care plan matters as much as the details of the plan. Each nurse should carefully decide how she or he can best maximize the health facilities available for each patient. It is useful to think of nurses in this case as *guides.* Nurses show patients the pathways to the various destinations of good health. As guides, they determine the pace and sequence of the trip; they help decide which route should be taken to achieve the desired end; and it is the nurse's responsibility to make the journey interesting and enriching for the patient traveler. The guide, with her or his own zest for the nursing profession, must awaken a desire in the patient travelers and instill in them the tenacity to complete the journey.

The nurse is also a *model* for patients to emulate, an example they can follow. This is one of the greatest responsibilities of the nurse and one from which she or he cannot escape. This part of the nurse's job is helped by cultural understanding. The impressions a nurse makes remain forever in the minds of her or his patients.

The nurse as a *counselor* bears much responsibility for advising patients. Patients continually are faced with major problems, many of which are personal. During times of crisis, some patients turn to their nurse for guidance. In this capacity a nurse is able to bend and shape patients into many forms of behavior. Insensitive nurses fail during these periods, and in so doing they fail to provide optimum health care.

The nurse is an *actor.* She or he fits Shakespeare's definition:

All the world's a stage
And all the men and women are merely players.
They have their exits and entrances,
And one man in his time plays many parts.

For example, an actor reads a script, decides he likes it, and studies it until he knows it. When he is competent, the actor goes on stage and portrays the character so that it communicates to the audience, and they come to know the content of the character before they leave the theater. It is much the same with an effective nurse. She or he learns the subject, goes into a health care setting, acts the role as care is given to patients, and before the performance ends, the patients come to know the nurse as a good or bad actor.

When the nurse guides patients, her or his chief work is helping them to learn how to better care for themselves. This means helping patients to define their own interests, needs, abilities, and problems; helping them to understand themselves and others; and otherwise helping them to become more healthy. Out of this process emerge specific goals each patient will want to achieve. The nurse's role is to help patients formulate and evaluate health goals in terms of their own values and those of the larger community. It is imperative to involve patients in as much of the health care process as possible. To best do this, each nurse must be in touch with herself or himself.

> One can master the facts, principles, and laws contained in a hundred books on psychology and still understand neither oneself nor others. Self-understanding requires integrity rather than mere cleverness. It involves emotion. To know oneself, one must be able to recognize feelings, act on them, and deal with them in constructive ways; and this is something quite different from reading or talking about them with detachment.[20]

An important factor hindering a cooperative relationship between nurses and patients is the fact that many patients view themselves as uneducated and incapable of understanding the explanations given by professionals, whom they frequently describe as talking among themselves and using Latin or Greek. A great many patients feel excluded from their own illnesses, convinced that physicians and nurses deliberately and needlessly withhold information from them. Embarrassed by their ignorance, patients often fail to ask their questions and instead act out their hostility at being pushed around and ignored as persons.

The job of the medical practitioner is further complicated by the belief of a significant number of patients in folk medicine concepts that are different from those of modern scientific medicine (see Part II). Such beliefs are particularly pervasive among Third World and poor patients, who are often operating in distinctly different cultural mores. Meaningful relationships between nurse and patient are further complicated by the marked increase in specialization. The nurse-patient relationship is also fractured by the need of Third World and poor patients to use health clinics, which means that patients frequently are cared for by different physicians and nurses on each visit.

> It appears that the degree to which the qualities ideally defined as essential to the therapeutic relationship, namely mutual trust, respect, and coopera-tion, will be present inversely with the amount of social distance. Conversely the greater the social distance the less likely the participants will receive each other in terms of the ideal type roles of professional and patient, and more likely they will perceive each other in terms of their social class status in the larger society.[21]

There is fairly general agreement that because of certain attitudes, the low-status patient has a markedly lower chance of obtaining optimal care than the high-status patient. Several generalizations are given for this discrepancy, including the following: low-status patients give less attention to symptoms, they are less willing to sacrifice immediate for future gain, and they display less initiative. When taken at their face value, these reasons stereotype low-status persons as being shiftless and lazy.

Knowing the effect of cultural conditioning on the behavior of both the care provider and the patient can do much to prevent inhumane aspects of health care. It can certainly reduce the negative human dimensions of our health care crisis.

CROSS-CULTURAL NURSING

Third World people who seek health care outside their family do so because neither they nor their families can help them. Ideally, the nurse will offer care that will minimize cultural conflicts. This type of reality-based caregiving is based on empathy (see Part III).

Nurses who are different from patients in terms of culture generally have more difficulty communicating empathy, congruence, respect, and acceptance than those who share or understand the patient's cultural perspective. To be more specific, non-Third World nurses who understand the social and psychological backgrounds of Third World patients are better able to work with such patients than their colleagues who lack this knowledge. Indeed, a meaningful relationship with a non-Third World nurse representing the dominant power society can do much to reduce hostile feelings of Third World patients. The act of giving care to another human being is a rare opportunity for understanding ethnic group similarities and differences. It is in this setting that the social science concepts discussed in this book are acted out.

Contrary to popular notion, little empirical evidence supports the assumption that race or ethnic group *per se* is related to the level of understanding between nurses and Third World patients. Generalizations about race and cross-cultural nursing should be made with great care. At best, the literature on the subject is inconclusive. Several studies suggest that cultural barriers make the development of successful cross-cultural nursing highly improbable. Yet other studies conclude that well-trained, empathic nurses can establish effective relationships with patients from other racial or ethnic backgrounds. It is this latter perspective that we advocate, and thus the articles we have selected for reading provide data and techniques for cross-cultural nursing.

Although the readings address specific issues, it seems appropriate here to provide an overview of areas in which it is important for nurses to be both knowledgeable and understanding. Bilingualism and biculturalism present a special kind of challenge. Spanish-speaking Americans are the largest number of bilingual-bicultural patients in American hospitals and clinics. Nurses must be aware that "language, culture and ethnicity play the most important role in the formation of the self-concept, and in the development of cognitive coping skills. The three concepts are analytically different, yet they are interrelated."[22]

Most bilingual-bicultural subcultures have not assimilated into the American melting pot because they prefer not to assimilate. Only black Americans (who are not bilingual-bicultural in the true sense of the terms) have mounted national civil rights campaigns to gain integration and assimilation with white Americans.

Nurses must be aware that Third World patients living in traditional families have to function according to the norms of their kinship network and also according to the norms of non-Third World institutions. This conflict was vividly captured by D'Arcy McNickle when he summarized the dilemmas of traditional Indians:

> The problem of being an Indian, and being obliged to function at two levels of consciousness, for many individuals reduces itself to this: They are aware that their communities, their people, their kinsmen are Indians and are held in low esteem by the general society. The young people especially recognize themselves as Indians, but they do not want the low-status equivalent. They look for some way in which they can share in the status ascribed to middle-class Americans without ceasing to be Indians.[23]

The lack of high status shows up when nurses mispronounce Third World names while taking ample steps to learn the pronunciation of equally difficult non-Third World names. Mispronouncing a person's name whether through carelessness or laziness can easily be interpreted as the nurse's lack of interest. In the case of Spanish, pronunciation is much more consistent than English because each vowel is pronounced the same way in all words. When in doubt about pronunciation, the nurse should ask the patient.

Ethnic group language shapes one's philosophy of life. Consider the following example: In English the clock runs; in Spanish *el reloj anda* (the clock walks); and for American Indians it just ticks. The former group is preoccupied with hurrying to be on time, whereas the latter two adopt a slower pace of life. Thus, acceptance of the concept of time and structuring relationships around clock-measured medical appointments vary according to culture.

The net result of ethnic people living outside their ancestral lands and maintaining their cultural heritage is a less than traditional culture. Black American culture is not African culture; the Mexican American culture is not Mexican culture; the mainland Puerto Rican culture is not island Puerto Rican culture; the Chinese American culture is not Chinese culture; the Japanese American culture is not Japanese culture. These cultures have become a synthesis of their own native and adopted American cultures. The derogatory terms *apple,* used to refer to American Indians who are red on the outside, white on the inside, and *banana,* used to refer to Asian Americans who are yellow on the outside, white on the inside, illustrate possible cultural conflicts growing out of assimilation.

As seen earlier, groups whose members share a common social and cultural heritage passed on to each successive generation are known as *ethnic groups.* Ethnic groups generally are identified by distinctive patterns of family life, language, and customs that set them apart from other groups. Above all else, members of ethnic groups feel a sense of identity and common fate. Ethnicity is frequently used to mean race, but it extends beyond race.

Nurses who do not know the various social class dimensions of ethnic minorities also are unlikely to know that despite common language, color, and historical backgrounds, all members of a particular minority group are not alike. It is presumptuous and counterproductive to talk about *the* blacks or *the* Indians or *the* Latins as if members of these and other groups have only one set of behavior characteristics. This text focuses on ethnic characteristics, but the reader is reminded that social class differences often are more determinant of a patient's behavior than ethnic background. Middle class-oriented Third World families tend to be much more ready to fit the hospital routine.

Finally, some thought should be given to nurses who ostensibly have everything in their favor when working with patients from their own ethnic group. Several factors frequently mitigate against them being effective nurses. First and most important, most Third World nurses are Anglo-Saxon in terms of their training and professional associations. They are, in short, carbon copies of their non-Third World colleagues. Of course, some Third World nurses are able to maintain their ethnic identities with a minimum loss in credibility. In terms of their verbal and nonverbal communication, however, many Third World nurses appear condescending to Third World patients.

In other instances, Third World nurses feel quite marginal—estranged from non-Third World persons and no longer comfortable with members of their own ethnic group. These nurses appear cold and detached to both Third World and non-Third World patients. Another problem is the possibility that Third World patients will displace to these nurses their hostility toward non-Third World persons.

A related issue seldom explored in depth is the lack of empathy and sensitivity nurses have for patients other than those of their own ethnic group. Indians, for example, display considerable hostility towards blacks, and Mexican Americans frequently reject Chinese Americans. No doubt you can think of other illustrations. It is worth repeating at this juncture that all Americans are products of institutionalized racism, and awareness of this fact will allow the nurse to better deal with her or his own racism.

Non-Third World nurses, who constitute the overwhelming majority of members in professional associations, are beginning to come to grips with their own racism and that of their colleagues. It is hoped such introspection will not lead to a repression or denial of hostile feelings. Nor should a nurse who is trying to understand her or his racism be immobilized by guilt. *Proactive nurses* rather than inactive nurses are needed if the vicious circle of racism is to be broken.

In the end, ethnic and sex similarities are not adequate substitutes for nurses who are (1) linguistically compatible with ethnic patients, (2) empathic, and (3) well trained. This means that the initial edge Third World nurses may have with Third World patients will be lost if the nurses cannot get beyond ethnic history and identity. These considerations should not, however, be interpreted as obviating the need for nursing programs to recruit and train considerably more Third World nurses, who comprise more than 50% of the nurse aides, less than 20% of practical nurses, and less than 10% of registered nurses.

References

1. *Health: United States, 1978.* 1978. Hyattsville, Md.: U. S. Department of Health, Education, and Welfare, p. xi.

2. Kennedy, E. 1972. *In critical condition: The crisis in American health.* New York: Simon & Schuster, Inc., p. 15.

3. DeBakey, M. June 20, 1974. Quoted in *Tulsa Daily World.*

4. Norman, J. C., editor. 1969. *Medicine in the ghetto.* New York: Appleton-Century-Crofts, p. 5.

5. *Health: United States, 1978.* 1978. Hyattsville, Md.: U.S. Department of Health, Education, and Welfare, p. 50.

6. *Health: United States, 1978.* 1978. Hyattsville, Md.: U.S. Department of Health, Education, and Welfare, p. 150.

7. Slater, J. June 1973. Hypertension: Biggest killer of blacks. *Ebony,* pp. 74-82. Also see Gaver, J. R. 1972. *Sickle cell disease: Its tragedy and its treatment.* New York: Lancer Books, p. 9.

8. Bullough, B.; and Bullough, V. L. 1972. *Poverty, ethnic identity and health care.* Des Moines, Iowa: Meredith Corp., p. 75.

9. See *Puerto Ricans in the continental United States: Uncertain future.* 1978. Washington, D.C.: U.S. Commission on Civil Rights.

10. Deloria, V., Jr. 1969. *Custer died for your sins: An Indian manifesto.* New York: Macmillan, Inc., p. 248.

11. Mosley, D. 1973. The nursing profession and the urban poor. *NCRIEED Tipsheet* 11:2-3.

12. Kohlberg, L. 1966. A cognitive developmental analysis of children's sex-role concepts and attitudes. In Maccoby, E., editor. *The development of sex differences.* Stanford: Stanford University Press, pp. 82-173.

13. For a model, see Orque, M. S. 1976. Health care and minority clients. *Nurs. Outlook* 24:313-316.

14. See Epps, E., editor. 1974. *Cultural pluralism.* Berkeley: McCutchean Publishing Corp.

15. For a comprehensive report of employment trends, see U. S. Department of Labor. 1979. *Employment and training report of the president.* Washington, D. C.: U. S. Government Printing Office.

16. Green, R. L. 1977. *The urban challenge: Poverty and race.* Chicago: Follett Corp., pp. 12-18.

17. Coles, R. 1970. *Uprooted children: The early life of migrant farm workers.* Pittsburgh: University of Pittsburgh Press.

18. Lyons, R. D. 1973. The coming crisis. *Colliers Yearbook.* New York: Macmillan, Inc., p. 76.

19. National Commission on Community Health Services, 1966. *Health is a community affair.* Cambridge: Harvard University Press, p. 2.

20. Jersild, A. T.; and Helfun, K. 1953. *Education for self-understanding: The role of psychology in the high school program.* New York: Columbia University, Teacher's College, p. 9.

21. Simmons, O. G. 1958. Implications of social class for public health. *Hum. Organ.* 16:16-18.

22. Sotomayor, M. 1977. Language, culture and ethnicity in developing self-concepts. *Soc. Casework* 58:195.

23. McNickle, D. 1968. The sociocultural setting of Indian life. *Am. J. Psychiatry* 125:119.

2

Gaining Awareness of Cultural Differences:
A Case Example

Raphella Sohier, R.N., M.S.N.

Ms. Sohier received her M.S.N. from the University of Illinois School of Nursing. Much of her graduate and post-graduate work was done in Scotland, Belgium, and the Netherlands. She is currently a lecturer on community health nursing at Wayne State University. Included among her memberships are the American Nurses' Association, the American Anthropological Association, the Society of Applied Anthropology and the American Public Health Association. Ms. Sohier has written articles on cultural awareness, homosexuality, and anthropological applications to nursing.

It is my opinion that the type of understanding which we call science can begin anywhere, at any level of sophistication. To observe acutely, to think carefully and creatively—these activities, not the accumulation of laboratory instruments, are the beginnings of science.[9]

During the last few years a core of nurse-anthropologists in the United States have given leadership to the development of the subfield Leininger[6] calls "transcultural nursing." This subfield had been generally ignored or perceived to be of little importance as a systematic field of study in nursing and health care. Growing interest in this essential area of study in contemporary nursing care is encouraging. A pioneer in the field, Leininger[3] states, "It needs active attention in research and educational endeavors." In one of her several works on the subject,[5] she asks the critical question: "Is it possible for any outsider who is not a member of that culture to become a helping person in a kin-based community?" This [chapter] will address this question by using a case example to demonstrate the phenomenon of cultural awareness and the transcultural nursing process and its implications.

Awareness of certain phenomenon can frequently develop quite independently in different parts of the world. It is of interest that at the time Leininger and other colleagues were laying the groundwork for the new subfield of transcultural nursing in the U.S.A., I was striving to find solutions to problems of a transcultural nature in Belgium in 1969 and 1970. My discovery of the importance of the nurse having an understanding of cultural factors in patient care seemed extremely important and unique. Since that time Leininger has published a book on the general subject of culture and nursing, is preparing another book, and has written many articles and given talks on the subject of transcultural nursing care since 1963. She has stressed the need to develop a body of transcultural nursing theory and concomitant skills to facilitate the delivery of optimal care to people of different cultures. Her writings provide a clear picture of nursing education's deficits in regard to cultural theory and the barriers to the acquisition of transcultural skills and knowledge. Most importantly, she contends that transcultural nursing is a legitimate field of specialized study and should be an essential part of all nursing and health care practices.

Unquestionably, many nurses working with patients whose cultural backgrounds differ from theirs, feel varying degrees of inadequacy in sensitively handling patients' cultural needs and problems. Patients outside of the dominant culture have often expressed their feelings that nurses do not comprehend their situation, needs, and concerns. Health care projects at home and abroad have often failed or had minimal success, which makes one realize that goodwill is not an adequate criterion for success in transcultural health projects. "Doc adapts modern medicine to the customs of the Cakchiquel. He feels that too often well-meaning missionary and other organized groups fail, precisely because they have tried to do it the other way round."[1] Few nurses have been prepared in the field of anthropology, but a growing number are awakening to the need for such knowledge. The fields of anthropology and nursing are quite complimentary, and this has been well documented in the writings of Osborne[7] and Leininger.[5]

A CASE STUDY

The Beginning of Awareness

I went in 1958 to live and work in Belgium. Having completed a program of study in nursing, I was ready to help others as a professional nurse. At this time I became aware of the need for transcultural nursing knowledge and skills. In the case study which follows I will explicate the development of transcultural awareness and the important place of cultural values in the provision of comprehensive nursing care, clarifying what occurred in a reciprocal nurse-patient transcultural experience over a span of time. Personal values, the subculture of nursing, patient values and attitudes, and psychophysical therapeutic care process will be highlighted. Indeed, mutual learning occurred, which provided one of the richest nursing experiences in my life and altered the course of my professional goals to focus more on transcultural nursing.

The Scottish Nurse and Nursing Education

Nursing education in Scotland in the 1950's was moving toward a new focus, and although it has not yet attained the degree of academic excellence of American nursing at university level, still the quality of nursing education and expectations were noteworthy. The average graduate of the Scottish nursing program emerged as a competent and confident nurse who was ready to learn new ideas. Accordingly, I envisioned myself as a competent and intelligent nurse with a desire to learn more about patient care.

When I went to live in Belgium, I brought my Scottish heritage and its subculture of nursing. My Scottish culture emphasized the values of equality, social justice, honesty, and industry. The subculture of nursing in Scotland emphasized the values of personalized care, support and respect of human dignity with ethical practices, and the right of every human being to receive quality care. Nurses were viewed with respect and even with awe. Babies were delivered by midwives with a high level of competence and their independent performance was not only accepted but expected. District nurses had cars, as did health visitors (community health nurses), which gave them a high degree of independence. In general, the nurse was viewed as having a spotless character or, if otherwise, the ideal values of Florence Nightingale in her public and professional endeavors.

I was born in Edinburgh, Scotland, and was socialized in a Scottish Presbyterian home. Our family culture was a highly disciplined one, but love was shared not only within the family and among friends but with all people as brothers. Racial prejudice was not evident. Family members were taught that other families lived differently and this idea was accepted and recognized.

As the only daughter, I was encouraged from an early age to choose an excellent profession, namely, nursing. I was not actively discouraged from pursuing other directions, and medical school was another possibility. I envisioned no great barriers to the delivery of optimal nursing care beyond that of language. Fortunately, my nursing instruction had stressed the importance of the patient as a total person with individual needs, and so I was aware that generalized care alone was not sufficient. Personalized care with careful observation and the ability to recognize conflict and different needs was part of my way of operating as a professional nurse.

The Problem

With these values and self-perception, I began working for the first time in my life in a large Jewish community. A few days were essential to recognize my own distress signals and my need to adjust to a new cultural group, the Jewish people. Indeed, these people appeared strange and different to me. I did not comprehend their values and behavior for some time, even when they spoke excellent English. I knew, however, that I was not meeting the needs of the Jewish family. While my nursing school in Scotland had taught me to provide physiological and psychological care to patients, this was not enough. I could not read their family signals, nor distinguish clearly between physiological and psychological needs of the people in relation to their cultural orientation and values. These Jewish people seemed overly solicitous of themselves, fearful, demanding, and unusually insecure. I could not understand why they did not respond to nursing practices which ordinarily brought favorable results in Scotland. Curiosity and professional idealism combined and I began to see the challenge as well as the reasons why this family was not being understood. Thus, the problem of understanding and responding to this Jewish culture became evident as a real challenge.

A New Culture to the Nurse

The Jewish community in Antwerp is very large and most of its members are traditional; some people are deeply religious and others less so. Most of the Jewish people are of Eastern European origin and use the customs of the traditional Shtetl communities which had their origins in Russia, Poland, and Hungary.[14] Almost all of these people speak several languages, an average being five.

After a few nursing encounters, I tried to evaluate the needs of the Jewish patients but found my lack of knowledge a barrier to understanding the people. In general, the most direct manner of learning about a culture is to become what anthropologists call a participant observer. So when I started as a private duty nurse to assist a Jewish gentleman in his home, I had a unique opportunity to become a participant observer and learn first hand the patient's culture, values, and lifeways in his familial environment.

Toshek, the patient I came to know, was a 54 year old diamond merchant who had a history of a recent, severe myocardial infarction and an aortic aneurysm. He suffered recurrent episodes of angina which were not always relieved by medication, and his prognosis was poor. I recognized the opportunity to take care of this man as a privilege and challenge and went to his home on the first day with apprehension. While attending to Toshek's physical needs the first morning, I invited him to tell me something about himself. He said, "I am a Jew, what more is there to tell." My only knowledge of Jews was what I had learned in Bible class and Toshek did not appear to be, or to live, like those people, and so Toshek's reply did not give me any insight. As the days passed, however, we began to communicate more freely and I could sense that he was also curious about me.

Toshek's wife, Malva, was a pleasant lady who talked freely from the beginning and so I gained from her some essential understanding of Toshek as a person. She also began talking about Jewish culture by explaining the values and attitudes which influenced Jewish thought. Jews, she said, had a great reverence for life and therefore with how life was used, and this extended to a reverence for people. Learning, she told me, had always had a central place in Jewish culture, especially Talmudic (religious) learning. The man of learning was treasured above all others and referred to as one of the "beautiful people."[13] The concept of the family is extremely important in the Jewish culture. In addition, industriousness and material success were considered important but always secondary to learning. Material success was perceived as a *mitsva* (blessing from God). Malva told me that even well educated Jewish women remain in an inferior position to men. The traditional Jewish man thanks God daily for the fact that he was not born a woman. Males have a social, economic, and political status over women in the traditional Jewish culture. Knowledge of these basic cultural values became of great importance to me in clarifying and maintaining a favorable family-nurse interaction. Evaluation of my performance depended on understanding and relating to these values.

The average Belgian Jew in 1958 had a poor concept of a nurse because the nurse's role was perceived to be subservient, and the nurse a person of minimal intelligence who relied heavily on the physician for direction. Scottish nursing education did not develop this type of nurse, and so I was a puzzle to Toshek. While I attended his needs with regularity, I did not perceive myself in the role of serving wench. Instead, to Toshek I displayed an alarming intelligence and made independent decisions about his care based on my own nursing values and observations. He was amazed to discover this behavior and that I also understood political and economic world affairs plus literature and music. So it was a cultural shock to his perception of a nurse and a woman.

Reciprocal Confusion

Shortly after my arrival in Toshek's home I perceived the importance of the family. Within a few days I was convinced that I was being spied upon by members of the extended family as they came to meet Toshek's nurse. It seemed there was never a minute when I was not being observed by one of the family members. I did not know that what I was experiencing was a cultural behavior pattern highly acceptable to a kin-based family. After an initial perplexed and slightly angry period, I asked Malva whether I was distrusted. She looked very embarrassed and asked what had given me such a strange idea. When I told her what was worrying me, she laughed and explained that traditional Jewish people believe that the act of charity performed by visiting a sick person mitigates his illness.

Every evening at about five o'clock (earlier on Fridays because Sabbath was about to begin) a handsome white-haired gentleman would come to visit the patient. He was a quiet and solemn man whom I often heard softly humming. He was introduced to me as Toshek's elder brother and was acknowledged as the head of the family, the patriarch, a deeply religious man. (I later discovered that his humming was praying.)

Learning More about the Patient's Culture

Most of my time was spent taking care of Toshek's needs, and I found he was a humble, friendly person despite his wealth. When he felt well enough he would listen to music or read books written in a strange script which I thought was Arabic but was in fact Yiddish, the language of the Shtetl communities, which is written in Hebrew characters. (Weinrich[13] has written an interesting article on this language which might be of further interest to some readers.) At times I enjoyed Toshek but often I felt inadequate to meet his complex emotional, spiritual, and intellectual needs. My abilities to comprehend or deal with these complex needs seemed meager, and I found myself limiting the time I spent with the patient in these early days.

Sometimes Toshek wept in self-pity or railed in anger at his fate. He denounced the eminent cardiologist who took care of him. He accused the family of neglecting him and yet they seemed almost overly attentive to him. Although we all cared for him, none could change his fate. I became more frustrated daily with my inability to help Toshek. My Christian background had taught me abnegation and resignation, but attempts to help Toshek accept his illness by explaining and using such concepts were rejected. The words which were appropriate to Christians and made sense in the light of my value system failed miserably. It is difficult to comfort a Jew by citing Christ as an example of patient acceptance. I tried to evaluate his needs from a Jewish viewpoint but was unable to achieve this goal. It was then I began to see clearly the important part culture plays in our life expectations and reactions to life's demands upon us.

Toshek's family belonged to a group of Jews who called themselves "modern traditional" since the second World War. Within this group traditions of culture are observed such as separation of meat and milk foods, including dishes and cooking utensils (*kosher*), and observations of religious ceremonies on Fridays, Saturdays, and special feast days. Food is prepared in advance of all holy days and only a minimal amount of necessary work is done on those days. Those who are deeply religious do not light fire nor use it on holy days. Most of the people in this group do not ride in trains or automobiles on holy days of religious observance. The men attend the synagogue accompanied by their sons. Women occasionally attend the synagogue, walking to and from it in the company of their female children. Men and women sit in separate areas in the synagogue according to the old tradition. Marriage ceremonies are observed in the traditional fashion with the bride preparing herself for marriage by taking ritual baths at the synagogue. A bridal contract is made in the presence of family members and the rabbi. The marriage takes place under a canopy in the synagogue, with the rabbi and cantor. Traditional family blessings are prayed over the young couple by the most revered family members. Traditional Jewish dances are still performed at the reception.

As Toshek's family observed and followed their traditions, I learned much about their rich cultural heritage. More and more I realized that lack of knowledge about Jewish culture limited the quality of health care I might provide, and so I made a formal request to the family to be instructed about their culture. The family was quick to respond for they too had a high regard for learning and they planned ways to help me learn. There is a strong oral tradition among Jewish people, and Toshek was a born storyteller. When he was feeling well enough, he would talk of Jewish history and explain their religion and ritual. We listened together to the great traditional cantors on records, and he explained the prayers and taught me to appreciate the free expression in the music. He also taught me modern Jewish history, culminating in suspense stories of the war years and the time he spent in hiding with the Maquis (the French underground army).

Edith, his daughter, became a friend as she shared her books with me and explained the trends of modern Jewish thought. I became familiar with Jewish literature and read avidly the lives of Jabotinsky and Hertzle, the giants and founding fathers of Israelian Zionism. Edith talked with me about contemporary Jewish problems in the areas of language and culture and occasionally shared with me her personal hopes and dreams.

Toshek's wife, Malva, who was keenly intellectual, explored with me the movement of European Jewry toward integration with the dominant culture stream prior to World War II. Particularly in Germany, Austria, France, Belgium, and Holland, many Jewish young people had chosen to integrate into the mainstream culture rather than embrace the ideals of Zionism. When Hitler's regime expanded to the development of a pure Aryan race, it became evident that the Jewish cultural heritage formed a barrier to integration. The family told me that a new wave of dedication to cultural and traditional practices occurred, in some cases with a deep religious component, and in others with simply a strong revival of traditional practice divorced from the religious component. This idea was difficult for me to comprehend since Jewish tradition has a religious base.

Malva also talked with me about Jewish political affiliations. We discussed music, art, and literature along with the problems and achievements of Jewish women. In time, Malva and I came to know each other well as she saw me trying to meet Toshek's needs. This helped her develop a trusting relationship with me. It seemed that each member of the extended family took an interest in helping me become acculturated. I learned much about Jewish culture including the dietary laws and their relationship to the patient's peace of mind. I took part in religious feasts and family festivals, and when the time came, I helped to prepare a clean passover (*Kosher Pesakh*). Indeed, I began to feel that I had been accorded a place in the family. If I were asked if it was necessary to become an integral part of another person's culture to fulfill a helping role, I would answer in the negative. From my experiences, it does not seem necessary (or even desirable) to "go native" in order to demonstrate one's willingness to accept another patient's cultural values, norms, and practices as part of his lifestyle. I believe it is necessary, however, to protect the patient's right in order to fulfill his important cultural obligations.

Developing New Nursing Skills

The nursing care required by Toshek was of course my central focus. He could be very demanding and challenged the effectiveness of traditional nursing care practices. In the beginning, Toshek showed anxiety and doubt as his cultural perceptions of my nurse's role conflicted with the behaviors he observed in me. Initially, when I made decisions about his care or management, he thought this was the prerogative of the physician, and he would become anxious or insist on Malva calling the cardiologist. When this had occurred on several occasions, the physician merely confirmed my decisions and Toshek ceased to be fearful.

Toshek was often very emotional. As I learned more about his culture I interpreted his behavior differently and began to see cultural significance in it. I perceived that at times his pain was not physical but rather emotional anguish arising from present and past life experiences. Sometimes it seemed to be the echo of a cry for help arising from the Jewish people, a cry which had gone unanswered in history. Sometimes his anger was not directed toward me but toward those other people who had unleashed pogroms on his ancestors or taken his family to the gas chambers. At other times, Toshek's frustrations were real and directed towards me. He would shake his head and say, "strange non-Jewish woman" (*Vreemd goyish meidl*). I understood his feelings and the conflict within him. It was unusual for a Jewish man to trust a non-Jewish woman, especially after the terrors of the war years. He also found it frightening to admit that he felt affection for me. His behavior placed real demands upon me but, as my knowledge of his culture increased, I found myself willing to risk the therapeutic use of myself.

In time, I could distinguish between physical pain and anguish. Toshek called both states pain. It was possible for me to test this phenomena as his physical pain was often greatly relieved, whereas his anguish could not be relieved effectively by medicine. In such moments I would listen and empathize with Toshek, and his anxiety would subside. There was no need for me to dissimulate interest, because I care about the welfare of the patient. I was moved by the history of his people and their agonies and impressed with their rich culture.

I came to realize that in a kin-based society, the children in the family play an important role, and sometimes a small service offered Toshek by a child of the family was more helpful than my professional care. I learned to channel care through the family to him, providing extra satisfactions for him. One of the happiest moments he experienced was when he learned that his daughter was pregnant. He said, "Now I can die in peace."

As the months passed, evidences that I was accepted and trusted became more frequent. For example, when decisions were made by the family which affected Toshek, I was included in the family conference. Again, when Toshek's condition deteriorated, the head of the family asked my advice about calling a consultant, and an eminent specialist from France was flown in by helicopter. Additional evidence was the growing extent of my influence within the extended family in that Malva and Edith talked about their conflicts regarding Toshek's condition with me. Other members of the family asked me to help solve their marital problems; I worked with a teenager who was having psychosocial problems and made suggestions about the management of the youngest member of the family, a child only a few weeks old.

Resolution

As Toshek became gravely ill, the family realized his approaching death, and I was integrated into the family. The men of the family would talk with me about management of Toshek and accepted the suggestions I made for his comfort. Although two other nurses were brought into the situation to assist with the care of Toshek, no decisions were made for him without consulting me. When Toshek became acutely ill for the last time, the cardiologist decided to hospitalize him. This happened on a Friday evening, the beginning of the Jewish Sabbath. I was not with him then, but he was transported to the hospital accompanied by six adult members of the family. He kept asking for me, and the family searched in the city until they found me. When I reached the hospital, it was nearly sundown and Toshek greeted me with the traditional *Shabbas* (which loosely translates, "We will celebrate this day together.") He had never before greeted me with this traditional greeting used among Eastern European Jews. He asked the time and when I told him, he sent all the members of the family home to prepare for Sabbath. This was a significant act with reference to the nurse-patient relationship. To choose to stay alone with me on the holy day of the week indicated again, that I was part of the family.

As the therapeutic process had developed, Toshek was occasionally able to speak of death in an abstract way with reference to others but seldom at this time of his own death. Later, however, he explained the traditional dying practices of the Jews in the Shtetl communities and asked whether I would arrange for him to die in the traditional manner, namely, lying on the floor, covered but naked. Because I expected Toshek to die in his own home I made a solemn promise to fulfill his wish. On the evening before his death he reminded me of this promise.

Within the nurse-patient relationship, I experienced a deep inner conflict between my own Scottish cultural values, the subcultural values of the nursing profession, and my desire to respect the patient's traditional values. It seemed cruel to have Toshek die on a hard terazzo floor and the subcultural values of nursing had imbued me with a desire to nurture and support dying people with physical comfort measures. Nonetheless, Toshek's cultural and religious values dictated that he should return to God as he was born, without the embellishments of the world. Part of my conflict lay in the judgment which I could expect from physicians and associates as I was certain that they would misinterpret my intentions and label the incident "bizarre." I worried about the fuss which I could anticipate from the hospital administrators. When the cardiologist and a group of consultants came to make their morning visit, I told them of the patient's desire. Some were appalled and others were so uncomfortable at the thought that they giggled. One house physician returned after the others left and said that if I called him when death seemed imminent he would help me put Toshek on the floor. Several members of the family were present when I decided he was close to death and with the help of the physician we laid him on the floor. Toshek had come to trust me and I felt a moment of great sadness when he could not respond to me when I asked if he knew I had kept my promise.

I had been Toshek's day nurse for a year and seven months at the time of his death. I grieved with the family. We departed from the hospital promptly leaving his body with four male family members who remained and prayed throughout the day. According to Jewish law, his body could not be moved until after sundown. His body was brought to his home in a sealed casket before the burial. Women do not go to the burial. Malva had a family member call and ask me to come and take part in the ritual mourning with her, to keep Shiveh in the idiom of the Shtetl. I was deeply moved by the request. It is very unusual for a stranger to be invited to keep Shiveh and almost unknown if the person is a Christian. Malva sat barefooted on a low stool, wearing a shredded garment (the sign of widowhood). The men of the family did not shave for at least a month after Toshek's death, indicating their dissociation from wordly things during the initial time of mourning.

RECAPPING THE NURSE-PATIENT RELATIONSHIP
PHASES AND THEMES

During the initiation phase of any nurse-patient relationship several main themes occur: (1) mutual sharing of knowledge about each other and the situation; (2) testing of the nurse by the patient, and (3) the emergence of a helping modality. In a transcultural situation, the first theme takes a longer period than in a situation between a nurse and patient of the same cultural background. This phase of initiation is one of great importance in all therapeutic relationships but particularly in a transcultural setting. Leininger has said, "The scientific and humanistic integration of culture into health practices is a relatively new undertaking for health practitioners. It is, however, an extremely important part of providing for optimal care to patients."[3] The nurse must, therefore, develop a cultural awareness. It is not realistic to expect a patient to divorce himself from his cultural background and to react in accordance with the norms of the dominant culture simply because he finds himself in the midst of the dominant culture. Instead, it is more reasonable to expect the nurse to learn to understand cultural differences in order to deliver optimal care. Nurses often label patients in transcultural situations as difficult, stubborn, strange, or impossible when, in fact, the patient is simply being himself, a person based on a tradition often not known or understood by the practitioner.

The discomfort which I felt in the early stages of the relationship had to do with my lack of knowledge of the patient and his culture. Toshek tested me on many occasions. He would tease me saying, "The British are shocked at everything," which I read as an attempt to make me retort unfavorably about Jewish culture. He would, also, tell stories of the inefficiency and lack of personal cleanliness he had observed in French nurses, an attempt to test me professionally. This was, also, the period during which he doubted my ability to diagnose his physiological problems, another lack of trust or testing situation.

During this initial phase of the nurse-patient relationship, it is necessary for the nurse to gain knowledge which will enable her to understand the patient by putting herself in his place. The helping process cannot be established until the nurse understands the patient's needs. Before reaching this understanding the nurse is no more than a general administrator of care. After this understanding is reached, the nurse becomes an essential part of the therapeutic process. In order to empathize with a patient, the nurse must understand his background. Travelbee says, "The ability to predict behavior or comprehend the behavior of another is limited by personal background,"[11] and "empathetic boundaries may be expanded by repeated contacts with individuals of varying backgrounds."[12] Mere contact is not enough, however. Without a realization that cultural values, attitudes, beliefs, and life styles vary and a willingness to explore the situation from the patient's place in the scheme, a therapeutic relationship is difficult to develop. Empathy cannot be achieved without understanding, which presupposes a knowledge of the patient's basic values. Glittenberg says, "Reading someone from another culture mandates understanding and acceptance of his way of thinking."[1] Therapeutic use of self is not without risk. The nurse, and especially the student, is open to possible discomfort in the interaction process, unless she is equipped with the appropriate cultural knowledge on which to build the nurse-patient relationship and develop it beyond the administrative phase. Therapeutic use of self is the ultimate in nursing process for the nurse who desires to assist the patient to find meaning in illness.

Therapeutic Maneuvers

During the continuation phase of the nurse-patient relationship many therapeutic maneuvers were employed in our attempt to help the patient uncover and deal with his feelings and eventually to find some meaning in his illness. Toshek was encouraged to express his feelings, and to cope with the hostilities he felt toward the world, his family, and fate. Occasionally, it was necessary to help him develop self-limiting techniques when his behavior caused his wife undue stress. After the therapeutic relationship had been entered into, I attempted to provide support for him in his depressed and anguished moments. One of the maneuvers which in retrospect I see as valuable to the patient was encouraging him to speak, when he wished, of his childhood. It seemed to me that in reviewing his entire life and expressing its satisfactions audibly he was better able to contemplate his approaching death. It was also during such sessions that I came to know much about the culture of the Shtetl communities.

Evaluation Modalities

Hofling, Leininger, and Bregg state: "Bringing a nurse-patient relationship to a close is as important as getting the relationship into action," but that "what actually occurs when the relationship between the nurse and the patient draws to a close is not so well-known, as the other previously discussed phases of the nurse-patient relationship."[2] Closure of nurse-patient relationships are certainly important. A therapeutic relationship is usually concluded by the patient leaving the hospital, the judging that the time is ripe, or determining if the personal commitment of the nurse to the patient is causing too much discomfort. How closure is achieved in many nurse-patient relationships is not known. Traditionally, the nurse has been charged with the task of developing a state of uninvolved involvement, a state which is a contradiction in terms and is particularly difficult in transcultural situations. It is difficult to pursue such an "uninvolved" relationship while learning to appreciate a new culture. This is even more difficult for the nurse in a transcultural situation as the nurse must be willing to risk herself therapeutically if she is to gain credence. Some degree of personal involvement is unavoidable and essential.

   Nurses engaged in psychotherapeutic relationships have been taught the dangers of continued interaction with the patient beyond a certain period of need. Some colleges of nursing teach the psychotherapeutic process with explicit criteria for the closure of relationships. I believe the establishment of explicit criteria for the closing of nurse-patient relationships could result in restrained relationships and patient doubt as to the authenticity of the nurse's caring attitude. In the case cited, criteria was based upon the health of the patient, and the relationship was continued beyond the usual period of time. The criteria used were (1) the desire of the patient or family for such continued interaction, and (2) recognition of a changing focus in the relationship. Thus I have continued my interaction with the family for fifteen years.

   Immediately after the death of the patient, I continued in a therapeutic role with the family members as they worked their way through the grief process. The contacts became fewer and fewer, and the focus of the relationship changed many times in the course of past years. Presently, the contacts are limited to occasional letters and phone calls. I evaluate, however, the continuation of interest in the family's well-being as a realistic result of affective and effective earlier nurse-patient-family exchanges. Although the nurse-patient relationship is essentially based on patient need, it is not possible to live through a deep human experience such as we do with some patients and their families and forget them. We as nurses also change our feelings and skills. We learn in each encounter something new about ourselves and are assisted in our "becoming."[10]

Rogers[8] in explicating patient-centered therapy has indicated that he has continued contact with clients for many years. To risk oneself in a transcultural nursing situation and in a therapeutic role is sometimes bewildering (even a little scary), but it is only in an atmosphere of genuine caring that the patient (especially the patient with terminal illness) can find some meaning in illness. I am confirmed in my thinking by the words of Rogers to a client, "All I know is what I am feeling and that is, I feel very close to you at the moment." This is a statement of genuine caring on the part of the therapeutic figure.

CONCLUSION

Returning at this point to Leininger's question as to whether one can become a helping person in a kin-based society other than one's own culture, I would answer in the affirmative. A skillful nurse willing to learn about a culture new to her and to risk herself in new kinds of nurse-patient relationships can fill such a role.

The nursing profession in the United States could be viewed as standing at the most exciting point in its entire history. The equal rights amendment to the Constitution and the impetus given to women's rights by the Women's Movement are creating opportunities for nurses to be heard. The traditional position of handmaiden has been rejected, and the nurse, male or female, is articulating freely about the profession and its goals.

Nurses are developing a body of knowledge which is peculiarly their own and impressing the public with their educational accomplishments. Innovative nursing practice legislation makes it possible for American nurses to practice legally roles which have been theirs for decades. An autonomy that has been surreptitious in the past has come into the open. Consequently, the nurse has a greater responsibility for the quality of care offered to patients and an increasing obligation to listen to consumer demands and serve as consumer advocates. We are at last free to make decisions about our professional needs in education, education which should equip us to deliver health care at a level of competence and relevance hitherto unknown.

Members of minority cultures across the country are demanding health care which meets their cultural needs, and since we are now free to plan health education curricula as we see fit, let us include the long neglected dimension of culture. Currently, there are a few nursing schools giving serious consideration to cultural deficits in the curricula. A very few have included basic cultural anthropology as an early prerequisite to the nursing major. Some schools are beginning to consider the development of undergraduate and graduate courses on the subject of transcultural nursing.

In this article I have tried to demonstrate that knowledge of cultural background, values and attitudes of the patient are indispensable for nurses who wish to deliver comprehensive health care. Total care can become a reality only when patients are seen in the framework of their individual cultural patterns.

References

1. Glittenberg, J. Dec. 1974. Adapting health care to a cultural setting. *Am. J. Nurs.* 74:2219-2220.

2. Hofling, C. K.; Leininger, M.; and Bregg, E. 1967. *Basic psychiatric concepts in nursing.* Philadelphia: J. P. Lippincott Co., p. 66.

3. Leininger, M. 1970. *Nursing and anthropology: Two worlds to blend.* New York: John Wiley & Sons, Inc., pp. 29-30.

4. Leininger, M. 1970. *Nursing and anthropology: Two worlds to blend.* New York: John Wiley & Sons, Inc., p. 45.

5. Leininger, M. 1972. *Using cultural styles in the helping process and in relation to the subculture of nursing.* Chicago: Nursing Papers, State of Illinois, p. 43.

6. Leininger, M. 1975. *Transcultural nursing: Theory and practice.* New York: John Wiley & Sons, Inc.

7. Osborne, O. H. 1969. Anthropology and nursing: Some common traditions and interests. *Nurs. Res.* 18:251.

8. Rogers, C. R. 1973. Client centered therapy. In Corsini, R., editor. *Current psychotherapies.* Itasca, Ill.: F. E. Peacock Publishers, Inc., pp. 162-163.

9. Rogers, C. R. 1959. A theory of therapy, personality, and interpersonal relationships as developed in the client-centered framework. *Psychology: A study of a science,* vol. 3. New York: McGraw-Hill Book Co., pp. 84-156.

10. Rogers, C. R. 1961. *On becoming a person.* Boston: Houghton Mifflin Co.

11. Travelbee, J. 1966. *Interpersonal aspects of nursing.* Philadelphia: F. A. Davis Co., pp. 16-19.

12. Travelbee, J. 1966. *Interpersonal aspects of nursing.* Philadelphia: F. A. Davis Co., p. 23.

13. Weinrich, M. 1953. Yiddishkayt and yiddish. *Mordicai M. Kaplan jubilee volume.* New York: Jewish Theological Seminary of America.

14. Zbrowski, M.; and Hertzog, E. 1952. *Life is with people.* New York: Schocken Books, Inc.

3

Countertransference and Ethnic Similarity

Mary L. Gottesfeld, M.S.S.

Mary L. Gottesfeld is Editor of the Clinical Social Work Journal *and has a private practice in psychotherapy and psychoanalysis in New York City. She is on the faculty and Coordinator of the Individual Therapy Certificate sequence of the Post-Master Program at Hunter College Graduate School of Social Work, City University of New York. A member of various scholarly societies, she received a certificate in hypnotherapy and hypnoanalysis from the Institute for Research in Hypnosis and has had an interest in the adjunctive use of hypnosis in psychotherapy. She has published clinical papers in* Psychoanalytic Review, Social Casework, *and* American Journal of Clinical Hypnosis, *among others.*

We tend to think of countertransference occurring when therapists cannot free themselves from strong ties of their archaic superegos and thus cannot be flexible with patients of different cultural backgrounds. Speigel (1965) says that "the experiences my colleagues and I have had, working with patients whose cultural backgrounds differed greatly from our own, is that the value discrepancy sets up a very complicated strain within the therapist" (p. 587). But the difficulties that

Source: Gottesfeld, M. L. 1978. Countertransference and ethnic similarity. Reprinted with permission from the *Bulletin of the Menninger Clinic,* Vol. 42, No. 1, pp. 63-67, copyright 1978, The Menninger Foundation.

occur when patient and therapist are ethnically similar can be just as complicated and, oddly, even more obscure than when their cultural backgrounds differ. In this paper I will attempt to describe the powerful effects on the therapist's ethnic identity when working intensively in psychotherapy with a patient of similar ethnic background.

One of my patients and I have similar backgrounds. Our forebearers came to this country from Italy; we both grew up in Italian communities, were reared as Roman Catholics, were born in the same year, had graduate education degrees, and grew up in extended families. But there are differences as well: My patient is a second-generation American, I am a third; she maintained her religion, I did not; she was the first member of her family to obtain a higher education, I was not; she speaks Italian fluently and grew up bilingual, I did not. Furthermore, while my forebears came from the south part of Italy (the area of greatest Italian immigration), her parents did not. By presenting her history and extrapolating from those parts of her therapy which are relevant to this discussion, I would like to show how certain countertransference reactions grew out of my own early ethnic (Italian) background and discuss some of my reflections about the influence of these reactions.

I came to a greater understanding of ethnicity through the writings of Giordano who said: "... ethnicity from a clinical point of view is more than a distinctiveness defined by race, religion, national origin, or geography. It involves conscious and unconscious processes that fulfill a deep psychological need for security, identity, and a sense of historical continuity. It is transmitted in an emotional language within the family and is reinforced by similar units in the community" (1974, p. 209).

CASE HISTORY

When I first saw the patient she was a forty-two-year-old single woman who had never been married. She was considerably overweight, but was attractive and neatly groomed. At that time she was completing a doctorate in library science and was on the faculty of a university. Her father had been dead for ten years; her mother died just six months ago. She was the youngest of nine children and resided with an unmarried brother and sister who were both in their sixties. Her social life consisted of family visits.

At the time she sought therapy, she complained of unbearable grief dating from her mother's death. She was unhappy with her job and had been unable to write her dissertation which had to be completed within two years or she would lose her candidacy. In addition, she felt considerable guilt over her habit of masturbation.

COURSE OF THERAPY

The patient's therapy lasted three years and was terminated at her request—she felt she had gone as far as she could go. She was quite verbal and motivated during this time. At the end of the second year she had changed her job from teaching to direct library service and was much more satisfied with her work. In her new position she had been able to make a few women friends with whom she socialized occasionally. She completed her dissertation on time and was awarded her degree. She had worked through her profound mourning and was no longer overwhelmed by it. The problem of masturbation remained, and it was over this issue that her therapy became considerably more complex.

During the first month of therapy, the patient, in talking about her early life and background, asked me if I had any knowledge of Italian heritage; I answered that I understood Italian families well because I was of Italian descent. Despite this comment, the patient often spoke as if I knew nothing about such things. When I asked her about this attitude, she insisted that "it must have been different for you." She never inquired as to what specifically was my Italian background, or what part of Italy my relatives came from. She rarely used any commonly known Italian expressions; in fact, she went out of her way to let me know that she spoke a most unusual Italian dialect understood by very few people. When I asked her to let me hear it, she would not use the dialect in sentences, but would give only single words as examples.

The patient was a virgin and had never had a date with a man. Although she indicated that her masturbation fantasies consisted of having sex with a man, she would not describe them. She wished to remain a practicing Catholic, despite some doubts about the modern church. She had gone from priest to priest over the years to confess her sin of masturbation but with no relief. At different times in the confessional she had received conflicting advice: Some priests told her that masturbation was a sin against God and that she must learn to control her "concupiscence" (her word) or risk eternal damnation; other priests told her she was in need of counseling, not confession.

At the beginning of the third year of therapy, the patient began to discuss her masturbation in more detail, but with a growing reluctance to do so. When this reluctance was pointed out to her, she raised the question as to whether therapy was for her an "occasion of sin," because after discussing her masturbation fantasies she was often left with a desire to masturbate which she could not control. I suggested to her that if having feelings here made the situation sinful, then indeed we were at an impasse.

About this time I became aware of some countertransference feelings which caused me to reexamine the therapy and eventually to understand the ethnic aspects of these feelings. Specifically, the patient spoke of needing a new car and of looking at one she was interested in buying. She arranged for the sister she lived with to go with her to see the car so the sister could "sit in the back seat and see if she liked it." Her sister pronounced the back seat—where she customarily sat—uncomfortable. With annoyance the patient remarked that although she wanted the car, she could not buy it. Without any thought at all I said, "You mean you didn't buy it for that reason?"

Within the transference the patient was describing the powerful bond between herself and the sister/mother. My question, therefore, would stand as therapeutic in that it might enable her to consider that buying her car does not have to be based on the relationship to her sister and all that implies. However, when I made the statement, this meaning is not what I thought of; instead I was aware of a strong feeling of incredulity which prompted me impulsively to say what I did. Later on, when I began to think about why I felt so incredulous, I realized it was because I thought she had acted in a way I imagined a recent immigrant from the old country would behave. From there I began to explore within myself why this "old country" feeling had been strong enough to remove me from my role as therapist and whether there were other ethnic feelings that were also affecting my work with the patient.

COUNTERTRANSFERENCE, ROLE, AND IDENTITY

The patient was diagnosed as an infantile personality in a borderline personality organization. Such patients suffer separation failures but have adopted life-styles which encapsulate the failure of individuation. In the case of this patient, her adaptations were reinforced and even exacerbated by some primitive ethnic feelings. Thus, she was permitted to live at home with her mother, remaining in the environment of and close to the person to whom she clung, with the approval of all those near to her. In fact, it was the death of the mother and the overwhelming grief of what was probably an abandonment depression that propelled her into therapy. Outside of her family and ethnic background, the patient would have had a difficult time accepting her level of adjustment and denying the conflicts that its awareness would create. By maintaining family secrets and having a secret life (masturbation fantasies), she retained control over the therapy and kept me outside her system (family). She managed this feat even in the face of my knowledge of Italian families because I was, by countertransference, in an ethnic collusion with her.

When I told her in the beginning that we had similar backgrounds, she moved away from me saying that her Italian background was "unusual" and never inquiring about mine. Her system and her secretiveness were so close to my own ethnic identity, that it was acceptable to me and I could barely see it. I recognized so many things from my own early childhood—speech inflections, words, foods, primitive ideas such as the evil eye (*malocchio*) and the horn (*cornuto*) for protection against it—that I shared with her a delicious sense of "our thing" (*cosa nostra*).

It is this powerful closeness with the family that remains at the heart of the

Italian experience, where "preservation of the family network is more important than the fate or goal of an individual" and where "children are trained for dependence on family relationships which must be preserved at all costs" (Spiegel 1968, p. 373). Unlike the Jewish experience, which is extensively articulated in an authentic way in literature (cf. contemporary writers such as Roth, Bellow, Malamud, Mailer, etc.), the Italian experience has not been similarly developed. I believe this fact to be part of the defense to maintain what is "ours." Even the mafia is a stereotype, a story for others to believe about Italians that is exaggerated, romanticized, and fictional (Rufus King's "Looking for the Lost Mafia" [1977]); but in believing this myth, "they" will never come to know about the family (*la famiglia*).

To some extent, I never went into this ethnic core with my patient. I had "passed," I was beyond it in my life; in reality, I had lived it. As to my comment about not buying the car, my ethnic identity had been touched by the tight relationship with the sister/mother. But, in studying this reaction, I became aware of how much I respected her system (family). Not knowing this aspect of my own identity had allowed me, in my role as therapist, to let her retain her secrets, her system, and her control. If I had encouraged her to find out about them, primitive ties might have been loosened. I realized she was not being withholding in a manipulative way because, during the course of therapy, she had willingly talked about painful feelings of inadequacy, shame, and guilt, and described numerous life experiences related to such incidents.

This awareness on my part permitted more openness and self-knowledge to become available to the patient. Some secrets were unfolded and discarded resulting in improved relationships and a better feeling on her part. She became aware of the secretiveness in the family; for example, her own birth was a secret since none of her siblings knew her mother was pregnant!

Thus my sense of psychological familiarity with the patient, usually so helpful with borderline patients, here became a case of too much psychic togetherness. The Italians' need to hold on to the family to the exclusion of outsiders caused us to reinforce each other: She was withholding family information and I, in turn, kept away from analyzing her secrets. Thus I was sometimes not able to entertain ego-alien responses which would have forced her to study her own feelings and reactions with a conscious ego. An example of this point was her sister telling her she could never be alone with the brother with whom they lived (the sister thus repeated the pattern of the original parents in which the father was stern and the children were tied to oversolicitious mother). The brother had been wounded in the war and was considered "nervous." The patient had always accepted her brother's "disturbance" but it colored their relationship. When I asked what was wrong with her brother and why their relationship was distant, she began to pursue this question with her sister. Eventually the patient was told that when she was an infant the brother was seen watching her very closely and was suspected of having sexual intentions toward her; hence, he was never to be left alone with her. This attitude continued into adulthood, binding them all to each other.

Finally, it was the Italian need for closeness to the sense of family that was, in part, a defense against the primary fixation the patient had with an archaic, unrewarding mother. Her mother was never affectionate with her but spoke only of "doing one's duty." Despite all her efforts, the patient could not get from her mother any of the preferential treatment reserved for the sons. The masturbation, therefore, was not only a pregenital fixation; but, more importantly, the sin of masturbation bound her to the critical, internalized mother from whom she sought forgiveness and love.

Although the patient made some overt changes during therapy, she could not give up the notion of masturbation as a sin; to do so would mean to renounce the ambivalent relation with the internalized mother, of sinning and seeking forgiveness. It was on this note, despite some valiant efforts, that the patient decided to terminate, having obtained what she wanted from therapy except for the resolution of her problems around masturbation. She did not think that any resolution could be reached by us.

We parted perhaps as therapist and patient should part, with each of us the wiser for working together. I agree with Giordano (1976) who said:

> The impact of ethnicity on the individual, though occasionally recognized, has been largely neglected in mental health research and literature. There are numerous reasons for this neglect, including a personal ambivalence toward ethnicity that is especially evident among upwardly mobile, middle-class professionals who have embraced universalist life-styles and value systems, leaving their own ethnicity behind (p. 4).

References

Giordano, J. 1973. *Ethnicity and mental health.* New York: Institute on Pluralism and Group Identity.

Giordano, J. 1974. Ethnics and minorities: A review of the literature. *Clin. Soc. Work J.* 2:207-220.

King, R. 1977. Looking for the lost mafia. *Harper's* 254:68-71, 74-75.

Spiegel, J. P. 1965. Some cultural aspects of transference and countertransferences. In Zald, M. N., editor. *Social welfare institutions: A sociological reader.* New York: John Wiley & Sons, Inc., pp. 575-594.

Spiegel, J. P. 1968. Cultural strain, family role patterns, and intrapsychic conflicts. In Howells, J. G., editor. *Theory and practice of family psychiatry.* Edinburgh: Oliver & Boyd, pp. 367-389.

4

The Language Barrier in Evaluating Spanish-American Patients

Luis R. Marcos, M.D., Med. Sc.D.
Leonel Urcuyo, M.D.
Martin Kesselman, M.D.
Murray Alpert, Ph.D.

Luis R. Marcos is Associate Professor of Psychiatry at the New York University School of Medicine and Director of the Department of Psychiatry at Gouverneur Hospital in New York City. He is also Adjunct Professor of Psychiatry at Bilbao University Medical School in Bilbao, Spain. He has served on several administrative and planning committees in New York City in the field of mental health and has been active in many professional societies and journals. His numerous publications, in both Spanish and English, reflect an intense interest in the relationship between bilingualism and psychiatry. He has also written several articles on psychiatric education.

Leonel Urcuyo is Associate Professor of Clinical Psychiatry at New York University School of Medicine and Director of Manhattan Children's Psychiatric Center of the New York State Department of Mental Health. He

Source: Marcos, L. R.; Urcuyo, L.; Kesselman, M.; and Alpert, M. 1973. The language barrier in evaluating Spanish-American patients. *Arch. Gen. Psychiatry* 29:655-659. Copyright 1973, American Medical Association.

has participated in numerous committees on transcultural psychiatry and has published several articles on the effect of bilingualism on psychotherapy.

Martin Kesselman is Director of Psychiatry at the Kings County Hospital Center in Brooklyn, New York. He is also Professor of Clinical Psychiatry, and Associate Chairman, State University of New York, Downstate Medical Center. His professional interests include transcultural psychiatry and the major psychoses, with an emphasis on schizophrenia.

Dr. Murray Alpert is Professor and Director of Psychology in the Department of Psychiatry, New York University—Bellevue Medical Center. He is on the Council of the American College of Neuro-Psychopharmacology and Secretary of the American Psychopathological Association. His research interests and numerous publications focus on the assessment of psychopathology and cognitive functioning in bilingual psychiatric patients.

In a previous report we described the effect of the language in which the interview was conducted on the assessed psychopathology of Spanish-American patients:[1] significantly more pathology was found when the patients were interviewed in English. These ratings were based on closed circuit television (CCTV) recordings of the interviews. The English and Spanish interview questions were identical in content, had been prerecorded, and were presented in a manner which minimized variables other than language. The ratings were made independently by separate pairs of English- and Spanish-speaking raters.

Although a contribution from rater prejudice (both negative and positive)[2] could not be excluded, there was evidence suggesting that the increment in psychopathology in the English ratings was unrelated to any difference in the clinical style or skillfulness of the two groups of raters. Nor was it simply a result of the patients' competence in English; even patients who were relatively fluent in English were evaluated as presenting more pathology in their English interview. It appeared reasonable to assume that the patients were, in fact, cuing the raters differently in the two languages.

Since the importance of the interview language on the psychiatric evaluation of foreign-born patients has been generally accepted, it is surprising that its effect on pathology assessment has received little experimental attention. In one report, Del Castillo[3] described clinical experiences in which Spanish-speaking patients appeared obviously psychotic during native-tongue interviews, but seemed much less so when the interview was conducted in English. In this report, however, no description of the patients' behavior was given. The interviews were part of pretrial examinations and the interviewer was free to conduct the interview in any manner he chose. Under these circumstances it is difficult to evaluate the extent to which the interview procedure, apart from the interview language, contributed to the difference in detected pathology.

We undertook the study of the effect of the interview language on verbal behavior utilizing the CCTV recordings that had been rated in our earlier study (i.e., standardized, prerecorded interviews conducted in counterbalanced order within a 24-hour period and recorded on videotape). We were concerned with uncovering the manner and extent to which the language of the interview produced changes in the patient's clinically relevant communications. Because our staff is largely limited to clinicians competent only in English, we also hoped to begin developing guidelines that would be useful in situations where a language barrier hampers communication. The availability of CCTV provided a reliable tool for minimizing interview variability and for attaining a permanent record that could be studied under well-controlled conditions.[4]

METHODS

Ten patients who were recent admissions to the adult service of Bellevue Psychiatric Hospital, New York City were selected for the study. The criteria for admission to the project were as follows:

1. Spanish as the mother-tongue, but sufficiently fluent in English to participate in English psychiatric interviews. In point of fact, all patients had received English-language intake interviews.
2. Diagnosis of schizophrenia made independently by two psychiatrists.
3. No evidence of organic brain disorder.
4. Willingness to volunteer for the study.

There were six men and four women of Puerto Rican birth ranging in age from 21 to 42. Their schooling averaged 8.7 years; the average stay in this country was 18.2 years. Each of the patients was receiving major tranquilizers and they were not informed as to the aim of the study.

CCTV recordings were made of standard psychiatric interviews in English and Spanish, half of the patients receiving the English version first. The two interviews were spaced no more than 24 hours and no less than 20 hours apart. During this period no change was made in the patient's medication. Although an English or Spanish-speaking clinician was present during the interview, his participation was minimal since the interview questions had been previously recorded on audiotape.

The English and Spanish questions were identical and presented in the same order. The questions were the items in the Psychiatric Evaluation Form[5] interview and are a distillate of the common problems used in psychiatric evaluations. The videotape recordings were independently rated by two English- and two Spanish-speaking psychiatrists using the Brief Psychiatric Rating Scale.[6]

To determine the differences between the English and Spanish interviews for each patient, two bilingual psychiatrists compare the verbal content and infra-content vocalizations of the English and Spanish interviews for each patient. The audio portion of the videotapes was re-recorded onto a high-fidelity audiotape. The two bilingual raters reviewed these tapes as well as verbatim transcripts of the interviews. Each pair of interviews was judged for differences and similarities in content, syntax, and infracontent (e.g., speech rate, silence quotient, and speech disturbances).

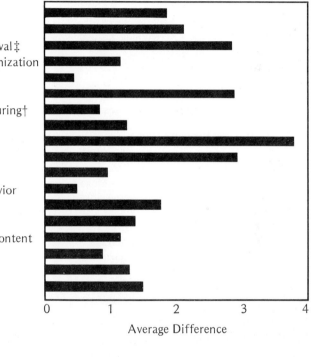

1. Somatic Concern*
2. Anxiety†
3. Emotional Withdrawal‡
4. Conceptual Disorganization
5. Guilt Feelings
6. Tension‡
7. Mannerisms & Posturing†
8. Grandiosity
9. Depressive Mood‡
10. Hostility‡
11. Suspiciousness
12. Hallucinatory Behavior
13. Motor Retardation
14. Uncooperativeness
15. Unusual Thought Content
16. Blunted Affect
17. Excitement
18. Disorientation

*P < .02
†P < .05
‡P < .01

Average Difference

Figure 4-1. Differences between pairs of English and Spanish pathology scores for each Brief Psychiatric Rating Scale subscale; all differences are positive English greater than Spanish.

RESULTS

For each patient clear and consistent differences were found between the English and the Spanish interviews. In [Figure 4-1] the differences between English and Spanish pathology scores for each BPRS subscale and their level of significance can be seen. It should be emphasized that the effect of the language of interview was similar despite the wide range in severity of pathology, age, education, length of stay in this country, and fluency in English.

Content Changes

A. *Changes in the Sense of the Response.* On numerous occasions the patients gave different responses to the same question in English and Spanish. Most often, the response in English suggested greater pathology, for example:

Question 7, Subject 1: "Do you get tired easily?"
ENGLISH RESPONSE: "Yes, yes, very tired, yes."
SPANISH RESPONSE: "No sir."

Question 9, Subject 2: "What about worries, do you have many worries?"
ENGLISH RESPONSE: "Yes."
SPANISH RESPONSE: "None."

Question 1, Subject 3: "Tell us something about your difficulties, and how they led to your coming to the hospital."
ENGLISH RESPONSE: "Ah, I really don't have any difficulties."
SPANISH RESPONSE: "Well, my name is _____ , I think that what brought me to the hospital was, well, trying to recall the past, I think that I was working too much, too many hours, and the free time instead of doing exercise and other similar things like reading, resting. I had too much of a good time, when I was young. I went out a lot, I didn't get enough rest, I used to drink too much ... [the patient continues talking about his past life, some marriage difficulties, and certain experiences he had prior to his being hospitalized] ... I believed that I was lost as if I had died and I was living a second life. I didn't tell anybody because nobody asked me, now I'm telling you, well, I think that's all."

Question 21, Subject 4: "Have you ever heard things and voices that other people can't hear?"
ENGLISH RESPONSE: Yes, I have, yes, voices, and I have seen people, but I must not argue, sometimes is very simple ... I am not a witch, but I believe in things, I've got to help people. . . ."
SPANISH RESPONSE: "No, no, well only once I heard somebody telling me that someone was destroying my family. . . . I couldn't figure it out."

Question 8, Subject 6: "What kind of moods have you been in recently?"
ENGLISH RESPONSE: "Ah, let me put it this way, I'm in a blue mood, I have been kind of sad. It is mainly caused by the reason that I have no way of finding a job. I am overworried, I have lately been sad, very sad, to the point that I have kept away from laughter, from enjoying conversation with other people, and I am being by myself."
SPANISH RESPONSE: "Lately I have felt better, because when I came to the hospital I was depressed, very sad. But as the days went by and with the treatment that I have received my mood has cheered up little by little, and I think I feel again as happy as I did before coming to the hospital."

B. *Length of Responses.* There was a striking tendency in our Spanish-American patients to answer the English questions with a short sentence, a word, or even silence. A total of 44 English questions were answered either with "I don't know," "I don't think so," or "no sir." In Spanish such simple negative responses occurred only seven times. Responses consisting of plain "yes," "yes sir," or "yes" followed by six words or less occurred 63 times in the English interviews and only 28 times when the interview language was Spanish. Thus there is a significantly higher number of short responses in English ($X^2 = 46.51$, df = 1, $P < .001$). The following are verbatim examples:

Question 19, Subject 6: "Do you take alcohol in excess, or any drugs?"
ENGLISH RESPONSE: "No sir."
SPANISH RESPONSE: "Well, no, when I am working, I don't drink, but when I find myself without a job I start to drink."

Question 21, Subject 7: "Have you ever heard things and voices that other people can't hear?"
ENGLISH RESPONSE: "Yes, I have, yes."
SPANISH RESPONSE: "Yes, it has happened many, well, not so many, on occasions. Once I was with my father, I was somewhat sick, I looked out of the window and I saw the Virgin of Saint Clares, dressed like in modern times, the Virgin was sitting on a branch, leaning against a fence. I was surprised, I waved my hand, like this [the patient continues giving more details of the hallucinations] . . .

C. *Translation Difficulties.* The effect of the longer response on the rater may be greater than the data suggest, since a patient's occasional attempt to expand on a particularly relevant subject gives the listener a sense of involvement and motivation for help with positive prognostic connotations. In addition to the obvious and expected difficulties in understanding questions and finding words to satisfy their communicative intent, our patients frequently showed a surprising amount of difficulty in using the past tense when interviewed in English. Usually they spoke in the present tense when interviewed in English, while their parallel Spanish response made it clear that they intended the past. An interviewer attempting to assess just how active a patient's symptoms are may be led astray.

Another related issue is the phenomenon of "language mixing": seven patients utilized Spanish words during their English interviews, some of them quite frequently. This language intrusion made their flow of thought sound less logical and more confused. Perhaps, not surprisingly, language mixing occurred in English in response to questions which were of special importance to the patient.

Question 16, Subject 1: "What sort of a person do you think you are, how do you feel that you compare with other people?"

ENGLISH RESPONSE: "Doctor Miller, Doctor Miller . . . el es el que me da las aspirinas [he is the one that gives me the aspirins] . . . I don't make what . . . [unintelligible sounds]."
SPANISH RESPONSE: "Well, in reference to the masculine sex, I am good."

In English we see an illogical and incoherent response. In Spanish, provided the interviewer is familiar with the concept of "machismo," the response can be viewed as relevant.

Question 2, Subject 8: "Have you been feeling well recently? Has anything else been bothering you?"
ENGLISH RESPONSE: "Some people are too bad [annoyed]."
INTERVIEWER (not prerecorded): "Who are they?"
PATIENT: "?? Los hijos del diablo [the devil's sons]." [At this point the patient attempts to leave the office.]
SPANISH RESPONSE: "No, sometimes I worry about my daughters, whether they got burns or what happened to them . . . the building caught on fire . . . I would like to know what happened to them [the patient starts crying] —I don't care what color they are, the only thing I care is to be with them."

This female patient was brought to the hospital by the police after having set fire to her apartment where she was living with her two daughters. In the English interview she appeared uncooperative and even attempted to leave the office, to a non-Spanish-speaking interviewer she would have sounded incoherent. In Spanish the patient was cooperative, relevant, and showed affect appropriate to the circumstance.

Infracontent Changes

A. *Speech Disturbances.* In working from the recorded material we were impressed with the frequency of speech disturbances such as the eight categories ("Ah," sentence correction, sentence incompletion, repetition, stutter, incoherent sound, tongue-slip, and omission) that Mahl has suggested as indicators of anxiety for native English-speaking patients.[7,8] We studied five minutes of parallel portions of the English and Spanish interviews; the two bilingual raters identified the various disturbances independently by listening to the audiotapes while simultaneously reading the transcripts. The interscorer reliability was .86 and .88 for the English and Spanish portions respectively (both correlations reject null at $P < .01$).

We computed the Speech-Disturbance Ratio

$$\left(\frac{\text{No. speech disturbances}}{\text{No. words spoken}} \right)$$

for the given language sample for each patient. The average Speech-Disturbance Ratio in the English and Spanish interviews were .132 and .041 respectively; the difference was statistically significant ($t = 2.43$; df = 9; $P < .05$). Among the speech-disturbances categories the most frequently found in the English interviews was incoherent sound and in the Spanish interviews, repetition.

We were unable to demonstrate a simple correlation between the Speech-Disturbance Ratio and the rater's impression of the patient's anxiety or tension, as Mahl had previously shown. However, our study should not be viewed as a replication of Mahl's because our patients were much sicker, and we had the additional variance due to the language factor. It seems likely that the Speech-Disturbance Ratio is more diffusely correlated with pathology in our sample, so that speech disturbances may contribute to the general increase in rated pathology level without a specific relation to anxiety.

B. *Speech Rate.* For English-speaking subjects increase in rate of speech has been shown to vary with increases in anxiety,[9-11] while decreases in speech rate have been associated with increases in depression.[10,12] Our subjects, who according to the speech-disturbance index might be expected to appear significantly more anxious during the English interview, showed a higher speech rate during the interview in Spanish. We determined the speech rate by a word count of the monologue that followed identical questions in each interview divided by the duration of the monologue in seconds.

The average speech rate was .582 words per minute for the English interviews and 1.025 for the interviews in Spanish; the difference was statistically significant ($t = 2.91$; df = 9; $P < .02$). The higher speech rate in Spanish suggests a greater fluency which may appear to reflect less anxiety, since many of Mahl's speech disturbances would tend to lower speech rate. But we cannot exclude the possibility that average speech rates in Spanish might simply be greater due to some nonpsychiatric characteristic of the Spanish language.

C. *Silent Pauses.* We calculated a Silence Quotient[10] for each patient by dividing the total duration in seconds of all pauses longer than one second by the total duration of the answer to question No. 1 in each language ("Tell us something about your difficulties and how they led to your coming to the hospital?"). The average Silence Quotient in the English interviews was .568 and in the Spanish interviews, .182; the difference was statistically significant ($t = 2.31$; df = 9; $P < .05$).

It appears from our material that speaking a second language may have a low activation effect on speech similar to what has been described in depression.[10,12] The English interview seems to evoke frequent and longer silences. Thus we see a number of infracontent aspects of talking behavior which may be interpreted as having clinical significance, whereas they derive from the special problems posed for patients when they are interviewed across the language barrier.

COMMENT

"People who speak different languages live in different worlds, not in the same world with different labels attached."[13] Anthropological linguists such as Sapir and Whorf have proposed that cognitive behavior is influenced by the semantic structure of languages and that men's minds are shaped by the language they speak.[14] Kolers[15] has suggested that bilinguals may have duplicate stores of meaning such that some information is readily accessible only via the language in which it was acquired. Clinically relevant processes may also suffer in the translation, so a patient's affect or anxiety may be bound to the language he is speaking.

We have attempted to explore the differences in the verbal component of behavior in a series of ten Spanish-American schizophrenic patients whose psychiatric ratings reflected significantly greater psychopathology when interviewed in English. The main finding of this study is that patients do, in fact, act differently in ways which the English-speaking clinician is likely to associate with increased psychopathology. A critical issue in the interpretation of these findings is whether this association is a real one or based on a misconstruction by the examiner. How much of this new behavior is a direct result of mental illness and how much is the result of the changed interview conditions?

Given the different levels of psychopathology found in the two languages, one might wonder which interview reflects the "true" condition of the patient. This question presupposes a pathological process existing independent of the behavioral manifestations through which we recognize the disease. It seems simpler to avoid this question by assuming that the environmental demands contribute to the manifest level of pathology and that under the lower demands of the Spanish-language interview the patients were in fact less sick.

When the patient attempts to speak a language other than his mother-tongue he creates problems both for himself and for the psychiatrist. Communicating his thoughts in a relatively unfamiliar language imposes an additional burden on the patient's already failing efforts to organize a fluid and chaotic subjective experience. Under these circumstances disturbances in fluency, organization, and integration occurred in English while they were absent in Spanish. These disturbances were not simply related to linguistic competence. It is possible that demanding the patient express himself in English acted as a distraction to cause further deterioration in his cognitive functioning. At points of affective arousal, patients frequently attempted to evade the linguistic constraints imposed on them by shortening their responses and lapsing into their native tongue.

An unexpected source of difficulty for the psychiatrist arose from the patient's lack of competence in English. Vocal cues serve as important sources of information in assessing psychopathology and there is a substantial body of work which attempts to articulate these cues. Such data has been developed from native speakers.

Another important finding of this study was the consistent tendency for changes in the expressive characteristics of the English-language interviews to overlap with just those vocal parameters which characteristically are associated with affective cues, e.g., those involving fluency, productivity, and rate of speech. It is likely that the psychiatrist's frame of reference, which is applicable to native English-speaking patients, cannot be directly applied to the evaluation of patient's behaviors which are influenced by psychopathology as well as cross-language factors.

It would be optimal if there were enough bilingual clinicians so Spanish-American patients could receive the attention of professionals competent in their language. Short of the optimal, it is important that clinicians be sensitized to the language-barrier effect, as well as to the culturally bound attitudes and beliefs of the Spanish-American population, e.g., "machismo," "ataque," black magic, spiritism, etc.[16-19] Speaking across the language barrier arouses a complex group of socially learned perceptions which color the patient's behavior.

When our patients spoke in English they showed a more uncooperative and guarded attitude toward the interviewer and the interview situation. This may reflect the cross-cultural antagonisms noted by previous workers;[20,21] perhaps, patients mistake linguistic differences for affective distance. In any case, patients were less communicative, more concise and formal, and more emotionally withdrawn in English than in Spanish.

As with all speech disturbances produced by speaking a foreign language, these may be compounded with indices of psychopathology. The patient's lack of linguistic competence may impede his flow of thought and lead him to evince what in an English-speaking patient could be interpreted as cognitive slippage involving mistaken interpretations, illogical, incoherent speech, concrete thinking, and impoverishment of thought not apparent in Spanish.

When a patient must be interviewed in a language in which he is less competent the clinician must make every effort to assure that the patient understands what is expected: he must introduce redundancy to facilitate communication and he ought not accept laconic responses as evidence of withdrawal or uncooperativeness. Furthermore, cues residing in the infracontent aspects of the interview should be carefully evaluated before considering them indicators of psychopathology. Finally, the English-speaking clinician should invest an extra effort in creating positive rapport and stimulating interview atmosphere.

References

1. Marcos, L. R., et al. 1973. The effect of interview language on the evaluation of psychopathology in Spanish-American schizophrenic patients. *Am. J. Psychiatry* 103:549-553.

2. Brody, E. B. 1966. Psychiatry and prejudice. In Arieti, S., editor. *American handbook of psychiatry* vol. 3, New York: Basic Books, Inc., Publishers, pp. 629-642.

3. Del Castillo, J. C. 1970. The influence of language upon symptomatology in foreign-born patients. *Am. J. Psychiatry* 127:242-244.

4. Alpert, M. Television tape for the evaluation of treatment response. *Psychosomatics* 11:467-469.

5. Endicott, J.; and Spitzer, R. L. What! Another rating scale? The psychiatric evaluation form. *J. Nerv. Ment. Dis.* 154:88-104.

6. Overall, J. E.; and Gorham, D. R. 1962. The brief psychiatric rating scale. *Psychol. Rep.* 10:799-812.

7. Mahl, G. F. 1956. Disturbances and silences in the patient's speech in psychotherapy. *J. Abnorm. Soc. Psychol.* 53:1-15.

8. Mahl, G. F. 1959. Measuring the patient's anxiety during interviews from "expressive" aspects of his speech. *Trans. N.Y. Acad. Sci.* 21:249-257.

9. Pope, B.; and Siegman, A. W. 1965. Interviewer specificity and topical focus in relation to interviewee productivity. *J. Verb. Learn. Verb. Behav.* 4:188-192.

10. Pope, B., et al. 1970. Anxiety and depression in speech. *J. Consult. Clin. Psychol.* 35:128-133.

11. Siegman, A. W.; and Pope, B. 1965. Effects of question specificity and anxiety producing messages on verbal fluence in the initial interview. *J. Pers. Soc. Psychol.* 2:522-530.

12. Alpert, M.; Frosch, W. A.; and Fisher, S. H. 1967. Teaching the perception of expressive aspects of vocal communication. *Am. J. Psychiatry* 124:202-211.

13. Sapir. 1971. Quoted by Edgerton, R. B.; and Karno, M. Mexican-American bilingualism and the perception of mental illness. *Arch. Gen. Psychiatry* 24:268-290.

14. Segall, M. H.; Campbell, D. T.; and Herskovitz, M. J. 1966. *The influence of culture on visual perception.* Indianapolis: The Bobbs-Merrill Co., Inc.

15. Kolers, P. A. 1971. Bilingualism and information processing. *Contemporary psychology.* San Francisco: W. H. Freeman & Co. Publishers.

16. Berle, B. B. 1958. *Eighty Puerto Rican families in New York City,* New York: Columbia University Press.

17. Fernandez-Marina, R. 1961. The Puerto Rican syndrome: Its dynamics and cultural determinants. *Psychiatry* 24:78-82.

18. Wolf, K. L. 1952. Growing and its price in three Puerto Rican subcultures. *Psychiatry* 15:401-433.

19. Rogler, L. H.; and Hollingshead, A. B. 1961. The Puerto Rican spiritualist as psychiatrist. *Am. J. Sociol.* 67:17-21.

20. Kline, L. Y. 1969. Some factors in the psychiatric treatment of Spanish-Americans. *Am. J. Psychiatry* 125:1674-1681.

21. Fitzpatrick, J. P.; and Gould, R. E. 1970. Mental illness among Puerto Ricans in New York: Cultural conditions or intercultural misunderstanding. *Am. J. Orthopsychiatry* 40:238-239.

Part I Review

SUMMARY

The dynamics of transcultural health problem-solving are threefold. First, the facts that constitute the problem must be understood. Such facts frequently consist of both folk and scientific medical definitions of good health. A major purpose of this book is to present basic facts pertaining to transcultural health care. Second, the facts must be thought through. Specifically, they must be probed into, reorganized, and recast for health care providers to understand as much of the total configuration as possible. Finally, a decision must be made that will result in resolving or preventing health problems. This usually involves changes in attitudes and behavior.

Problems and Solutions

Based on an analysis of the chapters in Part I, it is clear that problem resolution involves three operations: fact finding, analysis of facts, and implementation of conclusions. For greatest effectiveness, both patients and health care providers must be actively involved in efforts to define and solve health problems. It is possible for teachers and supervisors to define problems and prescribe solutions, but such a strategy weakens or destroys the patients' and care providers' sense of self-responsibility.[1] In solving health care problems it is helpful to keep certain principles in mind.

A problem cannot be solved if the necessary information is missing. A nurse, for example, may want to understand Third World people but may be unable to do so because she or he has inadequate information. It is not uncommon for care providers to find they know little about the ethnic groups with which they come in contact. Like any puzzle, missing pieces of information in a transcultural problem will render it insoluble. It is the task of the care provider to actively seek the knowledge needed.[2]

Information alone is seldom enough. Obviously memorizing words, phrases, or sentences from books will not of itself change attitudes and behavior. A few minutes of positive interaction with low-income or Third World people can do more to enhance a practitioner's cultural sensitivity than hours of reading about them. For example, rather than engaging in abstract discussions of folk medical beliefs and practices, interaction with an articulate folk healer will provide an invaluable education.[3]

Cultural sensitivity is the capacity to identify and empathize with the values, beliefs, and feelings of others. Ideally, all health personnel should be culturally sensitive. An inability to see other people as they see themselves, to dispel economic and ethnic group prejudices, and to communicate across cultural lines will turn health facilities into ideological and physical battlefields. Members of the various health professions may have difficulty imagining what it is like to be poor or to be a member of an ethnic minority group, but much of the difficulty will be overcome when care providers undertake a systematic study of cultural differences.[4]

Most health care providers need to learn how to explore new and contradictory ideas and facts. The greater the cultural distance between the care provider and the patient, the more likely the ideas and facts will be misunderstood. Knowledge of basic anthropological, sociological, psychological, and economic principles provide a basis for problem solving.[5] The need to understand religious and ethnic differences is not limited to Anglos. Non-Anglos need this knowledge, too.

Frequently, health care providers are either problems themselves or the causes of problems. The ability of health care professionals to achieve and maintain a humane stance is the key to the entire health plan. If the care provider remains wrapped up in her or his own cultural definition of good health, she or he will not be able to perceive clearly the feelings and needs of patients from other cultures. The challenge to health practitioners is awesome; they must act as feeling individuals without losing their objectivity. Transcultural health care requires accepting beliefs that may be counter to one's own.[6]

It is imperative that health care providers focus on transcultural problems that can be resolved within their health care setting. This is the most efficient and effective use of energies. Many transcultural problems acted out in health facilities have origins in the community and can be solved only there. In this text, we focus on health-related problems and solutions.

Socioeconomic Issues

An examination of the external and internal forces impacting on ethnic groups is vital to understanding their health behavior. It is a truism that socioeconomic phenomena influence health care. Relatedly, a group's ability to control or participate equally in community power relationships affects the quality of its health care. Furthermore, health knowledge is proportionally related to a group's technological advancement.

Health care should be viewed in relation to intervening socioeconomic variables because they significantly influence health beliefs and practices. For too long it has been erroneously concluded by some health care providers that only environmental conditions influence public health. The issue is much more complex than this simplistic analysis. The poor in particular have less health care knowledge and fewer economic resources to draw on in their battle against illness. However, even knowledgeable poor persons with minimally adequate financial resources or state-subsidized care plans are hesitant to take time from work for long-term treatment.[7]

The problem of poor health care cannot be attributed solely to lack of knowledge and economic deprivation. Structural differences also produce differences in attitudes and values. Health care providers consciously and unconsciously exclude the poor from active, peer participation in health-related organizations and activities. In turn, negative attitudes and social distance between themselves and affluent people prompt Third World poor persons to reject Western health care systems. Instead of narrowing the gap between poor and affluent citizens, increased technology has widened it. Yet, it is imperative to remember that because something has always existed does not mean that it must continue to exist.

Understanding and accepting another person's cultural reality are the beginnings of a helping relationship. Helpful, as opposed to harmful, relationships do not require either party to compromise his or her own values and beliefs. Often it is a lack of knowledge or understanding that leads to individual and group feelings of inadequacy and, ultimately, alienation. Successful transcultural involvement with another person requires considerable empathy. Ethically, health care providers ought to be committed to protecting their patient/clients' value systems.

The therapeutic process includes both delivery of services and protection of ethnic identities. Human relationships automatically involve risk taking, and sharing feelings and testing commitments are part of the helping relationship. Thus, although value conflicts are inevitable, they should not lead to individual ego or ethnic group destruction. The human relations lesson is quite clear; we can all be in the process of becoming more healthy and humane persons.

Cultural Barriers

One of the deficits in nursing education is the lack of systematic transcultural coursework and supervised transcultural experiences. A lack of understanding of culturally different patients is likely to result in health care providers feeling incompetent or inadequate. This feeling is not without foundation—optimum care delivery is impossible without cultural understanding. However, awareness of one's own cultural attitudes and values should precede knowledge of other cultures.

One way to gain knowledge of other cultures is to become a participant observer. If this is done, care must be taken not to view all people in other cultures as weird folks who need psychiatric treatment and a drastic change in values. A participant observer should not be a social voyeur. The kind of self we bring to the relationship will determine the quality of helping that occurs.[8]

Ethnicity affects the behavior of persons in both similar and different groups. There is the danger that health care providers will identify too much with the patient. Countertransference, the process of projecting one's own values on to the patient, must be dealt with for the therapeutic process to develop. Basic to dealing with countertransference is the need for care providers to examine their own feelings, attitudes, values, and behavior.

Verbal language can significantly effect psychopathological assessment of bilingual patients. The responses are cued differently, depending on whether or not interviews are conducted in the patient/client's native language. Factors such as the amount of content and expansion on a particular subject affect pathological assessment. For example, the tense used by a respondent may be incorrectly interpreted as a sign of activeness of a patient's symptoms; or language patterns may be incorrectly interpreted as signs of anxiety or depression. Clearly, language barriers pose special problems for diagnosis when patients are interviewed in a language other than their native one. Only recently have health care researchers noted that cognitive behavior may be influenced by the semantic structure of languages. Patients who do not act in ways acceptable to care providers may be judged as displaying signs of psychopathology by practitioners who are unaware of the patient's cultural norms.

Nurse-Patient Communication

Interviewing is a process that is carried out every day in almost every kind of health care situation. This exchange may be between a nurse and a patient, a physician and a patient, or another health-related person and a patient. The initial health care interview is designed to get and give information; therefore, the quality of this interaction is crucial to a patient's adjustment.[9] Third World persons coming to modern health institutions after being treated by traditional curers are likely to be extremely anxious and fearful. Hospitals are especially sensitive places.

For example, when a nurse admits a patient for treatment, she or he conducts an interview. This initial interview may result in valuable information that will be helpful in evaluating the patient and planning for subsequent medical care. Often, this opportunity is not used to its greatest advantage. Most nurses, especially those trained in less progressive schools, adhere strictly to the printed interview form, ask direct questions to make sure that all the blank spaces are filled, and usually fail to allow the patient time for self-expression.[10]

If a bilingual patient asks a question, a nonbilingual nurse usually gives long, detailed answers, which in most instances serve only to allay the nurse's fears or her feelings of inadequacy, thus leaving the patient floundering. In some hospitals the place for admitting a patient and conducting the interview is the nurse's station, where there is a continuous stream of traffic, or in the patient's room with an audience of one or more other persons. Obviously, these situations are not conducive to a good interview; they block the patient's desire to ask questions or to talk freely.

After the printed forms have been completed and the patient's vital signs taken, the nurse completes the written record. An example of an admission record is as follows:

Mrs. S, age 35, admitted to Ward 10 walking. Patient is to have a simple mastectomy in the A.M. B/P/150/100, T 98, P 120, R 28. The patient does not seem to be in acute distress, admission bath given. Patient to bed. Dr. M notified of patient's admission.

What does this record tell us? It merely tells us that Mrs. S is on the ward, what her vital signs are, that she had a bath, that she was put to bed, and that the physician was notified. If the patient showed signs of anxiety, if she seemed to be preoccupied, or if she had cultural or religious rituals that needed to be satisfied, we would not know it by reading this record. It is not surprising, therefore, that many patients after having been ushered through the admission assembly line, having been denied the right of self-expression and kept away from family and friends except for a few hours a day, generally feel that they have lost their identity and their individuality in the process of becoming just another number in an impersonal institution.

To conduct a successful interview, health care personnel must familiarize themselves with the purpose of interviewing and with methods of conducting interviews, including what to look for during the interview. The first consideration should be to put the patient at ease and to make him or her as comfortable as possible. This can be accomplished by the nurse introducing herself or himself and any other health care personnel who are present at the time. If available, the interview should be conducted in an unoccupied room or office.

Next, the nurse should explain to the patient what records will be needed to assist in the data gathering. Since the primary purpose of the interview is to elicit information about the patient's health, it is important to let the patient do most of the talking. The nurse may need to direct the interview to a certain extent, but the interview should not be dominated by the nurse. Self-expression on the part of the patient may uncover hidden problems and fears. It is important that these are uncovered early in the patient's confinement so that needed resources can be brought to bear before additional complications occur.

Much of what can be said about things nurses should observe in patients are just as important for nurses to know about themselves. Only by admitting personal fears, inadequacies, cultural biases, and so forth can nurses be optimally effective as care providers.

In addition to listening, nurses must be able to communicate with patients. The most effective communication is two way. This involves spoken language and body language. Frequently, a patient's spoken language is incongruent with his or her body language, and the reverse can be true. Congruence between words and gestures is the key to understanding the messages being sent and received.[11]

Questions for Further Study

1. How can a health care provider effectively remove himself or herself from the culturally biased value system likely to characterize his or her own culture?

2. How can one learn, understand, and accept a patient/client's cultural values, norms, and practices without them becoming an integral part of his or her culture?

3. Can an outsider ever be an effective health care provider for persons in a traditional kinship-based culture?

4. How can health care providers distinguish between helpful and harmful aspects of ethnic identity?

5. To what extent should health care providers and patients ignore their own ethnicity to embrace a nebulous "American" life style?

6. What are some effective ways of dealing with ethnicity in the therapeutic relationship?

7. What guidelines should be used in situations where language differences hamper communication?

References

1. See Burton, G. 1970. *Personal, impersonal, and interpersonal relations,* 3rd ed. New York: Springer Publishing Co., Inc.

2. Leininger, M. 1970. *Nursing and anthropology: Two worlds to blend.* New York: John Wiley & Sons, Inc., p. 20.

3. Leininger, M. 1970. *Nursing and anthropology: Two worlds to blend.* New York: John Wiley & Sons, Inc., pp. 120-121.

4. Martinez, R. A. 1978. *Hispanic culture and health care: Fact, fiction, folklore.* St. Louis: The C. V. Mosby Co.

5. Murphy, J. F., editor. 1971. *Theoretical issues in professional nursing,* Des Moines, Iowa: Meredith Corp.

6. Lantz, J. R.; and Meyer, E. A. 1979. The dirty house. *Nurs. Outlook* 27:590-593.

7. Fabrega, H., Jr.; and Roberts, R. E. 1972. Ethnic differences in outpatient use of a public-charity hospital. *Am. J. Public Health* 62:936-941.

8. Leininger, M. 1970. *Nursing and anthropology: Two worlds to blend.* New York: John Wiley & Sons, Inc., pp. 24-25.

9. Lewis, G. K. 1973. *Nurse-patient communication,* 2nd ed., Dubuque, Iowa: William C. Brown Co., Publishers.

10. Robinson, L. 1968. Psychological aspects of the care of hospitalized patients. Philadelphia: F. A. Davis Publishing Co., pp. 21-43.

11. Ramaekers, Sister M. J. 1979. Communication blocks revisited. *Am. J. Nurs.* 79:1079-1081.

EXERCISES

EXERCISE 1: Beliefs and Values

Respond to the following statements according to whether they are generally *true* or generally *false*.

I am someone who:

1. Accepts opinions different from my own.
2. Responds with compassion to poverty-stricken people.
3. Thinks interracial marriage is a good thing.
4. Would feel uncomfortable in a group in which I am the ethnic minority.
5. Considers failure a bad thing.
6. Invites people I don't like to my home.
7. Believes that the Ku Klux Klan has its good points.
8. Sets realistic life goals.
9. Would enjoy serving as a juror in a rape case.
10. Is concerned about the treatment of minorities in employment and health care.
11. Feels uncomfortable in low-income neighborhoods.
12. Prefers to conform rather than disagree in public.
13. Values friendship more than money.
14. Maintains high ethical standards as a professional.
15. Would not object to premarital sex for my children.
16. Usually spends a lot of time worrying about social injustices without doing much about them.
17. Believes that almost anyone who really wants to can get a good job.
18. Has a close friend of another race.
19. Would rather attend a concert than an athletic contest.

Exercise 2: Poverty

You have recently been hired by a large metropolitan hospital to provide assistance to home-bound patients. The hospital catchment area consists primarily of low-income persons: 70% black Americans, 15% Hispanic, 10% Anglo, and 5% Asian American.

1. What problems do you expect to encounter during your first home visits?
2. What "survival skills" will you need to succeed in your job?
3. Where could you go to find out more about the community? List ten community resources available in most metropolitan areas.

Exercise 3. Diet

While making a routine visit to a Chinese American patient's room, you discover that she has not been eating her food. The physician has left strict orders that the patient must eat her food to build up her strength. When you confront the patient with your discovery, she responds, "This food is too hot. I have been eating proper food brought from home."

1. What will you do? Why?

2. What do you know about Chinese folk medicine that will help you to understand the patient?

3. How do you feel about patients deviating from their diets?

PART II

Folk Medicine

Loudell Snow provides an excellent overview of black folk medical beliefs, especially as these beliefs compare with those of several other ethnic groups. Clarissa Scott's chapter focuses on patterns of health care of Bahamians, Cubans, Haitians, Puerto Ricans, and southern black Americans. She skillfully dispels the myth that all black people are alike in culture and customs.

George Foster traces Spanish folk medicine from Europe to the New World and its subsequent assimilation with Native American Indian cultures. On the subject of North American Indian medicine, Virgil Vogel's chapter is both succinct and authoritative. Because of distortions presented in movies and television, there are perhaps more misconceptions about Indian medicine than about any other kind.

Donn Hart focuses on folk medicine of ethnic groups frequently ignored in medical literature—Filipinos, Thai, and Burmese. Teresa Campbell and Betty Chang begin their chapter by refuting Chinese stereotypes. They then examine Chinese folk medicine as a contrast to Western medicine.

Although focusing on diverse cultures, the separate chapters bring out a similarity in indigenous medical beliefs and practices. But these data are not enough. Health care professionals would be wise to seek out other materials and experiences to clearly understand ethnic similarities and differences.

5

The Importance of
Folk Medicine

George Henderson, Ph.D.
Martha Primeaux, R.N., M.S.N.

Folk medicine, or Third World medical beliefs and practices, frequently is called "strange" or "weird" by health professionals who are unfamiliar with it. In reality, what is strange and what is not depends on familiarity. In most instances, Third World customs are not strange once health care providers become familiar with them. However, we could clearly distinguish between *familiar* and *desirable*. To become familiar with something does not mean that we must accept it as our own way of life. In its broadest sense, this form of tolerance is a two-way process; neither Third World nor non-Third World people should feel compelled to abandon their cultural beliefs and practices when they become familiar with modern medicine.

OVERVIEW OF HEALTH SYSTEMS

Third World cultures are non-Western in terms of medical beliefs and practices. Specifically, the cognitive world of traditional Third World people tends to be less compartmentalized than that of modern Western people. That is, traditional Third World people are not likely to separate the various medical aspects of life into neat mind-body dichotomies.[1] Chapter 5, as well as those that follow, focuses on medical systems that differ from the Western medical system. In this section we have subsumed traditional Third World beliefs and practices under three topics: magic, witchcraft, and religion.

A person's world view largely determines his or her beliefs about disease and appropriate treatment. For example, the belief in magic leads to assumptions that disease is the result of human behavior and that the cure is achieved by sorcery. A religious belief of the world leads to assumptions that disease is the result of supernatural forces and that the cure is achieved by successfully appealing to supernatural forces. A scientific view leads to assumptions that disease is the result of cause-effect relations of natural phenomena and that the cure is achieved by scientific medicine. Western disease etiologies give little credence to supernatural theories of causation; whereas most Third World disease etiologies are based on beliefs in magic and supernatural forces.

Medical Systems

Both Third World and Western medical practices are social systems, and both have interdependent parts or variables that, in the words of Thomas Weaver, include "the whole complex of a people's beliefs, attitudes, practices, and roles associated with concepts of health and disease, and with patterns of diagnosis and treatment."[2] Every medical system is based on ideas about or a philosophy of survival: what constitutes health and what constitutes illness. Frederick L. Dunn described the adaptive nature of a medical system as the pattern of cultural traditions and social institutions that evolves from deliberate behavior to improve health, whether or not the outcome of particular aspects of behavior is ill health.[3] To achieve good health, people must have some idea about what constitutes disease with its concomitant conditions of pain and suffering. Horacio Fabrega, Jr., succinctly described the social dimensions of defining disease:

> The social character of disease is revealed by the fact that its elements consist of changes in the way people function, behave, define themselves and/or report their feelings. Deviations from the typical are what prompt people to seek medical help and to follow or reject the advice. Furthermore, such deviations serve as the basis for allowing observers (be they scientists, shamans, or others) to construct what they judge to be meaningful regularities in line with sociocultural conventions, whether they are chemical, physiologic, or supernatural. These regulations become codified as disease entities and groups then certify and legitimate them.[4]

Once a philosophy of health is adopted, various health roles are delineated. These roles require specific health care practitioner initiation rites and training. Broadly speaking, practitioner status is given by medical societies or supernatural forces. As we review Third World and Western medical systems, we shall discuss the elaborate hierarchies that exist among diagnosticians, curers, and care providers. Relatedly, we shall consider some of the equipment or materials used in the two medical systems. Because the body is an integral aspect of each individual, all medical systems use body parts or excreta for diagnostic purposes. And all systems prescribe medicines to rub in the skin, to irrigate the body, or to anoint the sick. Thus, we shall focus on three components of health systems: ideas of health, prescribed roles of health practitioners, and equipment used by practitioners to cure people.

Ecological and Religious Models

Closely related to the medical system model of health care are the ecological and religious models. Margarita Kay defined ecology in terms of three foci: "biological (that branch of biology that deals with the relations of organisms and their environment), social (the relations of people and institutions and their interdependence), and cultural (the relation of culture and environment, which includes the other cultures and societies that are in the environment)."[5] Ecological dimensions of health care can provide plausible explanations for certain people contracting specific diseases and communicating them in specific ways.

Within the past decade, health care practitioners have become increasingly concerned with the ecological dimensions of racial and ethnic minority group health problems. Several textbooks have been devoted to this topic but few have provided broad transcultural analyses.[6]

Differences in foci are seen when comparing Western and Third World health care practices. Some of these differences are more significant than others. For example, Western societies usually have dyad relationships, such as physician-patient and nurse-patient. Third World societies usually have multiperson health care networks. The latter relationships consist of parental and nonparental, relatives and nonrelatives as caretakers. Multiperson networks are no longer dismissed by Western practitioners as being irrelevant. Slowly, the Western system is shifting to include the multiperson perspective.

Ethnic diets are another aspect of human ecology that health care providers are beginning to understand and utilize. Each ethnic group must consume enough food to meet its nutritional requirements for energy, fat, protein, vitamins, and minerals. Cheryl Rittenbaugh wrote, "Relatively little is known about the range of human biological variability both among and within human populations with regard to such common parameters as nutritional requirements, physiological response to malnutrition, and digestive capabilities."[7] This lack of knowledge has resulted in Western-oriented care providers prescribing nonacceptable diets for Third World patients. As we shall see in Part III, geographical biological adaptations of Third World people have rendered some of them physiologically incompatible with certain Western foods.

Third World people are likely to explain their illnesses in terms of imbalance between the individual and his or her physical, social, and spiritual worlds. In short, health and illness come from the supernatural. Although all medical systems focus on preventive and curative medicine, good health among most Third World people centers on personal rather than scientific behavior. From this perspective, it makes sense to burn incense or to avoid certain individuals or cold air or evil eyes.

> However, one person's religion is another's magic, witchcraft, or superstition. Traditionally, a fascination of anthropologists and folklorists, the study of religion, magic, and witchcraft is difficult for health professionals to see as directly relevant to their practice. It is equally difficult for them to realize that for some groups religion is an equivalent of science.[8]

All religious systems have elaborate rules that determine appropriate and inappropriate health care behavior. This includes rules for giving care and receiving care. Religious experiences include blessings from spiritual leaders, apparition of dead relatives, and miracle cures. Furthermore, healing power may be found in animate as well as inanimate objects. The key concept in religious systems is "faith." It is important to note that the distinction between the shaman, whose powers derive from the supernatural, and the priest, who learns a codified body of rituals from other priests, is not always easy to make. Both may engage in similar behavior.

In traditional Third World societies some of the most significant religious rituals are those that mediate between events "here" in this world and those "out there" in the nether world.[9] To mediate these worlds, folk practitioners may effect cures and work protective and evil magic. As we shall see, there are many names given to individuals who utter charms, spells, supplications, and incantations.

Strengths and Weaknesses of Third World Medical Systems

Both Third World and Western medical systems are functional systems. However, certain strengths and weaknesses of Third World medical systems should be remembered.

For example, Third World medical systems are comprehensive. They include an individual and his or her family and community environment. The curer tries to maintain a balance between humans, their society, and their physical environment. Relatives and friends are part of the curing rites. When effective, Third World therapeutic techniques relieve pain, and frequently they provide emotional catharsis and a sharing of guilt. Thus, one does not suffer alone. By removing the line between physical and mental symptoms, indigenous therapies often achieve remarkable results.

Regarding weaknesses, however, Third World pharmacopeias are relatively ineffective when compared with scientific pharmacopeias. Third World health orientations are interanlly oriented and subjectively based, thus they have for the most part not led to the development of rational and effective medicine. For example, because geographical differences are found in foods considered hot and cold, it is impossible to empirically validate the health concept of hot and cold foods. Indigenous cures tend to be based on trial and error and passed on by oral tradition. It is not surprising than that the same illness may be treated by greatly different potions depending on the herbalists involved.

The efficacy of a medical system is not easily evaluated. For, as George M. Foster and Barbara Gallatin Anderson point out, "There are no universally agreed on units to be measured, and the personal biases and expectations of those who evaluate may differ greatly. There is not even agreement as to what is being judged."[10] Even so, when using the criterion of consumer satisfaction in terms of the religious, legal, social and psychological functions they fulfill, Third World medical systems compare favorably with the Western medical system.

Whichever system one prefers, all medical systems provide (1) a rationale for treatment, (2) an explanation for the "why" of health and illness, and (3) a rationale for social and moral norms. Folk beliefs offer little resistance to modern medical practices; however, preventive medicine tends to be resisted by poorly educated Third World people who have difficulty comprehending theoretical injunctions that do not lend themselves to easy empirical observation.[11] Foster and Anderson believe that people modify preexisting health care practices only if (1) they perceive economic, social, health, or other advantages in so doing; (2) they can economically afford to change; and (3) the social costs do not outweigh the perceived medical advantages.[12]

HOLISTIC APPROACH TO HEALTH

Sometimes a physician will report that an operation was a success but the patient died. That is, the technical procedures were correctly followed but the patient needed something more to recover. Intangibles such as faith in the medical personnel, the will to live, and the ability to heal are the areas in which most American health professionals seem poorly educated. Western medicine carves the patient into territorial pieces, and few health professionals are taught to handle the intangible portions.

Conversely, most non-Western cultures tend to adopt a holistic approach to health care. The mind-body dichotomy gives way to viewing the patient as a biological, psychosocial, and spiritual whole existing in a specific environment. From this perspective, epidemiology rests side by side with folk medicine. For this reason, many Third World people feel comfortable with modern curers who understand, for example, that hypertension and cirrhosis of the liver are more than physiological conditions: they are also manifestations of stresses that accrue at a higher rate to people of low social status than to those of high social status.

Although they focus on the whole patient and have effected some miraculous cures, we should also be aware of the less medically sound aspects of folk medicine. Modesta Orque provides the following succinct illustration of such practices:

In both traditional Chinese and the Spanish cultures there exists the belief
that a woman, during postpartum convalescence, should refrain from taking
showers and baths. . . . This is consistent with the Chinese belief that during
the postpartum periods, the Yin energy forces or "cold" in the body must
be decreased to bring back some balance of Yang or "hot" air. In
Spanish-speaking patients there is a similar belief that during the . . .
postpartum period, the woman should avoid exposing herself to any
condition which could cause bad air (*mal aire*) to enter through the
vagina.[13]

HISTORICAL DIMENSIONS

Some cultures believe in *bad medicine*–spells, evil eye, and other harmful magic. To
counter bad medicine, *good medicine*–taboos and magic–are used. A taboo is an
injunction to do or not to do something. Indian medicine men are believed to be
the original folk healers in this country. Currently taboos are employed by shamans
or medicine men and witch doctors. (Both men and women administer folk
medicine as shamans and witch doctors, but in most societies the man's medicine is
believed to be stronger than the woman's medicine.) Any ill luck or misfortune can
be attributed to the breaking of a taboo.[14]

Lest you attribute taboos only to primitive people, we call your attention to
modern social taboos such as women wearing high heel shoes that deform their feet
or men wearing too much clothing to conform to beauty taboos. Or we can cite
religious persons who would not leave home without a miniature cross. Nor should
we overlook people who believe that broken glass or walking under a ladder will
bring bad luck. Generally, nonprimitive people call their taboos "etiquette,"
"customs," and "conventions."

Blacks from Africa and the West Indies also brought magical rites to this
country. Black magic, *obeah*, was once a widely practiced form of healing in the
West Indies, the Guianas in Latin America, and the southeastern part of America.
Male and female obeah doctors used plants, ground fibers, and ground glass among
other things to instill fear in their followers.

Obeah is not the same as Voodoo, which is a form of African religion or
serpent-god worship requiring an animal sacrifice.[15] Obeah has little to do with
religion. Rather, it is a form of witchcraft or black magic. There have been instances
when obeah doctors have been able through autosuggestion and fear to perform
remarkable feats. For example, they have been able to put pins, needles, and other
objects in the flesh of their subjects without drawing blood or causing pain.
Conversely, they have been able to cause a person to exhibit painful medical
symptoms without being touched. In extreme ire, an obeah doctor can frighten to
death an otherwise healthy follower.

Early humans believed that illness was caused by the entrance of devils or evil
spirits into a person's body. Using charms, incantations, chants, and dances,
medicine men tried to drive out the spirits. If a person died, it usually was

considered a sign that the medicine man's magic was not strong enough to cast out the devils. Through indigenous efforts to heal people, many important cures have been developed. American Indians employed sassafras, arnica, sarsaparilla, viburnum, liverwort, gentian, mullein, and hundreds of other plants for curing diseases long before white people started using them.

Incan and pre-Incan Indians had surgeons who performed delicate trepanning operations, amputations, and removal of damaged eyes. The remarkable nature of these feats becomes even more apparent when we realize that these operations were performed with crude stones and bronze instruments. Quinine was used by Peruvian Indians several centuries before white explorers set foot on American soil. The Chinese provide another illustration. After minimizing acupuncture for hundreds of years, Western medical doctors are finally learning to use needles to relieve pain.

Some of the so-called primitive methods of expelling evil spirits from the body were based on what we now know is consonant with physical laws. For example, sweating, inducing emesis, and cauterizing were medically sound practices used by the primitive people in many appropriate instances. Of course, some of their other practices, such as beating and blistering inflicted persons, were quite harmful. The tendency of many Americans to think of Indian and Latin American medical systems historically irrelevant overlooks several other facts, including the following:

1. As early as the eighteenth century, Spanish explorers observed Indian tribes using inoculation with cowpox, *vaccinia,* to prevent small pox.

2. In 1570, Francisco Bravo published in Mexico the first medical book, *Opera medicinalia,* to appear in the western hemisphere.

3. Hospital de Jesus Nazareno, built in the 1500s, was the first public welfare institution in the western hemisphere.

4. Autopsies for medical research purposes were performed in Hospital de Jesus Nazareno during the last quarter of the sixteenth century.

5. Hospital de Amor de Dios, built in 1535, specialized in care of patients with contagious diseases, especially venereal diseases.

6. In 1578, the medical school of the University of Mexico was founded.

Certainly the early medicine men, witch doctors, and scientific health professionals had ample patients to cure. With this large pool of subjects, medicine improved. For example, Indians were inflicted with smallpox, venereal diseases, typhus, and measles by white explorers. Later, African slaves were inflicted with dysentery, tetanus, hookworm, yaws, and smallpox. These few examples only scratch the surface of this topic.

SPIRITUALISM

Spiritualism is an integral part of folk medicine, especially among Hispanics, Indians, and black Americans. For the purpose of our discussion, spiritualism is defined as the belief that the visible world also includes an invisible world inhabited by good and evil spirits who influence our behavior. Spirits make their presence known through *mediums*. Failure of health care professionals to acknowledge and understand the importance of spiritualism for millions of Americans can be detrimental to a health plan.

> In addition to conferring protection and enabling the medium to function, spirits can both cause and prevent illness. One's spiritual protection acts as a shield, turning away evil spirits and hexes while at the same time bringing one good luck. If one loses spiritual protection . . . one can become ill. The illness may be manifested by such signs as pain, lethargy, nervousness and bad luck.[16]

The belief in supernatural forces is also expressed in magic, witchcraft, and religion. Several years ago, anthropologists observed that there is virtually no incompatibility between religion and spiritualism. Religion, like spiritualism, is based on the belief in spirits. Furthermore, like the medium, a religious leader's authority is of a spiritual nature. Both magic and religion offer relief from suffering by the use of ritual and belief in supernatural forces; thus it is easy to understand why the Roman Catholic church and Hispanic spiritualism have appealed to overlapping populations.

Mediums treat both emotionally related and physical illnesses. Unlike Western-based approaches to health, Third World cultures (Africa, Asia, and Latin America) do not distinguish sharply between physical and mental illnesses. Consequently, mediums treat the whole person. For example, in Puerto Rican culture psychological symptoms are frequently expressed as somatic illness. Most American physicians and nurses tend to ignore psychosomatic illnesses. Mediums do not ignore such complaints but instead take for granted their dual nature.

Herbal medicine is another aspect of folk medicine. Like physicians, mediums often prescribe herbs as part of the cure. Herbal medicine, which dates back further than any other form of medicine, has magical and symbolic connotations. More than 150 drugs that are presently listed in the *Pharmacopeia of the United States of America* were used by North American Indians of Mexico, and 50 were used by Indians of the West Indies, Mexico, and Central and South America. Sociologists have observed that the medicine chests of low-income ethnic minorities are well stocked with herbal remedies.

Mediums have a distinct advantage when compared with physicians and nurses. This advantage is due to the fact that most mediums share the ethnic background, language, social class, and community of their followers. Also, mediums are not bogged down with bureaucratic red tape. Perhaps the essence of their success resides in the faith that their followers have in them.

SOCIOCULTURAL ASPECTS

Folk medicine does not exist in a vacuum. Rather, it is an integral part of other sociocultural conditions. For this reason, a brief review of sociocultural aspects of several ethnic groups should be of value to health professionals who want to better understand these groups.[17] We have elected to focus on black Americans, Mexican Americans, Puerto Ricans, American Indians, and Asian Americans. Together these groups comprise more than 20% of our nation's total population and more than 80% of its Third World population. Black Americans number about 25 million, Mexican Americans number 7 million, Puerto Ricans number 1.7 million, Asian Americans number more than 2 million, and American Indians number 900,000. (See also Table 5-1 for selected characteristics of these groups.) Remember, however, that the following comments are broad generalizations, many of which may not be applicable to specific situations.

TABLE 5-1. Selected characteristics of six American ethnic groups.

Ethnic group	Approximate time of United States population influx	Estimated population (1979)	Traditional family structure	Expression of pain	Folk healers
Black Americans	1600s	25,000,000	Extended/ matriarchal and egalitarian	Open, public	Hoodoo men and ladies Root doctors Blood doctors
Mexican Americans	400 B.C.	7,000,000	Extended/ patriarchal	Open, public	Curanderos
Puerto Ricans	1900s	1,700,000	Extended/ patriarchal	Open, public	Espiritistas
American Indians	13000-18000 B.C.	900,000	Extended/ patriarchal and matriarchal	Closed, private	Medicine men
Chinese Americans	1700s	500,000	Extended/ patrirachal	Closed, private	Herbalists Herb pharmacists Acupuncturists
Japanese Americans	1800s	700,000	Extended/ patriarchal	Closed, private	Herbalists

Black Americans

Black children begin life facing higher survival odds than white children. They are more likely to die in infancy than white babies. If a black baby lives, the chances of losing his or her mother in childbirth is four times as high as the white baby. The black baby is usually born into a family that lives in the inner city (over 70% of the black American population does). It is a family that is larger than its white counterpart, and it is crowded into dilapidated housing—quarters structurally unsound or unable to keep out cold, rain, snow, rats, or pests.[18]

With more mouths to feed, more babies to clothe, and more needs to satisfy, the black family is forced to exist on a median family income that is barely half the median white family income. When the black youngster goes to school, he or she usually finds it no avenue to adequate living, much less to fame or fortune. And because black children are generally taught in slum schools, with inferior teachers, equipment, and facilities, the educational gap between black and white students of the same age often approaches 5 or 6 years.

In most communities heavily populated by black Americans, low- and middle-income groups live in extremely close proximity to each other. This situation is not caused primarily by a natural selection process but rather by *de facto* housing segregation. Consequently, the plight of poverty-stricken black Americans is distorted if only census tract data are examined. Black "haves" appear less affluent, and black "have nots" seem less disadvantaged than they actually are. There is, in short, a much wider gap between black middle and lower classes than is statistically apparent. Both groups closely approximate their white counterparts in income and living styles. Low-income black Americans are a minority within a minority.

Black Americans are the most difficult ethnic group to categorize. The difficulty stems mainly from slavery, where African heritages were almost entirely lost through assimilation with non-African cultures. Even so, the following generalizations typify black American cultural conditioning.

Extended Family. The black family is sometimes extended bilaterally, but often it is maternally oriented. The black extended family is a closely knit group, frequently consisting of grandparents, aunts, uncles, nieces, nephews, and cousins. Within the black family roles are interchanged more frequently than in most non-black families. This sharing of decisions and jobs in the home stabilizes the family during crisis situations.

Kinship Bonds. Children born in and out of wedlock are loved. Legitimacy refers to parents; it has little to do with black children being accepted. Children are proof of an individual's manhood or womanhood, and caring for them is proof of an individual's humanity. When children marry or otherwise reach adulthood, they leave home but often settle close to their parents or other relatives. Family unity, loyalty and cooperation are part of the black life style. (These values are also strongly held by the other ethnic groups discussed in this book.)

Authority and Discipline. Childhood in the black community revolves around assertive behavior and challenging authority. There is a constant crossing of wills.

Through this process the black child learns the acceptable limits of his or her behavior. Discipline tends to be harsh, strict, and preoccupied with teaching children respect for their elders, respect for authority, responsibility for oneself, and an understanding of what it means to be black in America.

Religious Orientation. On the whole, black Americans are highly religious. Most black Americans are Protestant. The church offers spiritual hope to many persons who live in oppressive environments. The church also offers a facility for conducting nonreligious activities, such as Boy Scout and Girl Scout meetings.

Achievement and Work Orientations. Contrary to popular notion, most black parents pass on to their children high achievement aspirations. However, many black homes lack middle-class role models for children to emulate. The desire to survive has forced many black families to internalize a strong work orientation that makes palatable the unskilled and semiskilled jobs available in the discriminatory job market within which most black Americans must work.

Folk Medicine. African health practices make little distinction between physicians and nurses; both attend to the physical, emotional, and spiritual health of the patient. According to traditional black African beliefs, both living and dead things influence an individual's health. In addition, health is directly related to nature. To be in harmony with nature is to have good health, whereas illness reflects disharmony with nature.

The secret to good health among many black Americans is maintaining a balance between the forces of good and evil. Voodoo doctors or conjurers cast out evil spirits or demons. Several methods—including putting pins in dolls and applying heat and cold to an afflicted person's body—have been carried over from ancient African history. Extensive use is made of roots, minerals, and plant mixtures.

Faith healers, root doctors, and spiritualists are still used in some black communities; however, like other ethnic groups, as black Americans become middle class, they tend to abandon folk cures. Affluent minorities are likely to utilize modern health facilities and take medicine only if it is prescribed by a physician.

Mexican Americans

Mexican Americans reflect a variety of cultural patterns that are influenced by their parental heritage and the length of time their families have been American citizens. Second- and third-generation descendants of early Spanish settlers are usually affluent, but second- and third-generation descendants of agricultural workers tend to be poor. Still a third group is formed by the first generation children of *braceros*—farm workers who have recently migrated from Mexico. The first two groups are likely to be Americanized; they have little knowledge of their Spanish heritage, and they speak little or no Spanish. Children of migrant workers speak fluent Spanish and hold tightly to Mexican customs and traditions. All Spanish groups are discriminated against by the Anglos—the white American majority. In fact, in some communities Mexican Americans are the victims of more discrimination and segregation than black Americans.[19]

Census projections indicate that the total Hispanic American population may soon exceed the black American population. In addition to Mexicans and Puerto Ricans, a sizeable number of legal and illegal immigrants come from Argentina, Peru, and Venezuela. Part of the difficulty in accurately counting and classifying Hispanic immigrants is due to the tendency of non-Puerto Rican Hispanics to list themselves as Puerto Rican to gain full rights as American citizens. In Texas and California it is estimated that 1 million illegal immigrants enter from Mexico.

In many ways Mexican Americans epitomize both racial integration and cultural separatism. This duality is clearly seen in a brief review of Mexican history. The Aztecs were intermarried with their Spanish conquerors and with Indian tribes hostile to the Aztecs. The children of these mixed marriages were called *mestizos*. *Creoles,* pure-blooded Spanish people born in Mexico, largely disappeared through intermarriage. Blacks from Africa, brought into Mexico during the colonial period as slaves, married Indians, and their offspring were called *zambos. Zambos* and *mestizos* later intermarried, causing the so-called Negro blood to disappear.

Although they are a racially mixed people, the heritage of Mexican Americans is quite similar. Some Mexican Americans prefer to be called Chicanos. The word "Chicano" stems from the Mexican Indian Nahuatl word "Mechicano." The first syllable was dropped, and "Chicano" is left. It is an old term for the American of Mexican descent. The Chicano movement (or Chicanismo) represents a commitment to the improvement of life for all Spanish-speaking Americans and Americans of Mexican descent.

Programs that work well for Mexican Americans may not work well for other Latino persons because of subcultural differences. For example, knowing that a patient speaks Spanish may be inadequate cultural knowledge. There are qualitative differences in the language of Latinos who are monolingual Spanish or bilingual Spanish-English. Furthermore, Spanish has many dialects—those brought to the United States by Latino immigrants and several that have developed in this country. A discussion of some of the common characteristics of Mexican Americans follows.

La Raza (The Race). All Latin Americans are united by cultural and spiritual bonds believed to have emanated from God. Because God controls all events, Mexican Americans tend to be more present oriented than future oriented. The influence of the Roman Catholic Church on La Raza is pervasive—Mexican Americans are born, get married, work, die, and are buried under the auspices of religious ceremonies.

Family Loyalty. The familial role is the most important, and the family is the second most cherished institution in Mexican American society. A Chicano owes his or her primary loyalty to the family. The worst sin is to violate one's obligations to God, and next comes the family.

Respect. The oldest man in the household is the family leader. Respect is accorded on the basis of age and sex. The old are accorded more respect than the young, and men are accorded more respect than women. Latino families are based on family solidarity and male superiority.

Machismo. Mexican culture prescribes that the men are stronger, more reliable, and more intelligent than women. *Machismo* dictates that the man will show a high degree of individuality outside the family. Weakness in male behavior is looked down on.

Compadrazgo. The Mexican American family is extended by the institution of *compadrazgo,* a special ceremonial bond between a child's parents and godparents. Often the bond between *compadres* is as strong as between brothers and sisters.

Folk Medicine. Humoral pathology is an important aspect of Latin American and Spanish folk medicine. Their simplified form of Greek humoral pathology was elaborated in the Arab world, brought to Spain as scientific medicine during the period of Moslem domination, and transmitted to America at the time of the Spanish Conquest. According to humoral medical beliefs, the basic functions of the body are regulated by four bodily fluids, or "humors," each of which is characterized by a combination of heat or cold with wetness or dryness. For example, blood is hot and wet, yellow bile is hot and dry, black bile is cold and dry, and phlegm is cold and wet. Most foods, herbs, beverages, and medicines are classified as "hot" (*caliente*) or "cold" (*fresco* or *frio*). As we shall see in later chapters, the secret to good health is to balance hot and cold humors. The wet-dry conditions are less important. The hot-cold syndrome has been reported operative in most of Latin America, including Chile, Colombia, Guatemala, Mexico, and Peru. It also is prevalent in Puerto Rico, Haiti, and Jamaica; however, there is tremendous intercultural variation in the assignment of hot/cold qualities to foods, medicine, and so forth.

Puerto Ricans

Puerto Rico is an island in the Caribbean approximately 1,000 miles from Miami and 1,600 miles from New York. Puerto Rico's population of over 3.5 million represents a density greater than that of China, India, or Japan. As a result of the Jones Act of 1917, all Puerto Ricans are American citizens. The island population is a mixture of Taino Indians, Africans, and Spaniards; Puerto Rican skin colors range from white to black, with shades and mixtures in between.[20]

Mainland (American)-raised Puerto Ricans are sometimes called Neo-Ricans. Neo-Ricans are mainly English speakers; few speak fluent Spanish. Despite dissimilar backgrounds, Puerto Ricans tend to be labeled black and subjected to the same prejudices inflicted on black Americans.

Many Puerto Ricans are reluctant to adopt American life styles. The following characteristics typify Puerto Rican culture.

Sense of Dignity. Respeto demands that proper attention be given to culturally prescribed rituals, such as shaking hands and standing up to greet and say good-by to people. A sense of dignity is present in all important interpersonal relationships.

Personalismo. Personal contact is established by Puerto Ricans before beginning a business relationship. It is important to exchange personal life data (such as size of family, their names, and their ages) before talking business.

Individualism. Puerto Ricans place high value on safeguarding against group pressure to violate an individual's integrity. This makes it difficult for Puerto Ricans to accept the concept of teamwork in which the individual relinquishes his or her individuality to conform to group norms. This characteristic reduces the importance of the Roman Catholic Church in the lives of Puerto Ricans, most of whom are Catholic.

Cleanliness. Great emphasis is placed on being clean and well dressed. To Puerto Ricans, looking good includes wearing bright colors and, frequently, styles rich in ornament.

Fear of Aggression. Puerto Rican children are discouraged from fighting, even in self-defense. A Puerto Rican idiom describes this conditioning: *juegos do mano, juego de villano* (pushing and shoving, even in play, makes one a villain). Survival in urban slum neighborhoods forces many Puerto Rican children to be villains.

Ataques. This form of hysteria is characterized by hyperkinetic seizures brought on by acute tension and anxiety. The *ataque* is also called "the Puerto Rican syndrome." It is not a terminal mental disorder but, instead, a culturally acceptable reaction to situations of extreme stress.

Compadrazgo and Machismo. Compadrazgo and machismo are operative in Puerto Rican culture in the same manner as in Mexican American culture. Like black Americans, Puerto Ricans love children, and illegitimacy is neither frowned on nor punished.

Folk Medicine. For a discussion of Puerto Rican folk medicine, see the section pertaining to Mexican Americans. Both cultures are quite similar.

American Indians

There are approximately 400 Indian tribes in the United States. Some are bilingual and others are not. Nor is there a common tribal language. This is why sign language became the chief means of intertribal communication. Currently, American Indians and Alaskan Natives are at the bottom of the economic ladder in the United States. They have the highest rates of unemployment and school dropouts, live in the most dilapidated housing, and in some parts of the country are accorded the lowest social status. These conditions reflect both what white Americans have done to the Indians and what the Indians have not been able to do for themselves.[21]

Unable to realize that we do not have an Indian problem but rather an *American problem,* the federal government has established government-controlled Indian bureaus, reservations, and assistance programs—including hospitals and clinics. Each of these short-sighted solutions has contributed to the psychological emasculation of Indian men, the demoralization of Indian women, and the alienation of Indian children. In other words, most government programs have failed to assist Indians in their efforts to maintain individual dignity and cultural identity while achieving success in the larger society.

Half the Native American population lives on 40 million acres of reservation in 30 states. Part of their plight is revealed in the following statistics. Indians have 100 million fewer acres of land today than in 1887. Their average life expectancy is 45 years. Nearly 60% of the adult Indian population has less than an eighth-grade education. Infant mortality is more than 10% above the national average. The majority of Native American families have annual incomes below $5000; 75% have annual incomes below $4000. Indian unemployment is almost ten times the national average.

Conflicts between white and Indian cultures are found on reservations, in small towns, and in big cities. The strain shows up in many ways, including juvenile delinquency, adult crime, and alcoholism. Historically, non-Indians have looked at Indian tribes but have failed to see the deplorable social, psychological, and physical deprivations. Some non-Indians tend to think that because an exceptional Indian has managed to succeed, the others should also. Generally, the following characteristics apply to traditional American Indians.

Present Oriented. Indians are taught to live in the present and not to be concerned about what tomorrow will bring. Non-Indians tend to be future oriented; they are constantly destroying the past and building the future.

Time Consciousness. Many earlier Indian tribes had no word for time. Thus, historically, the emphasis was placed on doing as opposed to going to do something or being punctual. Unlike non-Indians who rush to meetings to be punctual, Indians try to finish current activities. (Black Americans and Latinos have similar time consciousness.)

Giving. The Indian who gives the most to others is respected. In many tribes, saving money or accumulating goods resulted in ostracism.

Respect for Age. Like the other ethnic groups discussed in this book, respect for the Indian increases with age. Indian leadership is seldom given to the young.

Cooperation. Indians place great value on working together and sharing resources. Failure to achieve a personal goal is believed to be the result of competition.

Harmony with Nature. The Indian believes in living in harmony with nature. He or she accepts the world as it is and does not try to destroy it. Along with this belief goes a belief in taking from the environment only what is needed to live.

Extended Family. The American Indian family network is radically different from other extended family units in the United States. The typical non-Indian extended family includes three generations within a single household. American Indian families include several households representing relatives along both vertical and horizontal lines. Grandparents are official and symbolic family leaders. In addition, namesakes, formalized through a religious ceremony, become the same as parents in the family network.

Folk Medicine. The Indian medicine man is a vivid reminder that long before physicians, nurses, social workers, and counselors intruded into their lives, Native Americans had folk cures for physical and mental illnesses. Upon reflection, it is no more logical to believe in germs that we cannot see than in spirits whom we cannot see.

An example of Indian folk medicine is seen in traditional Navajo culture that asserts that illness is a sign that a person is out of harmony with nature. Indian religion and medicine are virtually indistinguishable. Medicine men, singing, rituals, and chants are important aspects of treatment for illness. Furthermore, for rehabilitation to become a reality, the patient's extended family must be part of the nursing plan.

Asian Americans

The plight of poverty-stricken Asian Americans is vividly captured in Los Angeles and San Francisco Chinatown statistics: more than one third of the Chinatown families are poverty stricken; three fourths of all housing units are substandard; rents have tripled in the past 5 years; more than half the adults have only a grade school education; juvenile delinquency is increasing; and the suicide rate is three times the national average. Most Asian Americans, however, are neither poverty stricken nor poorly educated.[22] Many of the following values that characterize traditional Chinese are applicable to most traditional Asian cultures.

Filial Piety. There is unquestioning respect for and deference to authority. Above all else, there is the expectation that each individual will comply with familial and social authority.

Parent-child Relationship. Children defer to their parents, especially in communication, which is one way from parents to children.

Self-control. Strong negative feelings are seldom verbalized. Assertive and individualistic people are considered crude and poorly socialized.

Fatalism. Resignation and pragmatism is the manner in which Chinese Americans deal with change in nature and social settings.

Social Milieu. Chinese Americans are other directed and therefore greatly concerned with how their significant others view and react to them. Social solidarity is highly valued.

Inconspicuousness. Taught to avoid calling attention to themselves, Chinese Americans are likely to be silent in public settings.

Shame and Guilt. Since Chinese Americans are taught to respect authority and maintain filial piety toward their parents and their ancestors, a violation of this cultural norm results in feelings of shame and guilt. The Chinese family is a continuum from past to future whose membership includes not only the present generation but also the dead and the unborn.

Folk Medicine. Asian folk medicine and philosophies have a strong Chinese influence. This is the result of early Chinese migration throughout Asia. We need only to compare Chinese, Japanese, Filipino, and Korean medicine to see the similarity. All four have similar philosophies concerning nutrition, acupuncture, and herbology. The art and science of Chinese medicine goes back at least 5000 years to Emperor Huang Ti (2697-1597 B.C.). Unlike Western medicine, which emphasizes disease and cure, Asian medicine focuses on prevention.

The theoretical and philosophical foundation of Chinese medicine is the Taoist religion, which seeks a balance in all things. From a Taoist perspective, humans are microcosms within a macrocosm. Human energy of the microcosm interrelates with the universe. Both energy (*Chi*) and sexual energy (*Jing*) are vital life energies, with Chi and Jing kept in balance by Yin and Yang. Yin is feminine, negative, dark, and cold; whereas Yang is masculine, positive, light, and warm. According to Chinese medicine, an imbalance in energy is caused by an improper diet or a strong emotional feeling. Balance or good health may be achieved through the use of appropriate herbs. Finally, the universe and humans are susceptible to the laws of earth, fire, water, metal, and wood.

Vietnamese folk medicine is an example of how Southeast Asian nations have adapted Chinese traditional medical concepts. According to Vietnamese folk medicine, health depends on maintaining a balance of bodily elements; therefore, cure of illness is predicated on restoring the balance. Many Vietnamese foods and illnesses are believed to be hot or cold in nature; thus, Vietnamese pregnant women avoid certain hot and cold foods in an attempt not to disturb the body's balance of forces, which in turn would make them susceptible to illness.

It is wise to remember that in all ethnic communities both Western and traditional non-Western medicines are used. To be aware of which medicines are accepted is to be able to care effectively for patients.

References

1. Morley, P.; and Wallis, R., editors. 1978. *Culture and curing.* Pittsburgh: University of Pittsburgh Press, p. 2.

2. Weaver, T. 1970. Use of hypothetical situations in a study of Spanish-American illness referral systems. *Hum. Organ.* 29:141.

3. Dunn, F. L. 1975. Transcultural Asian medicine and cosmopolitan medicine as adaptive systems. In Leslie, C., editor. *Asian medical systems: A comparative study.* Berkeley: University of California Press, p. 135.

4. Fabrega, H., Jr. 1975. The need for an ethnomedical science. *Science* 189: 970. Copyright 1975 by the American Association for the Advancement of Science.

5. Kay, M. 1978. Clinical anthropology. In Bauwens, E. E., editor. *The anthropology of health.* St. Louis: The C. V. Mosby Co., p. 6.

6. See Alland, A. 1970. *Adaptation in cultural evolution: An approach to medical anthropology.* New York: Columbia University Press; Branch, M. F.; and Paxton, P. P. 1976. *Providing safe nursing care for ethnic people of color.* New York: Appleton-Century-Crofts; Brink, P. 1976. *Transcultural nursing.* Englewood Cliffs, N. J.: Prentice-Hall, Inc.; Landy, D., editor. 1977. *Culture, disease and healing: Studies in medical anthropology.* New York: Macmillan, Inc.; and Spector. R. E. 1979. *Cultural diversity in health and illness.* New York: Appleton-Century-Crofts.

7. Rittenbaugh, C. 1978. Human foodways: A window on evolution. In Bauwens, E. E., editor. *The anthropology of health.* St. Louis: The C. V. Mosby Co., p. 113.

8. Kay, M. 1978. Clinical anthropology. In Bauwens, E. E., editor. *The anthropology of health.* St. Louis: The C. V. Mosby Co., p. 7.

9. Morley, P.; and Wallis, R., editors. 1978. *Culture and curing.* Pittsburgh: University of Pittsburgh Press, p. 40.

10. Foster, G. M.; and Anderson, B. G. 1978. *Medical anthropology.* New York: John Wiley & Sons, Inc., p. 124.

11. Erasmus, J. C. 1952. Changing folk beliefs and the relativity of empirical knowledge. *Southwestern J. Anthropology* 8:418.

12. Foster, G. M.; and Anderson, B. G. 1978. *Medical anthropology.* New York: John Wiley & Sons, Inc., p. 244.

13. Orque, M. S. 1976. Health care and minority clients. *Nurs. Outlook* 24:315.

14. Hand, W. The folk healer: Calling and endowment. *J. Hist. Med.* 26:263-275.

15. Snow, L. F. 1978. Sorcerers, saints and charlatans: Black folk healers in urban America. *Culture Med. Psychiatry* 2:87-91.

16. Fisch, S. 1968. Botanicas and spiritualism in a metropolis. *Milbank Mem. Fund* 41:378.

17. See Devereux, G. 1958. Cultural thought models in primitive and modern psychological theories. *Psychiatry* 21:359-74.

18. Henderson, G., editor. 1979. *Understanding and counseling ethnic minorities.* Springfield, Ill.: Charles C. Thomas, Publisher, pp. 29-30.

19. Samora, J., editor. 1966. *LaRaza: Forgotten Americans.* South Bend, Ind.: University of Notre Dame Press.

20. Maldonado-Denis, M. 1972. *Puerto Rico: A socio-historic interpretation.* New York: Vintage Books.

21. Deloria, V., Jr. 1973. *God is red.* New York: Grosset & Dunlap, Inc.

22. Sue, S.; and Sue, D. W. 1973. Understanding Asian-Americans: The neglected minority. *Personnel Guid. J.* 51:387-389.

6

Folk Medical Beliefs and Their Implications for the Care of Patients:
A Review Based on Studies Among Black Americans

Loudell F. Snow, Ph.D.

Loudell F. Snow is Associate Professor of Anthropology at the College of Human Medicine, Michigan State University. The information in this chapter was taken from her doctoral dissertation, revised and published under the title, "Popular Medicine in a Black Neighborhood," Ethnic Medicine in the Southwest. *The main focus of her professional research has been the health beliefs and practices of low-income black Americans. She is particularly interested in those areas where folk belief interferes with good health practices. Her articles have appeared both in medical and social science journals, including* Journal of the American Medical Association, Journal of Family Practice, Journal of American Folklore, *and* International Journal of Women's Studies.

In 1967 a conference on the health status of black Americans was held. It was concluded that the gap between black and white mortality and morbidity was widening and that this was true for most of the important public health indexes used in the United States.[1] A 1968 survey reported that two thirds of urban blacks usually "feel sick" and that more than half believe that their health is worse than

Source: Snow, L. F. 1974. Folk medical beliefs and their implications for care of patients. *Ann. Intern. Med.* 81:82-96.

that of their parents or grandparents.[2] More recently, interviews with several hundred Harlem adolescents showed that three fourths of them believe an individual can expect a lot of sickness during his lifetime, and more than half think that there is not much to be done about it.[3] Few would deny that, as a group, low-income blacks, rural or urban, have received little professional health care until the last few years. The key word here is *professional,* however, and it would be fallacious to assume that a lack of professional health care means no health care at all. Health is of prime concern in all societies, and no group has yet been found that did not have some systematized way of dealing with illness. It is not surprising, therefore, that a viable folk medical system is part of American black culture. Most of the information in this paper is based on the ethnographic study of this system in a poor black neighborhood in Tucson, Arizona.

METHODS

A preliminary investigation of the neighborhood used historical sources, U.S. Census data, mapping techniques, and information from the Tucson City Directory.[4-6] The neighborhood is a small, residential backwater that has been surrounded on all sides by the city's urban expansion. Most of the inhabitants were at the lower end of the economic continuum, many on welfare. There were 223 households in the neighborhood, 114 (51%) of which were headed by women, 38 (17%) by men, and the remaining 71 (32%) by married couples.[6] In all, 47 individuals were interviewed, members of 29 separate families living in 37 households; 15% of each head-of-household category is represented.

The ethnographic portion of the study included the collection of life histories, preparation of geneologies, and in-depth interviews; additional data on each informant include date and place of birth, length of time lived in Tucson, marital status, household composition, rental or ownership of home, occupation, amount and source of income, education and religious affiliation. Informants were from 36 to 85 years old, and with one exception, none were born in Arizona. Most had been born and reared in rural areas of the border south, particularly Oklahoma, Texas, Arkansas, and Kentucky. The level of formal education of informants was rather low. One woman has a college degree, and one other has had 1 year of college training. Six other women have high school diplomas and all other informants reported only some primary schooling. None of the men in the sample had completed high school. The occupations of neighborhood residents reflect the low educational level, usually requiring few skills.

Persons formally interviewed were seen at least twice, and these interviews were taped whenever possible. Those informants with special knowledge of health system were interviewed several times. Several neighborhood women are considered expert in home remedies, for example, and others are thought to possess special healing power. One woman is a Voodoo doctor and thus able to cure diseases caused by witchcraft. Although her office is not in the neighborhood,

neighborhood residents sometimes consult her, so she too was included in the sample.[7] Some interviews were not taped, and in these instances notes were taken instead: those who do some folk curing are aware of licensing laws, and some were afraid of getting into trouble if "they" heard the tapes.

Information was also collected informally at such public gatherings as Model Cities Neighborhood Task Force meetings. Religious services were attended at neighborhood churches and, on other occasions, special ceremonies as well: healing night at a Pentecostal church; message night at a Spiritualist chapel, where mediums bring word from loved ones in the spirit world; a revival; a baptism by immersion; and Mother's Day services at a Voodoo temple.

Further information has also been collected in Lansing, Michigan, that has corroborated the Tucson study and in some instances extended the findings to persons who are both younger and much better educated than the Arizona informants. Four individuals are working women, one a nurse's aide and the others in clerical positions at Michigan State University; six others (two women and four men) are either undergraduate students at Michigan State or medical students at the university medical schools.

A study of folk healers in the Chicago area is being carried out at the present time, and a final report is not yet ready. Preliminary findings indicate, however, that beliefs concerning the allocation of the ability to cure, who is able to cure what, and the techniques used are the same as those in the Tucson study. A survey of the literature yielded further information, which is included where pertinent.

FOLK MEDICAL BELIEFS AS A SYSTEM

In general, however, the information presented in this paper is meant to illustrate the beliefs found among lower-class blacks who have been socialized in the rural South or maintain kin ties in the South, or both. Black folk beliefs concerning maintenance of health, the causes of illness, the allocation of the ability to cure, and the curing techniques commonly used will be described. Although folk medicine is a fascinating topic in its own right, this report focuses on those areas where the contrast with orthodox scientific medicine might produce conflict. Knowledge of potential conflict does not guarantee its resolution, of course, but practitioners should be aware that patients' behavior may be adversely affected by their commitment to a different belief system.

The system is a composite of the classical medicine of an earlier day, European folklore regarding the natural world, rare African traits, and selected beliefs derived from modern scientific medicine. The whole is inextricably blended with the tenets of fundamentalist Christianity, elements from the Voodoo religion of the West Indies, and the added spice of sympathetic magic. This mixture of cultural elements has formed, in folklorist Richard Dorson's phrase, "a rich complex of unified folklore whose parts intertwine in a many-veined, dazzling filigree."[8] It is a coherent medical system and not a ragtag collection of isolated superstitions. If the underlying premises are accepted, it makes just as much sense to the believer as the principles of orthodox medicine do to the graduate of an accredited medical school.

The folk medical system under scrutiny here is not, however, restricted to black Americans. Portions of it are to be found among groups as diverse as the Pennsylvania Dutch, the Hutterites, and Amish, Appalachian whites, the Cajuns of Louisiana, Kansas farmers, Puerto Ricans in New York and the Midwest, and Mexican-Americans wherever they are found.[9-33] Similar beliefs are to be found from rural Florida through the Ozarks and from California to the Upper Peninsula of Michigan.[34-39] They are, therefore, characteristic of a great many people, and a secondary aim of this report is to compare and contrast the beliefs of the different groups.

Three major themes emerge from the data, particularly that collected from black informants—first, that the world is a hostile and dangerous place; second, that the individual is liable to attack from external sources; third, that the individual is helpless and has no internal resources to combat such attack but must depend on outside aid. That the world is seen as hostile and dangerous for poor black people has been reported in studies by anthropologists, sociologists, psychologists, and psychiatrists.[40-47] The behavioral adaptations this produces are perhaps best seen in the fictional and autobiographical works of black authors, in poetry, and blues songs.[48-54]

The individual as potential victim of attack must be wary of the world of nature, of a punitive God, and of the malice of his fellow man. This latter is embedded in a pessimism about the nature of human relationships and "the bedrock conviction that most people will do ill when it is in their interest, that doing ill is more natural than doing good."[42] This distrust may be extended to friends and relatives as well as strangers.[41,43,55] Life is a constant hustle, and success in interpersonal relationships may be seen as the ability to manipulate others.[49,56]

Feelings of emptiness and helplessness are reflected in the content of much religious music and a dependency on supernatural aid. The use of magic is also prominent and is commonly found when what is wished for is of great emotional significance, the outcome uncertain, and other means to the end are not available.[57-59]

There is a tendency to lump events as to whether they are desirable or undesirable, resulting in a mixture of conceptual domains confusing to the science-oriented professional. Good health is classed with any kind of good luck: success, money, a good job, a peaceful home. Illness, on the other hand, may be looked upon as just another undesirable event, along with bad luck, poverty, unemployment, domestic turmoil, and so on. The attempted manipulation of events therefore covers a broad range of practices that are carried out to attract good, including good health, or to repel bad, including bad health.[60]

NATURAL AND UNNATURAL PHENOMENA

The folk medical system described here depends largely on the classification of happenings as "natural" or "unnatural." This division of the universe into natural and unnatural phenomena is common among New World blacks. It has been reported in Haiti, in Trinidad, and wherever in the United States black people are found.[58,61-66] It is also common to Spanish-speakers in Mexico, in the West Indies, and the United States.[13,28,31,67] Although the terminology is slightly different, this idea is expressed by Southern whites when they differentiate between the natural and the supernatural.[20,23,35]

Perhaps the simplest way to describe this division is to state that natural events have to do with the world as God made it and as He intended it to be. Natural laws therefore allow a measure of predictability for daily life. Unnatural events, in contrast, imply just the opposite: by their very existence they upset the harmony of nature. At best they interrupt the plan intended by God; at worst, they represent the forces of evil and the machinations of the Devil. They are frightening because they are not predictable. They are outside the world of nature and, when they do occur, they are beyond the abilities of ordinary mortals to control.

Pertinent to this tendency to view phenomena in terms of oppositions such as good versus evil and natural versus unnatural is the belief that everything has its opposite. This is expressed in health terms by proverbs stating that for every birth there is a death, every illness has its cure, every poison an antidote, every herb a healing purpose.[36,63,68] This belief is largely responsible for the lack of acceptance of the chronicity of some diseases; most informants feel that all illnesses are curable. If every illness has its cure, then what one must do is find it: a new medicine, another treatment, a different doctor, faith healing perhaps—and the search is on.

Illnesses are also classified as natural or unnatural, which affects the type of cure or practitioner sought. All illnesses represent disharmony and conflict in some area of the individual's life and tend to fall into three general categories: environmental hazards, divine punishment, and impaired social relationships.

Natural Illnesses

In this first category the individual has come up against the forces of nature without suitable protection. Dangerous agents are cold air, which may enter the body, and impurities in the air, in food, and in water, which may enter the body to cause illness; they will be more fully discussed later. Such problems are considered natural because the source is natural. For example,

> Well, in other words, it's *exposure*, that you get sometime when you're young in your body. Through your system as you get older, it takes effect ... dampness and not takin' proper care of yourself. Goin' out in bad

weather and rainy weather, you expose yourself. Pores are open. You're subject to takin' a complaint in through the blood . . . kind of grows into the system, and as you get older it works with you. [Excerpt from tape recording, December 1970.]

Second, it is commonly believed that illness may be sent by God as punishment for sin. It is believed in Trinidad, where the "powers" may punish wrongdoing with sickness, in Haiti, when the *loa* send misfortune as a "chastisement," and death is the will of *le bon Dieu*.[65,66,69] Mexican-Americans see natural illnesses (*males naturales*) as God's will and, in some cases, as a direct punishment, or *castigo*.[33] Among Appalachian whites "the wrath of God" may be the final explanation for sickness.[20] Such illnesses may take any form but are often sudden and severe enough to give the individual time to reflect on his or her transgression. A paralytic stroke, for example, allows the sinner time to think over past behavior and repent. Retardation in children is commonly cited as punishment to the parents, who then spend the rest of their lives contemplating the result of their misdeeds. The punishment of the parent by inflicting illness, injury, or death on the child is a common theme, and one which cross-cuts social class and educational level. One college-educated informant considers a younger sister's death from meningitis as a punishment to the father for "drinking and running around with women." The bacterial etiology was also fully understood but did not preclude the supernatural explanation as well. More often, when asked what sins are thought to bring on such retributions, informants cite pride and "thinking you are better than other people." Fear of such punishment therefore operates as a social leveler, that is, to insure that individuals do not blatantly exhibit feelings of superiority or flaunt material possession. To do so is to invite divine displeasure:

So many times the Lord gets vexed with us when we do things. Like sickness I would say sometimes is a whup to us, just like whuppin' a child. So many times we have to be taught a lesson, a sickness sometime bring us down to make us serve the Lord's will. Sometime we don't know how to praise the Lord and thank Him for things He did for us. You can invite it in yourself. If you live a real good life for God, it's just like children: if you got good children you don't have to punish 'em. Sickness and different things is like a whuppin'. A reminder. The Lord would heal all the people if they would ask the Lord to heal 'em. But the people, they forget God. [Excerpt from tape recording, January 1971.]

Such punishment, whatever its nature, is considered natural because it is the will of God.

It is believed that the doctor is unable to help the patient whom God is punishing. Thus a Baptist minister admonishes his congregation that the doctors cannot cure many people because "medicine cannot reach the mind, nor a heart diseased by sin."

On the other hand, God may intercede in the favor of the individual—one woman, a Pentecostal evangelist, spends much time at a local hospital praying for the sick. She understands that there are illnesses caused by microorganisms but believes that while she is making her hospital rounds God puts an invisible barrier around her that germs cannot penetrate. Preventive measures may also be taken that illustrate the powerlessness of the individual and the emphasis on possession of some tangible sign of protection. Such measures range from the asafoetida bag worn around the neck to keep away illness to the printed prayer given me by an informant to keep me safe, which assures that the possessor will never burn or drown, poison will have no effect, 82 accidents will be averted, childbirth will be eased, and epileptic seizures precluded. It is an exact duplicate of one sent to William Black nearly a century ago, as reported in his classic treatise on folk medicine.[70]

Unnatural Illnesses

In extreme cases the individual may be so grave a sinner that the Lord withdraws His favor. An unprotected person is easy prey to demons and evil spirits and in some instances may be possessed by them. The presence of such beings, which lurk about waiting to pounce on the sinner, is usually referred to as evil influence, or, among Spanish-speakers, *malas influencias.* If this does occur and the Devil takes over, the illness is no longer natural but unnatural. The following passage illustrates the feeling that one may be buffeted by opposing external forces and the idea that alone one may do nothing.

> Evil influence mean the *Devil* which name is Satan. He is Evil, he can put evil thought in your mind. Also the Devil can work in the frame of anyone mind, cause you to do things you don't want to do. Our body is made up of Evil and of Good. If we are not close to God in spirit, the Devil take control of us. God guide me each day and teach me wisdom and knowledge how to cope with my problem and people around me. Sometime I have so many burden on my shoulder I don't know which way to turn to. I learn to work them out by talking to Jesus and forget about them, and before long He work them out because I can't do anything for myself. [Excerpt from letter to author, January 1974.]

Evil influences may be blamed for any sort of problem, from nightmares to tuberculosis.[71] Like those illnesses that result from divine punishment, the physician is unable to help the patient afflicted by evil because you cannot fight the Devil with drugs. This may create real treatment problems: a diabetic black woman in Grand Rapids, Michigan, for example, has consistently refused to inject herself with insulin because she believes her illness is one that the Devil has "put on" her because of a sinful youth. It is now 18 months since the initial diagnosis, and she is called on daily by a visiting nurse who gives the injection.

Most commonly, however, unnatural illnesses refer to those caused by witchcraft. Here, too, it is believed that the physician is unable to treat such illness, and a prime symptom is that the more you go to the doctor the sicker you get. Witchcraft is based on the belief that there are individuals with the ability to mobilize unusual powers for good and evil. The use of such abilities is based on the principles of sympathetic magic, and because they underlie so much of folk medical practice a brief description is in order. Sympathetic magic is based on the assumption that everything in the universe is connected and that events can be interpreted and directed by an understanding of these connections. There is a division into imitative and contagious magic. Contagious magic has to do with the premise that things once physically connected can never be separated and that what you do to the part you do to the whole. Many witchcraft practices are based on contagious magic, and an enemy need only obtain a lock of the victim's hair, fingernail clippings, worn clothing, or a used menstrual pad to do harm. Thus, says a coed, "I'm a little skeptical of letting just anybody use my comb or borrow too many of my personal possessions." Imitative magic depends on the assumption that like follows like, and you imitate what you wish to achieve: a knife under the bed will cut pain or the effect of medicine, or an evil charm put on when the moon is waxing will increase with the moon.

Belief in witchcraft as a cause of illness is widespread; it is found among Haitians, Trinidadians, Puerto-Rican Americans, American blacks and Mexican-Americans.[13,27-29,31,33,58,61,64,66,69,72-75] It does not seem prominent in the folk nosology of Southern whites, although belief in nonmalign magic certainly is. It is estimated that one third of the black patients treated at a Southern psychiatric center believe that they are the victims of witchcraft, and a Spanish-speaking physician in California reports that this is true for one fourth of his patients.[39,76]

Among blacks, the terms commonly used to describe such occurrences are roots, rootwork, witchcraft, Voodoo or Hoodoo, a fix, a hex a mojo—the evil has been "put on" or "thrown at" the victim.[75] Among Spanish-speakers, comparable terms are *mal puesto* (literally, "evil put on"), *mal ojo, mal artificial, brujería, hechicería,* or *enfermedad endañada,* the illness of damage. Regardless of the term used, the idea is that someone has done something to cause another illness, injury, or death. The fear of such attack is very great and may contribute to what Engel has called lethal life situations.[77] A classic case at Baltimore City Hospital describes how such fear is believed to have contributed directly to a patient's death.[78]

A recurring theme in witchcraft belief is that animals are present in the body, introduced by magical means. Animal intrusion as a cause of illness has a long history in European and American folk lore, usually from accidental ingestion of the creature: spring water might contain a "spring lizard," river water contains eggs that can be swallowed while swimming, a garden hose might harbor a small reptile and should not be drunk from, and sleeping in the grass should be avoided lest a snake or lizard crawl into the mouth.[70,79] In witchcraft, however, the magical component is obvious, in that the animal has been dried and pulverized, sprinkled on food, and then reconstituted in the body of the victim. Lizards, snakes, toads, and spiders are most commonly mentioned, and "satanic worms" kept in milk, frog eggs hatching out in the blood, and canned corn or the victim's own hair turning to snakes or worms in the stomach have all been reported.[15,28,58,64,72] A Tucson informant told me that a rival in a love triangle had placed an octopus egg in his beer; it had than hatched, and the baby octopus had to be removed from his bladder. The main symptom seemed to be hematuria, and I have puzzled since as to what the problem actually was; whatever he was told, he interpreted it in culturally acceptable terms. Although the offending beast is almost always a reptile, amphibian, or insect, in one rare instance a gopher was reportedly served up in a dish of hopping john.[75]

Symptoms of witchcraft are often described as reptiles crawling over the body or wriggling around in the stomach.

> I've heard of people with snakes in their body, how they got in there I don't know. And they take 'em someplace to a witch doctor and snakes come out. My sister, she had somethin', a snake that was in her arm. She was a young woman. I can remember her bein' sick, very sick, and someone told her about this healer in another little town. And I do know they taken her there. This thing was just runnin' up her arm, whatever it was, just runnin' up her arm. You could actually *see* it. And we would have to hold her in the bed. And someone told her about this healer, and my parents did take her there. And this actually came out of her arm. You could actually see it when she would go into one of her spells, it was in her left arm. Some woman they said didn't like her [had done it]. [Excerpt from tape recording, October 1973.]

Because of the fear of adulterated food there is often anxiety about eating in other people's homes or in public places, and some people refuse to do either. It is not surprising that presumed symptoms of unnatural illnesses are often associated with eating, so that the appetite is lost, there are pains in the stomach, food doesn't taste right, or that food eaten does no good. This latter is a particularly frightening symptom, since it isn't natural to lose weight while consuming the usual amount of food. As continued weight loss may be symptomatic of serious illness, the observation here may be correct if the interpretation is not.

Perhaps more commonly, behavioral changes—anything that is perceived as "crazy"—will be seen as the sign of fix or hex. This idea is illustrated in the following passage, as well as the idea of external control by another person.

> Well, I've heard people can take your clothes, take your underclothes or your menstruating [pads] or anything that you wear on your body. I heard that they could put stuff in your food, or they could come to your house and put something down for you. Yeah, I hear talk of it. Yeah, I hear about a few people, someone have control of 'em. They *do* act rather *peculiar,*

they doesn't act normal, or sensible. Well, for instance, I've heard of men fixin' their wives and wives fixin' their husbands, stuff like that, you know. Well, if this *happen* to you, they say you would be the last person to suspect; anyone could tell you and you wouldn't believe it. Well, [lowers voice] I don't know why, but I hate the thought of a person takin' control of you if they want to. [Excerpt from tape recording, March 1971.]

A Tucson informant who was hospitalized for "nerves" (professional diagnosis, acute anxiety state) was greatly relieved to afterwards dig up a pair of underpants buried with a snapshot of herself, the date she was to die was printed on the back of the picture. Finding it supposedly broke the spell—but in a burst of eclecticism she started attending church more regularly, continued to see her physician, and began training classes at a Spiritualist temple to learn to visualize herself "in the white light of protection." Rubel[32] also states that dramatic mania is the one symptom nearly always attributed to *mal puesto* by Mexican-Americans, with the understanding that the victim is controlled by someone else.

Any symptom that is seen as unusual may be frightening, however, and the mere fact that an illness has not been cured may signal to believers that it is unnatural in origin. In one recent instance in Lansing a man had a skin rash that the physician was unable to clear up immediately. The rash reportedly occurred "only where it showed," which was seen as being strange—the combination of chronicity plus the unusual symptom was enough to make him call in a root doctor.

Even when the patient does not think the illness is the result of malign forces, the practitioner may inadvertently plant this fear. So simple an act as telling the patient to return in a few days when the results of tests are completed may be interpreted as uncertainty on the part of the physician, and therefore the illness may be unnatural.[58]

The most commonly cited reasons for witchcraft attack are sexual jealousy and envy, among both blacks and Spanish-speakers. It is dangerous to be one of the "higher-ups," or to have anything that someone else might want—a new car, money, a pretty face, a faithful husband. Like divide punishment, fear of witchcraft can act as a leveling device—if you've got it, don't show it off. When I accepted a teaching position in another state, one woman warned me against going to and accepting refreshments at social gatherings:

Witchcraft is real, it can be did; you can be hypnotized. You hafta be careful where you eat and drink. Parties is not good; you know some ladies is looking at that man of yours. You is new there so don't be so fast in going to parties and eating and drinking, it isn't good. [Excerpt from letter to author, January 1972.]

Among Mexican-Americans the power of envy is believed to be so strong that the mere glance of an envious person can kill pets or house plants.

Although such beliefs may be bizarre to the scientist, they are understandable in their cultural matrix. Witchcraft beliefs are the most extreme example of distrust and unease in social interactions. They are the magical expression of the fear that strangers, friends or relatives may wish you harm. In a survey in a federal slum housing project in St. Louis, 91% of black respondents agreed with the statement, "It's not good to let your friends know everything about your life because they may take advantage of you," and 69% agreed that it was also unwise to trust your relatives.[42] As one man put it, "You know yourself, man, when you walk out in the streets you have got to be ready. Everybody walking out there is game on everybody else."[42] When the discussion shifts from the theoretical to the concrete, however, the malice of unknown others is replaced by accusations of individuals in the immediate social network. In virtually every case reported in the literature and in my own data as well, the evildoer is specifically identified and is usually girlfriend or lover, husband or wife, a parent, a sibling, or an in-law. This is true for both blacks and Spanish-speakers, and there is no more graphic example of personal inadequacy and the deep distrust and ambivalence that many feel in their social ties. The possibility of external control is matched by the belief that magical means are *needed* to bring about desired behavior in others: charms must be used to get what you want, and to keep it.

The need for visible protection is also exhibited, and a silver dime is often worn somewhere on the body in the belief that it will turn black if someone is attempting to do evil to the wearer.[80] Oils, incenses, candles and aerosol room sprays may be used to repel evil, and such items may be ordered by mail or purchased at specialty stores; in a Spanish-speaking neighborhood they are available in the *botanica*.[13,60,81,82]

Perhaps most individuals who believe themselves the victims of witchcraft do not turn up in the clinician's office because they believe that only a person with special powers can remove the spell. Occasionally they do, however, and there is a growing number of reports in the medical literature giving actual case histories; physicians interested in knowing how such a patient presents himself in the clinical situation are urged to consult these.[27,72-74,77,83]

If illness is seen in terms of attack from without, cures may be described in equally dramatic terms: demons can be exorcised, the cold driven out, God can lift up those He has struck down, and, if one can find a powerful curer, the fix or hex that was put on can be taken off again. The view of illness as something that can be driven out of the body *en masse* holds true for both natural and unnatural categories. Thus a white Southern mountain woman reports, "Over in Kentucky, they prayed for a woman who had cancer of the stomach. They was holiness people and they prayed for her and anoited her with oil and laid hands on her, and before she left the church, she vomited that thing up."[18] This view of illness as a *thing* that strikes the unprotected individual is clearly expressed in the following passages; the speaker, an evangelist in the Holiness Church, has given up praying for the sick.

"I don't pray for 'em, though, cause I picks up their ailment. See, you could have something wrong with you and I could pray for you, and I'd take it." "Would I get well [Author]?" "Yeah, you'd be all right. But I'd be sufferin' with it! It'd go in *me*! And then somebody's have to come along and pray it out of me! Lots of times people won't accept it; it's the way you have to pray for the sick people to keep from takin' it. Reverend ―――――――, he stopped me from prayin' for people down there. Ever' *time* I'd take it. Pick it up, take it like that. And they had to come right on and pray it off of me. And so they kinda stopped me." [Excerpt from tape recording, December 1970.]

Although the separation of illness into natural and unnatural categories is useful as a descriptive device, in reality it is not always so clear-cut. Since the emphasis is on presumed cause rather than effect, illnesses that are identical to the clinician may be variously interpreted: a stroke may be blamed on divine punishment, on improper diet, or on the entry of cold air into the body of a menstruating woman. Treatments, as will be seen, also reflect an intermingling of pragmatism, religious belief, and magical practice, so that a nosebleed might be handled by packing the nose with cobwebs, the recitation of a biblical verse, or placing broom straws crosswise in the hair to cross up the flow of blood.

Although the physician should be aware of these beliefs regarding witchcraft and divine punishment, most health problems occur because the individual is no longer in harmony with the forces of nature. Good health is primarily based on such harmony, and this requires that the rules of nature must be known and followed. If not, "Nature will kill you, you won't kill it."

The individual is responsible for knowing the rules of nature that thus govern life, and if a lapse results in illness it is his or her own fault. On the positive side, this creates an atmosphere in which preventive medicine can flourish, since people are necessarily concerned with monitoring their health. It may have negative repercussions, however, in that the wise individual in incessantly dosing himself or herself to prevent illness. Self-treatment for illness is common, and in one study nearly 40% of the people in the sample reported treating all illnesses at home in the previous year.[84] In another study *every* respondent disclosed that they deliberately withheld use of "old timey" remedies from physicians.[34] Some of these practices are extremely dangerous in the light of orthodox medical practice. Laxative abuse is legion, and other oral medications include kerosene, turpentine, moth balls, and carbon tetrachloride.[76,85,86]

ATTAINING AND MAINTAINING GOOD HEALTH

There is safety in harmony and balance and danger in anything done to the extreme. It is bad for the body to eat too much, drink too much, stay out too late at night, and so on.[87] In a study in Harlem 90% of black adolescents believe that good health is largely a matter of "looking after yourself."[3] The results of excess may not be immediately visible but will certainly affect the individual sooner or later because the body has been weakened. Older people in poor health usually attribute it to the rash behavior of youth, whereas older people whose health is good look back on a life of moderation:

> I feel that it's the care that they take of theirselves. That's what I think I don't know. I feel like they exposes theirselves too much, and don't take enough care of theirself like they should. That's one reason that I can get around and do things now at my age! Now I've worked hard all my life, ever since I started at ten years old. But otherwise, I've taken care of myself. And I never was the goin' kind! I didn't work all day and then goin' half the night and all like that ... I taken my rest and taken care of myself. [Excerpt from tape recording, November 1970.]

Strength and Weakness During the Life Cycle

There is an age/sex differential associated with strength and weakness, strength being correlated with greater ability to withstand illness and weakness with heightened susceptibility. There is an explicit correlation with strength and sexuality, and the very young and the very old, seen as asexual, are constitutionally weak. Females are considered weaker than males, and weakness is part of the ideal female role for both Latin women and women in the rural South.[35] This sex-correlated weakness means that women are more prone to illness, primarily because of functional blood loss and anatomical differences:

> There's somethin' about a girl gets a disease quicker than a boy. On account of her different sex. She's easy to catch or she's eager to catch ever'thing. Because she'll get it in her breast. Different things come through the breast, through your vagina too, you know. There are two things you have a man don't have, that make you easily [get sick]. [Excerpt from tape recording, December 1970.]

The unborn infant is the weakest of all, and the fetus is at the mercy of the mother's prenatal behavior. Harmony and moderation are again the watchword, and the pregnancy period is one of many behavioral prescriptions and taboos. This doctrine of maternal impressions is nearly universal, and in the United States is found among Spanish-speakers, the Amish, the Hutterites, and both whites and blacks in the South.[9,16,88] The mother's emotional state may affect the baby, whether pity, fear, mockery, or hate is experienced. Feelings of hate for a particular individual may cause the baby to resemble that person, one young mother told me, adding ingenuously, "It's usually the father." A child may suffer seizures because the mother saw someone having a seizure and felt pity; worrying about a loved one with a particular health problem may cause the infant to have the same problem. The theme of divide displeasure again appears for blacks, Southern whites, and Mexican-Americans; it is reported that if a pregnant woman makes fun of someone with a physical afflication the baby may be born with the same thing, punishing the mother for lack of charity.[16,33] Dietary cravings are also potentially harmful to the fetus, and if the pregnant woman desires a particular food she must not touch herself until the craving is satisfied. Otherwise the baby will have a birthmark resembling the food she wanted, located on the spot corresponding to where she touched herself.

The young infant is still prey to external conditions because of its inherent weakness. Many of the folk diseases unique to Mexican-American culture occur during childhood, when the child is seen as being in delicate balance with life. The folk illness *mal ojo* (evil eye), for example, occurs when an infant or small child is admired by an adult with "strong vision."[28] There is a widespread belief that a newborn child should not be handled by a menstruating woman; among black women that belief is that it will cause the infant "to strain."[80] In Tucson, Mexican-American women blame umbilical hernia on the handling of the new baby by a menstruating women or another new mother. According to Foster, this belief is found in some and perhaps all Spanish-American countries, from El Salvador to Peru.[26] In accord with the principles of imitative magic, the cramping of the menstruating woman affects the baby in the same way, and strain or hernia is the result.

Natural Forces

Sympathetic magic is also incorporated in the notion that there is a direct connection between the body and the forces of nature. Here the basic premise is that natural phenomena, such as the phases of the moon, position of the planets, season of the year, and so on, directly affect the human body and its processes. Since these phenomena are observable, and man is a direct part of nature, the maintenance of health is directly associated with the ability of the individual to read "the signs." As one woman says, "Lotta doctors stand around on their butts laughin' at the signs; they'd do better if they paid attention." Dependence on the signs to regulate behavior is found all over the rural South among both blacks and whites, in northern and western cities where southerners have migrated, and in other parts of the country as well.[17,23,24,36,38,64] The clearest exposition of how the signs are read is to be found in *The Foxfire Book*.[24]

A farmer's alamnac is the repository of much of this nature lore and is an instructional guide that reports the best days to plant crops, to set hen's eggs, to destroy weeds, wean babies, and go fishing. The almanac is consulted for the best times to have teeth extracted (during the increase of the moon) or filled (during the moon's decrease). It is also used to pick the optimal time to have surgical procedures done, as will be shown. The almanac is not used by rural people alone, and I recently purchased one in a store on Chicago's south side. The proprietor described it as a very popular item, pointing out that it had been written by an M.D.; first edition 1897.[90] Many people who use the zodiacal signs to manipulate their own health regimens do not mention this to health professionals for fear of being laughed at. They are, however, the basis for a constant and lively practice of self-medication, dietary regulation, and behavioral modifications, and the physician should be aware of these beliefs. Some are harmless, some neutral; others, however, are potentially damaging, as will be shown. Again, they illustrate how external forces are brought to bear on the individual, who must learn to manipulate them for his or her own well being. . . .

THE ART OF HEALING

The mixture of natural, magical, and religious domains seen in ideas about illness causation, treatment, and prevention is also found in views on who has the ability to cure. Practitioners are classified according to the methods used in healing and how they received the ability to heal.

In the first instance it is said that "medical" doctors give medicines, "surgical" doctors cut, "rubbing" doctors manipulate the body, and so forth. It may not be generally understood that surgeons are also trained in general medicine or that there is any real difference between the chiropractor and the M.D. or D.O., other than the type of treatment used.[21,23,36] In some instances the chriopractor is considered superior because he prevents illness, whereas the medical doctor can only cure it; in others, the chriopractor is sought after other, orthodox medical services have been used without success.[10] In some cases, in fact, the physician may be considered inferior to the nurse or pharmacist in health matters.[34] Because the "medical" doctor gives medicines he or she is in the same class as the herb doctor, the housewife, or the neighbor who happens to know a lot of home remedies. This gives rise to a great deal of hostility toward professional practitioners, and they are often seen as motivated by cupidity; likewise, the feeling that doctors are not interested in having poor people as patients is very widespread.[2,25,47] Southern mountain women in Detroit complain that doctors think they are "poor white trash."[23] Black people in New Orleans have even reported belief in the "gown man," or "needle doctor," characterized as a student physician who lurks in dark alleys at night to fall upon hapless victims, kill them with an injection, and then take them away to dissect at leisure.[43,89] A Tucson woman who had just been released from the hospital noted bitterly that the physician just looked at her without touching her when he made rounds, which she interpreted as meaning he didn't want to put his hands on a black person. The behavior of the low-income patient is often just as frustrating to health personnel.[21,108,109] In an extreme case, medical personnel have categorized Appalachian whites as abnormal, and "one group, the 'cultural primitives,' is described as characterologically similar to schizophrenics and the other group, the 'traditional farmers' as having character structures similar to psychoneurotics."[110]

The synthetization of medications in the past few years also contributes to misunderstandings, and informants frequently mention items formerly available in the pharmacy that they cannot now obtain or that requires a prescription. The pharmacist is blamed for collusion with the physician in seeing that the patients have to use prescription medicine; one woman complained that the pharmacist had laughed when she asked for buzzard grease. The fear of not knowing what is in prescription medicine has already been mentioned. It is also believed to be quite strong, so that if it is taken it should produce practically instantaneous results. Another frequently mentioned complaint, therefore, is that the doctor only gives you enough medicine to keep you alive until the next office visit, implying that he could give you enough to cure you if he wished but prefers to keep the patient returning until the money is gone.

The ability to heal is seen as being a gift from God, and the gift is differentially bestowed. Healing practitioners, that is, can be ranked according to how much "power" God has given them to cure. There are three ranks of healers graded in this way, the lowest including those who learned their craft from others, whether one's grandmother, a talented neighbor, or a medical school—M.D. or D.O., therefore, is classed along with the herb doctor and neighborhood healer. Above these are those individuals whom God thought fit to receive the gift of healing, during a religious experience later in life; evangelist Oral Roberts is a well-known example of this kind of healer. The individual with the greatest ability, however, is the person born with the gift of healing, which is evidence of special divine approbation literally from birth. The sorts of illnesses dealt with are also correlated with the amount of power the individual healer is thought to command.

The conferring of expertise by education is, of course, a particularly middle- and upper-class phenomenon, and is relatively meaningless to those who have little education or for whom education does not guarantee upward mobility. There is marked ambivalence on the part of informants concerning education. On the one hand, it is highly valued and seen as the key to success—realistically, however, most poor people do not have any expectations of advanced training, and both envy and resent the "higher ups" who have it. For blacks the fact that most "higher ups"—including physicians—with whom they come in contact are white compounds feelings of helplessness and anger. Since such avenues to advancement are largely closed, they fall back on the cultural system where religion and magic allow them to deal with a hostile world. This was succinctly expressed from the pulpit of a Pentecostal church one morning when the pastor, a janitor during the week, stated, "Mrs. Snow is learning a lot of things from books. We didn't have that opportunity, so God helps us and shows us the way." Thus any ability, including the ability to learn, is seen as a divine gift. I was frequently told that an atheist would be unable to cure anyone, irrespective of the number of years in medical school. The gift is more important than the training, therefore, and the individual whose healing ability was gained by training—whether M.D. or neighborhood healer—is only able to cure the simplest kinds of illnesses, those natural problems caused by the entry of cold or impurities into the body. Such individuals are not able to deal with problems resulting from divine punishment or those which result from witchcraft activity.

A more powerful practitioner is the man or woman on whom God has bestowed the gift of healing during a religious experience later in life. It is commonly stated that "the gift" was put into the hands, and curing techniques are prayer and the laying on of hands. The cure seems, like electricity, to flow directly from God through the hands of the healer into the patient. It is obvious that education or training is completely irrelevant in this sort of situation.

> I was called by God! Darlin', He called me one morning and give me my position to visit the sick and to preach and to help save the laws. And I heard this and I didn't believe it! I went on back to sleep, and then he woke me up again. And this mellowtoned voice, you know, waked me again. And I wasn't frightened, it wasn't a frightenin' voice, it was a *glorious* voice! I don't know whether you ever felt the Lord or not. When I felt the Lord, it just woke me out of sleep, just seem like it touched me all over. And called me by my name: "Erma! Go ye therefore!" I said, "Yes, Lord." . . . It was one morning afore day. God called me to a ministry. And to visit the sick and pray for the sick, and pray for the hands that handles them and so forth . . . that night when He called me to a ministry here, it meant somethin' in life to me. I mean it *meant* that I couldn't stop, wherever I go. If I went to Kansas, I went in the hospitals there, too. He gave me somethin' in my hands that I could touch the peoples that they may be healed. [Excerpt from tape recording, February 1971.]

Such individuals are able to deal with all natural illnesses, including those caused by punishment for sin. Since spiritual healing, as it is usually styled, gives the healer additional power, such a practitioner may be sought out when a physician tells a patient that an illness is incurable.

> See, now, if you have cancer, the doctors can't cure cancer! But if they go prayin' for you, and you have lots of faith, the Lord will cure that cancer! The Lord heals a whole lot of people of things the doctors gone give up! While the doctor may give you up, the Lord can come in and deliver you! Put you on your feet! Then whenever the doctor come back and examine you for that particular thing and he don't see it, why, he'll say, "Well, I know it was there, but I don't know what became of you now!" They'll be amazed theirself; they want to know what happened! [Excerpt from tape recording, January 1971.]

Another good example of such magico-religious healing techniques is the belief that bleeding can be stopped by reciting a charm or prayer. One informant who is such a "blood doctor" told me how she stopped the bleeding from a deep cut by reciting a passage from Ezekiel while also applying an ice pack. When I inquired as to whether the ice pack might have had something to do with the cessation of bleeding, I was reprimanded gently with, "God sewed it with *His* needle, darlin'." Such treatment has been in use since the 13th century, and "blood stoppers" or "blood doctors" are found from Florida to the Upper Peninsula of Michigan among blacks, Southern whites, and the Pennsylvania Dutch.[11,12,23,24,35,36,37,70]

To be born with the power of curing is a sign of God's highest approval, a sign that the individual is to have special powers throughout life. It of course implies that the infant must be identifiable at birth as special. The birth order may be important, and special powers have been attributed to a seventh son or seventh daughter for centuries, and today this accounts for special abilities for blacks, Southern whites, Cajun *traiteurs,* and Puerto Rican healers in the Chicago area.[12,26,68,70,111] The child born after a set of twins is powerful, a West African belief found as well in Haitian Voodoo.[65] A variation is that the child who has never seen his father can cure specific ailments. It is said, for example, that such a person can cure a child of oral moniliasis ("thrash" or "thrush") by blowing into the mouth; this belief is found in the United States today among both blacks and whites.[12,39,87,89,112] The birth itself may be seen as unusual—one centuries-old belief still extant is that the child born with a caul ("the veil") has special abilities. This has been reported worldwide since the Chaldeans and is found today in the United States among Louisiana Cajuns, Appalachian whites, and blacks from the Sea Islands of South Carolina to Michigan. It may confer healing ability, "second sight," or just good luck.[12,16,23,59,68,112] In even rarer cases, the infant itself signals before the birth his or her special ability.

> Some people say that I have the gift because I was born behind two twins. But I don't know, I always had the *urge* that I could cure anything! I've always felt like that. But my grandmother knew it *before* I were born. I cried three times in my mother's womb *before* I were born. Then she said, "That's the one. That's the one what's gonna be exactly like me!" I was fortunate, I was born just exactly with the gift.[7]

The person born with power can cure all illnesses: natural or unnatural they often report the ability to "see" or "hear" the diagnosis of illness, usually with spiritual aid.[7] The cure may be sent by air, and, in some cases, the healer may not even have to see the patient; simply thinking about the illness heals it. It is easy to see how such people outrank the ordinary physician in the assessment of curing ability.

CONCLUSIONS

The folk medical system described in these pages reflects a view of the world as a dangerous place. The individual must be constantly on guard against the vagaries of nature, the potential hostility of his fellow man, and possible punishment from God.

It is a world view that teaches that the individual had better look out for himself, that mistrust is wiser than trust, and that safety lies in not calling attention to oneself. It is not, unfortunately, a world view in which the physician is readily seen as the altruistic healer come to dispense medicine to the poor.

The presence of an alternate medical system which at best is different from and at worst is in direct conflict with that of the health professional can only complicate matters. It is not simply a matter of offering health care in place of no health care at all, or even of offering *superior* health care in the hope that such superiority will be patently manifest to the clientele. Deeply ingrained beliefs about how to attain and maintain health affect behavior whether or not the individual ever becomes a patient in a modern health setting. These beliefs about the intricate network linking man to the natural and supernatural world may greatly color the doctor/patient relationship and influence the decision to follow—or not—the doctor's orders.

When a low-income black, Southern white, Puerto Rican American or Mexican-American finally *does* arrive for professional health care, it probably may be assumed that every home remedy the patient knows about has already been tried. It is important that the physician know what the patient has been using to combat the illness—if it is harmless, it might be left in the treatment plan and the physician's own suggestions added. A harmful practice might be more readily eliminated if the physician simply suggests that since it has apparently *not* worked something else should be tried. Laxative use and changes in food habits should be inquired into, and, if possible, the physician should make suggestions that can fit into the patient's belief system. The numbers three and nine might be used to advantage, for example, as they are important in the folklore of every group that has been considered here.

As more and better health care is made available to the poor patient, some of these beliefs will gradually begin to die out. Those intimately tied to religious belief will probably not, however, and others, such as the belief in witchcraft, may continue to be operative as long as the status of the Spanish-speaking or black American is economically and socially marginal. For some time to come, therefore, physicians practicing in the inner city or rural areas will need some knowledge of folk medicine to be able to assess how the diagnosis and subsequent advice is likely to be interpreted by patients.

References

1. Cornely, P. B. 1968. The health status of the Negro today and in the future. *Am. J. Public Health* 58:647-654.

2. Wiener, J. 1969. Mental health highlights. *Am. J. Orthopsychiatry* 39:530-531.

3. Brunswick, A. F.; and Josephson, E. 1972. Adolescent health in Harlem. *Am. J. Public Health* (suppl.), p. 9.

4. United States Bureau of the Census. 1963. *U. S. census of housing, 1960,* vol. 1, part 2. Washington, D.C.: U.S. Government Printing Office.

5. United States Bureau of the Census. 1971. *U. S. census of population, 1970: Number of inhabitants, final report PC (1)–A4 Arizona.* Washington, D.C.: U.S. Government Printing Office.

6. *Tucson (Pima County, Arizona) city directory.* 1970. Dallas: R. L. Polk and Co., Publishers.

7. Snow, L. F. 1973. I was born just exactly with the gift: An interview with a Voodoo practitioner. *J. Am. Folklore* 86:272-281.

8. Dorson, R. M. 1959. *American folklore.* Chicago: University of Chicago Press, p. 198.

9. Eaton, J. 1958. Folk obstetrics and pediatrics meet the M.D.: A case study of social anthropology and medicine. In Jaco, E. G., editor. *Patients, physicians and illness.* New York: The Free Press, pp. 270-271.

10. Hostetler, J. A. 1964. Folk and scientific medicine in Amish society. *Hum. Organ.* 22:269-275.

11. Jones, L. 1949. Practitioners of folk medicine. *Bull. Hist. Med.* 23:480-493.

12. Dorson, R. M. 1964. *Buying the wind.* Chicago: University of Chicago Press, pp. 115, 265.

13. Fisch, S. 1968. Botanicas and spiritualism in a metropolis. *Milbank Mem. Fund Q.* 46:377-388.

14. Harwood, A. 1971. The hot-cold theory of disease: Implications for treatment of Puerto Rican patients. *J.A.M.A.* 216:1153-1158.

15. Dorson, R. M. 1971. Is there a folk in the city? In Paredes, A.; and Stekert, E., editors. *The urban experience and folk tradition.* Austin: University of Texas Press, pp. 26, 41.

16. Hand, W. D., editor. 1961. *Popular beliefs and superstitions from North Carolina,* vol. 6, Durham, N.C.: Duke University Press, pp. 17-52.

17. Hand, W. D., editor. 1964. *Popular beliefs and superstitions from North Carolina,* vol. 7. Durham, N.C.: Duke University Press, pp. 3-97.

18. Kahn, K. 1973. *Hillbilly women.* New York: Doubleday & Co., Inc., pp. 141-142.

19. Osgood, K.; Hochstrasser, D. L.; and Deuschle, K. W. 1966. Lay midwifery in southern Appalachia. *Arch. Environ. Health* 12:759-770.

20. Pearsall, M. 1959. *Little smoky ridge.* University, Ala.: University of Alabama Press, pp. 106, 119-120, 154-157.

21. Pearsall, M. 1962. Some behavioral factors in the control of tuberculosis in a rural county. *Am. Rev. Respir. Dis.* 85:200-210.

22. Secrest, A. J. 1964. Contemporary folk medicine. *N.C. Med. J.* 25:481-482.

23. Stekert, E. Focus for conflict: Southern mountain medical beliefs in Detroit. In Paredes, A.; and Stekert, E., editors. *The urban experience and folk tradition.* Austin: University of Texas Press, pp. 95-127.

24. Wigginton, E., editor. 1972. *The foxfire book.* New York: Doubleday & Co., Inc., pp. 215-232.

25. Wigginton, E. 1973. *Foxfire 2.* New York: Doubleday & Co., Inc., pp. 269, 282-290, 383.

26. Foster, G. M. 1953. Relationships between Spanish and Spanish-American folk medicine. *J. Am. Folklore* 66:201-217.

27. Galvin, J. A.; and Ludwig, A. M. 1961. A case of witchcraft. *J. Nerv. Ment. Dis.* 133:161-168.

28. Madsen, W. 1964. *The Mexican-Americans of South Texas.* New York: Holt, Rinehart & Winston, pp. 70-86.

29. Martinez, C.; and Martin, H. 1966. Folk diseases among urban Mexican-Americans. *J.A.M.A.* 196:161-164.

30. Romano, V. O. 1965. Charismatic medicine, folk healing and folk sainthood. *Am. Anthropologist* 67:1151-1173.

31. Rubel, A. 1960. Concepts of disease in Mexican-American culture. *Am. Anthropologist* 62:795-814.

32. Rubel, A. 1971. *Across the tracks: Mexican-Americans in a Texas city.* Austin: University of Texas Press, p. 168.

33. Samora, J. 1961. Conceptions of health and disease among Spanish-Americans. *Am. Cath. Soc. Rev.* 22:314-323.

34. Murphree, A. H.; and Barrow, M. V. 1970. Physician dependence, self-treatment practices, and folk remedies in a rural area. *South. Med. J.* 63:403-408.

35. Murphree, A. H. 1968. A functional analysis of southern folk beliefs concerning birth. *Am. J. Obstet. Gynecol.* 101:125-134.

36. Randolph, V. 1947. *Ozark superstitions.* New York: Columbia University Press, pp. 92-124, 150.

37. Dorson, R. M. 1956. *Bloodstoppers and bearwalkers.* Cambridge, Mass.: Harvard University Press, p. 150.

38. Withers, C. 1966. The folklore of a small town. In Scott, W. R.; and Volkart, E. H., editors. *Medical care.* New York: John Wiley & Sons, Inc., pp. 233-246.

39. Clark, M. 1970. *Health in the Mexican-American culture,* 2nd ed. Berkeley: University of California Press, pp. 127, 164-172.

40. Turner, C.; and Darity, R. 1973. Fears of genocide among black Americans as related to age, sex, and region. *Am. J. Public Health* 63:1029-1034.

41. Kardiner, A.; and Oversey, L. 1962. *The mark of oppression.* Cleveland: World Publishing Co., pp. 67-68.

42. Rainwater, L. 1970. *Behind ghetto walls: Black family life in a federal slum.* Chicago: Aldine Publishing Co., pp. 69, 222.

43. Davis, A.; and Dollard, J. 1964. *Children of bondage.* New York: Harper & Row, Publishers, Inc., pp. 41-45, 86, 201.

44. Clark, K. B. 1967. *Dark ghetto.* New York: Harper & Row, Publishers, Inc., pp. 63-64.

45. Ladner, J. A. 1972. *Tomorrow's tomorrow: The black woman.* New York: Doubleday & Co., Inc., p. 75.

46. Greier, W.; and Cobbs, P. 1971. *The Jesus bag.* New York: McGraw-Hill Book Co., p. 171.

47. Coles, R. 1971. *Migrants, sharecroppers, mountaineers.* Boston: Little, Brown & Co., pp. 145, 427.

48. Wright, R. 1966. *Black boy.* New York: Harper & Row, Publishers, Inc., pp. 83-85.

49. Mitchell, G. 1973. *I'm somebody important: Young black voices from rural Georgia.* Urbana, Ill.: University of Illinois Press, pp. 31-32, 62.

50. Angelou, M. 1971. *I know why the caged bird sings.* New York: Bantam Books, Inc., pp. 21-27.

51. Oliver, P. 1963. *The meaning of the blues.* New York: Collier Books, pp. 231-257.

52. Guffy, O. 1971. *Ossie: The autobiography of a black woman.* New York: Bantam Books, Inc., pp. 18-31.

53. Haley, A. 1964. *Malcolm X: The autobiography of Malcolm X.* New York: Grove Press, Inc., pp. 1-22.

54. Brooks, G. 1971. *The world of Gwendolyn Brooks.* New York: Harper & Row, Publishers, Inc.

55. Liebow, E. 1967. *Tally's corner.* Boston: Little, Brown & Co., p. 180.

56. Abrahams, R. 1970. *Deep down in the jungle: Negro narrative folklore from the streets of Philadelphia,* 2nd ed. Chicago: Aldine Publishing Co., p. 19.

57. King, S. 1962. *Perceptions of illness and medical practice.* New York: Russell Sage Foundation, pp. 129-130.

58. Whitten, N. 1962. Contemporary patterns of malign occultism among Negroes in North Carolina. *J. Am. Folklore* 75:311-325.

59. Forbes, T. R. 1966. *The midwife and the witch.* Cambridge, Mass.: Yale University Press, pp. vii, 95.

60. Winslow, D. J. 1969. Bishop E. E. Everett and some aspects of occultism and folk religion in Negro Philadelphia. *Keystone Folklore Q.* 14:59-80.

61. Kiev, A. 1962. Psychotherapy in Haitian voodoo. *Am. J. Psychotherapy* 16:469-476.

62. Kiev, A. 1961. Folk psychiatry in Haiti. *J. Nerv. Ment. Dis.* 132:260-265.

63. Courlander, H. 1960. *The drum and the hoe.* Berkeley, Calif.: University of California Press, pp. 9-10, 336-337.

64. Puckett, N. N. 1926. *Folk beliefs of the southern Negro.* Chapel Hill, N.C.: University of North Carolina Press, pp. 167-310.

65. Metraux, A. 1959. *Voodoo in Haiti.* New York: Oxford University Press,

pp. 39-40, 146, 285-286, 305.

66. Simpson, G. 1962. Folk medicine in Trinidad. *J. Am. Folklore* 75:326-340.

67. Kelly, I. 1965. *Folk practices in North Mexico.* Austin, Tex.: University of Texas Press, pp. 7, 22-23.

68. Parsons, E. C. 1923. *Folk-lore of the Sea Islands, South Carolina.* Cambridge, Mass.: American Folk-Lore Society, pp. 192-198.

69. Bourguignon, E. 1959. The persistence of folk belief: Some notes on cannibalism and zombis in Haiti. *J. Am. Folklore* 72:36-47.

70. Black, W. G. 1883. *Folk-medicine: A chapter in the history of culture.* London: Elliot Stock, Publisher, pp. 76-85, 136-138, 162.

71. Rohrer, J. H.; and Edmonson, M. S. 1960. *The eighth generation grows up.* New York: Harper & Row, Publishers, Inc., pp. 150-151.

72. Wintrob, R. 1972. Hexes, roots, snake eggs? M.D. vs. occult. *Medical Opinion* 1:55-61.

73. Snell, J. 1967. Hypnosis in the treatment of the "hexed" patient. *Am. J. Psychiatry* 124:311-316.

74. Tinling, D. 1967. Voodoo, root work, and medicine. *Psychosomatic Med.* 483-490.

75. Hurston, Z. N. 1935. *Mules and men.* Philadelphia: J. B. Lippincott Co., p. 232.

76. Michaelson, M. March 1972. Can a "root doctor" actually put a hex on or is it all a great put-on? *Today's Health,* p. 39.

77. Engel, G. 1971. Sudden and rapid death during psychological stress: Folklore or folk wisdom? *Ann. Intern. Med.* 74:771-782.

78. Clinocopathologic conference: Case presentation (BCH #469861). 1967. *Johns Hopkins Med. J.* 120:186-199.

79. Arner, R. 1971. Of snakes and those who swallow them: Some folk analogues for Hawthorne's "egotism: Or the bosom serpent." *South. Folklore Q.* 35:336-346.

80. Hyatt, H. M. 1970. *Hoodoo, conjuration, witchcraft, rootwork,* vol. 1. Hannibal, Mo.: Western Publishing Co., Inc., pp. 484-493.

81. Claremont, L. 1960. *Legends of incense, herb and oil magic.* Dallas: Dorene Publishing Co., Inc., pp. 70-81.

82. Gamache, H. 1942. *The master book of candle burning or how to burn candles for every purpose.* Highland Falls, N.Y.: Sheldon Publications, pp. 74-96.

83. Kimball, C. P. 1970. A case of pseudocyesis caused by "roots." *Am. J. Obstet. Gynecol.* 107:801-803.

84. Cowles, W.; and Polgar, S. 1963. Health and communication in a Negro census tract. *Soc. Prob.* 10:228-236.

85. Saphir, J.; Gold, A.; Giambrone, J., et al. 1967. Voodoo poisoning in Buffalo, N.Y. *J.A.M.A.* 202:437-438.

86. Hughes, W. T. 1963. Superstitions and home remedies encountered in present-day pediatric practice in the south. *J. Ky. St. Med. Assoc.* 61:25-27.

87. Cornely, P. B.; and Bigman, S. K. 1961. Cultural considerations in changing health attitudes. *Med. Ann. D.C.* 30:191-199.

88. Bauer, W. W. 1969. *Potions, remedies and old wives' tales.* New York: Doubleday & Co., Inc., pp. 112, 175.

89. Webb, J. Y. 1971. Louisiana voodoo and superstitions related to health. *H.S.M.H.A. Health Rep.* 86:291-301.

90. *MacDonald's farmers almanac 1974.* 1973. Binghamton, N.Y.: Atlas Printing Co., unpaginated.

[References 91-107 have been omitted from this chapter.]

108. Strauss, A. L. 1969. Medical organization, medical care and lower income groups. *Soc. Sci. Med.* 3:143-177.

109. Strauss, A. L. 1973. Medical ghettos. In Jaco, E. G., editor. *Patients, physicians and illness,* 2nd ed. New York: Free Press, pp. 371-378.

110. Goshen, C. E. 1970. Characterological deterrents to economic progress in people of Appalachia. *South. Med. J.* 63:1053-1061.

111. Shryock, R. H. 1966. Medical practice in the old south. *Medicine in America.* Baltimore: The Johns Hopkins University Press, pp. 49-70.

112. Dorson, R. M. 1956. *American Negro folktales.* Greenwich, N.Y.: Fawcett Publications, Inc., pp. 62-63.

7

Health and Healing Practices Among Five Ethnic Groups in Miami, Florida

Clarissa S. Scott, Ph.D.

Clarissa S. Scott is Assistant Professor of Social Anthropology in the Department of Psychiatry, University of Miami School of Medicine. She is currently on the faculty of the Cross-Cultural Training Institute, an organization funded by NIMH to train health professionals to provide culturally sensitive and appropriate care to ethnic patients. Prior to this experience, Ms. Scott was field coordinator of the Health Ecology Project, a four-year investigation of health beliefs and practices among Bahamians, Cubans, Haitians, Puerto Ricans, and American blacks in inner-city Miami. Her primary interests include the influence of cultural beliefs about health in relation to therapeutic regimens; and the use of alternative, non-medical therapies such as spiritual healing and herbal teas. She has published articles which examine the relationship between ethnicity and healing practices, health care systems, gynecology, and medical management.

Ethnic groups from the Bahamas, the West Indies, and Central and South America converge in large numbers in Miami, Fla., and most of these peoples retain their vigorous, indigenous health cultures. The term health culture is used here to refer to "all of the phenomena associated with the maintenance of well-being and problems

Source: Scott, C. S. 1974. Health and healing practices among five ethnic groups in Miami, Florida. *Public Health Rep.* 89(6):524-532.

of sickness with which people cope in traditional ways, in their own social networks."[1] Evaluating the importance of this concept, Weidman and Egeland[1] note that use of this definition sets out the sphere of health belief and behavior as "one of the basic social institutions of a society" and raises it to the same order of classification as the economic or political system.

THE HEALTH ECOLOGY PROJECT

Preliminary findings of the Health Ecology Project, which is conducting comparative research on the health cultures of the five largest ethnic groups in the inner-city area of Miami, reveal that many members of these groups are not moving resolutely away from traditional health beliefs and practices toward scientific (orthodox) medicine. Rather, they are holding fast to numerous prescriptive health beliefs and practices, combining the two systems (orthodox and traditional) in different ways and to different extents. The five groups being studied are Bahamian, Cuban, Haitian, Puerto Rican, and southern U.S. black.

The project is concerned with illness of both physical and psychological origin. It has two important goals within the context of this paper. The immediate goal is to describe the beliefs and practices relating to health, illness, and healing among the ethnic groups. The second goal is to determine the patterns of use of both the orthodox and traditional healing systems among these populations. Ultimately, the hope is to develop models for more appropriate health care delivery.

The project is using a combined sociological-anthropological methodology. Our six field assistants, who collect the majority of the data, are women who are members of the ethnic communities in which they work. Each community has one full-time fieldworker, except the Puerto Ricans; in this population, two women share one full-time position. The fieldworkers include a Bahamian who uses the services of faith healers and sorcerers, a Haitian whose aunt was a prominent voodoo priestess, and a Cuban who was a practicing attorney in Havana before coming to Miami as a political refugee. Thus, training of these women has been highly individualized, based on both the weaknesses and strengths of each as well as her background.

As part of the research protocol, each field assistant administers a sociological-type questionnaire to 100 families in her ethnic group, and then she selected 30 to 40 families from the 100 to work with on a long-term basis. The families selected are asked to keep a health care calendar for 4 consecutive weeks, and the mother (or whoever cares for the family members) records any symptoms of illness or conditions which appear in family members and the precise action taken in response. In this way, we are obtaining a description of health problems as seen by members of each ethnic group, rather than according to scientific medical terminology. During the long period of contact, the assistants attempt to gain more understanding (from the mother's point of view) of the etiology of the problems and the family's reasons for engaging in certain health behaviors in place of or before others.

Much of the data in this article are based on the techniques that are closely associated with anthropological fieldwork—participant observation and in-depth interviewing over a long period of contact. The bulk of the fieldwork was done by the indigenous assistants and by me in company with them. We are fortunate in also being able to share field data and observations with five behavioral scientists, each of whom acts as a "culture broker" for his or her respective ethnic group and who, in turn, has a team of indigenous workers under her or him. A culture broker, as defined by Weidman[2] in general terms, is a "bridging" person between two health cultural systems confronting each other. More specifically, within the setting of the University of Miami School of Medicine, this person is a medical anthropologist or behavioral scientist with specialized knowledge of a local ethnic group who works to establish linkages between that ethnic community and in-house psychiatric services.

Although the broad overview and statistical data which derive from the questionnaire and other sociological types of field instruments are invaluable in telling us *what* is happening, it is the months and years of daily contact in the communities which provide us with the insight and data to interpret the *whys* and *hows* of the statistical picture.

For further clues and insight into health beliefs and practices, we use behavioral-science literature pertaining to the ethnic groups' country of origin as well as to counterpart ethnic enclaves in other U.S. cities. This must be done with great circumspection because each local ethnic community is unique in some ways while sharing certain commonalities with their opposite ethnic number elsewhere. Unfortunately, virtually no literature describing Miami's ethnic communities has yet appeared in scientific journals.

PATTERNS OF HEALTH CARE

Each of the five populations (Bahamian, Cuban, Haitian, Puerto Rican, and southern U.S. black) tends to use available health systems somewhat differently. The following descriptions of health care patterns were obtained in a pilot study within the overall health Ecology Project.

Bahamians. Folk remedies and healing techniques thrive among the Bahamians. There is constant traffic between Miami and Nassau (only 30 minutes by plane) and numerous Bahamian herbs and concoctions are brought in by friends and relatives. Many Miami residents retain close relationships with their relatives in the Bahamas by returning for visits, telephoning, and so on. There are several Obeah men in Miami, and at least one commutes between Miami and Nassau to see patients in both countries. Bahamians sometimes "cross the water" (return to Nassau) which automatically removes any effects of Obeah from them. Many use the services of southern black root doctors and spiritual doctors, as well as southern black faith healers.

In anthropology, there is a technical distinction between witchcraft and sorcery. Wittkower and Weidman[3] define witchcraft as involving "innate and extraordinary power which is inherited and is exercised as a psychic act," and sorcery as being "learned" and involving "the use of power which resides in resources outside the individual." Obeah is the term used by Bahamians to indicate sorcery; the southern black term for sorcery is rootwork, and those who practice it are root doctors.

The health calendars of our Bahamian sample indicate chronically poor health. They frequently use the orthodox health system only for crises or in conjunction with folk therapy, for obvious reasons such as language barriers, transportation problems, and "social distance"—the distance between ethnic "consumers" and health "providers" who subscribe to a different set of values. In addition to these manifest reasons there is lack of cultural "fit," which probably also pertains to the four other ethnic groups. This lack occurs when two or more health cultures are dissimilar in crucial ways that make it impossible for a member of one health cultural tradition to accept certain beliefs and behaviors of another. The result is dissatisfaction by both the health care provider and the consumer.

Furthermore, all the ethnic groups in our study attribute certain symptoms and conditions to social and interpersonal conflict and supernatural activity. Their feeling is that "everybody knows" that these are health problems which medical doctors are incapable of curing, therefore it is useless to expect remedial treatment from an orthodox medical practitioner. Among the Bahamians particularly, a person seeks an Obeah man or crosses ethnic lines to use the services of a southern black counterpart, a root doctor. Finally, the intensity with which the Bahamians in the study group practice folk therapy may be related to the closeness of the Bahama Islands to Miami. Visiting and communication can be maintained easily, and there are ample opportunities to replenish home remedies and to reinforce Bahamian health beliefs and practices.

Cubans. Cubans have come to Miami in such numbers that they have been able to duplicate their entire former health care system, including the manufacture of patent medicines previously produced in Cuba. Only a few families in our sample had used a hospital emergency room during the previous 12 months—a significant difference between this group and the others. One possible reason is that a majority of our study families attend 1 of the 23 or more private Cuban clinics, which are operated like a health maintenance organization and are open around-the-clock. Also, according to our data, Cubans seem to be highly motivated toward preventive medicine.

Some Cuban druggists guardedly continue the Latin American practice of selling prescription drugs without prescriptions. Simultaneously, they sell traditional medical plants to their customers. Small churches which include faith healers are found throughout "Little Havana." Large numbers of espiritistas and santeros ply their trade. An espiritista is a practitioner of Espiritismo—a religious cult of European origin based on an ethical code—which is concerned with communication with spirits and the purification of the soul through moral behavior.[4] A santero is a practitioner of Santeria, a syncretic product of African beliefs and Catholic practices. The santero takes no moral position, as does the espiritista; he works solely in behalf of his client. His activity can be beneficial, of no import, or harmful to others.[4]

The Cuban business district has many botanicas; these religious-articles stores sell herbs, lotions, sprays, and other items prescribed by espiritistas and santeros. Home remedies, such as punches, teas, and salves, are used in most of the households in our study.

According to our questionnaire and health calendar data, the Cubans seem to be making full use of the medical resources available to them. Also, at this point in our research, their calendars indicate that they experience less illness than do the other groups. The Cubans who came to Miami on refugee flights are eligible for free care at the Refugee Center, which is staffed by Cuban health personnel; however, the center is being terminated because the Cuban Airlift of refugees has ended. The Refugee Center is not as conveniently located as are other facilities. Families often use it in conjunction with private clinics and physicians, according to their financial status and time available. Cuban health professionals and paraprofessionals have entered the United States orthodox health system in such great numbers that even when a Cuban goes to the public health clinics or to Jackson Memorial Hospital, the university teaching hospital, he is often cared for by Cuban nurses, physicians, technicians, or social workers.

Haitians. The Haitians are relatively recent arrivals to Miami; our pilot study respondents have been here an average of 2.2 years. Medicinal preparations and elements of the traditional Haitian health care system are limited in Miami, possibly because their population is not yet large enough to support more than a handful of indigenous healers.

We know of two priests (*Houngan*) and one priestess (*Mambo*) of the Vodun cult in Miami. Herskovits[5] defines Vodun, or voodoo, as "a complex of African belief and ritual governing in large measure the religious life of the Haitian peasantry. . . ." In addition to these, two men represent themselves as spiritual doctors. They use the title "Reverend" and use the power of the holy spirit to cure. Finally, we have knowledge of five "Readers" or "Diviners" (men and women who read cards and hands) who predict and cure. They cure by means of being possessed by a spirit (*mystère*) which sometimes touches the patient and gives directions for cure.

The Haitian pattern of health care which emerges from our preliminary data is to treat first with herbs and home remedies. When Haitians move into the orthodox system, three characteristics dominate their use of it: (a) frequent use of the emergency room, (b) the names of the same few private physicians and one private clinic appear again and again, and (c) the types of facilities used are more limited in range than those used by the other four groups. These characteristics indicate that the Haitians do not know the territory and thus rely on each other for recommendations of health facilities. Their economic status is generally low on arrival in the United States. The emergency room at Jackson Memorial Hospital (the only public hospital in Miami) does not demand immediate payment, and therefore it accommodates the needs of the Haitians who lack money.

Catholic Haitians tend to be Catholics in name only and still retain their Vodun beliefs. They are likely to attribute certain illnesses to supernatural causes and, in such cases, many seek out those few native healers who are available in Miami. Baptist Haitians who believe that illness is not responding as it should to either home remedies or the orthodox system are likely to pray (either alone or with their pastors) for God's help in effecting a cure. They have been converted to a belief in a protective God who is powerful enough to conquer evil with good and to help the doctors cure both natural and supernatural illnesses.

When home remedies and techniques fail, alone or in conjunction with the orthodox system, Haitians sometimes return to Haiti at great expense to use the services of the types of healers who are not yet available in Miami.

Puerto Ricans. Of the five groups, the Puerto Ricans have consistently shown the least use of the orthodox health care system. Compared with the other ethnic groups, a significantly smaller percentage used the services of an emergency room or saw a private physician during the previous 12 months. Checkups were rare. This infrequent use of the orthodox system and the health calendar data indicating extensive poor health lead us to hypothesize that this group may be isolated from its own healing system as well as from the orthodox system and for the following reasons specific to the Puerto Ricans:

1. Their lifestyle is such that many wives and mothers remain close to their homes and neighborhoods and rarely feel comfortable venturing outside these boundaries. Submissive and protected, the Puerto Rican woman in Miami takes direction from her husband. The father in one of our study families forbids his wife to leave home during the day, even for a brief time to have a cup of coffee with the next-door neighbor.

2. When Puerto Ricans do reach a hospital or clinic, they are usually assigned to Cuban staff because they are Spanish-speaking. There is considerable antagonism between Cubans and Puerto Ricans in Miami, and the Puerto Ricans believe that Cubans treat them in an offensive manner, without respect (*respeto*). To treat and be treated with respect is a fervently held value. Seda, a Puerto Rican anthropologist, has said that a Puerto Rican possesses "an almost fanatical conviction of his self-value."[6] While Puerto Ricans are especially sensitive to lack of respect by Cubans, this may also be a negative factor in their contact with health

care personnel from any ethnic or cultural group.

3. Puerto Ricans in Miami do not have as diverse and powerful a folk healing system as they do in New York or Puerto Rico. Although there are several espiritistas in Miami, our information indicates that their following is not large. Puerto Rican and Cuban espiritistas are similar in that they are both practitioners of Espiritismo. However, Garrison[7] characterizes Puerto Rican Espiritismo as a folk-healing cult, as Sandoval[4] describes the Cuban counterpart.

Cuban santeros and espiritistas are thought to be more powerful than the Puerto Rican healers in Miami. When Puerto Ricans believe that "a thing" (*hechizo*) has been done to them, they often believe that it has been effected by a Cuban santero. They fear that there is little chance of "taking it off" because (a) if they go to a santero, he probably will not work anything against a fellow Cuban and (b) if they go to a Puerto Rican espiritista, he will not have sufficient force for the task. Thus, they often do nothing about this situation.

Puerto Ricans in Miami rely heavily on herbs and folk remedies, which they grow in their yards or purchase from Cuban groceries. Our health calendar data from the pilot study indicate that Puerto Ricans are less likely than any group but the Haitians to take action in response to a symptom. Our preliminary findings concerning Puerto Ricans support those reported by Suchman[8] for New York City: they are most socially isolated as a group and the most deviant from a standard response to illness.

Southern Black. In Miami, the southern blacks show a greater range of variation in their traditional healing system than do either the Haitians or the Puerto Ricans. Home remedies lean more to materials such as vinegar and rubbing alcohol than to herbs. Faith healers appear on radio, television, in revival tents, in churches devoted in large measure to healing, and in "galas" attended by thousands and directed by nationally known figures. There are many spiritualists—those who engage in spiritual healing—who operate out of "temples," "churches," and "candle shops." Root doctors, sometimes known as Hoodoo men or Hoodoo ladies, are numerous. These therapists advertise openly in the local newspaper published by and for blacks; one even focuses attention on his ad with a large drawing of the roots of a plant. If Miami folk therapists are not powerful enough to bring about a cure, southern blacks may travel to Georgia or South Carolina where the reputation of the local root doctors is legendary.

In their use of the orthodox health care system, southern blacks appear to have numerous, but superficial, contacts. Approximately 50 percent of our sample attended public clinics during the previous 12 months and 23 percent were seen in an emergency room. Nevertheless, the health calendars kept by the families and the accompanying interviews indicate that symptoms and conditions continued week after week, month after month, and are rarely cured. A characteristic of the southern blacks' use of the orthodox system is that private physicians and public clinics are often used within the same family, sometimes at the same time.

USE OF MULTIPLE RESOURCES

Preliminary data suggest that the five ethnic groups have unique patterns for using their own health systems as well as the orthodox system. However, the use of multiple resources—that is the use of different therapies or healers serially or concurrently—is one overall feature that cuts across the five individual patterns. Evident in our study are four types of usage within and among systems. In each of these types, the remedies or healers, or both, are used one after the other or at the same time, as illustrated in the following examples:

Healers and therapies in the orthodox system. A Puerto Rican mother takes her baby who has symptoms of a cold to a public health clinic, and the physician prescribes cough medicine and pills. The mother is not satisfied because she believes that an injection is necessary for a cure. She takes the baby to a succession of private physicians until one finally gives the child the anticipated injection.

Among the local black populations, many families report seeing a private physician when they can afford to ("because they treat you better") but relying on emergency room treatment when they lack money for private care.

Healers and therapies within a folk system. A 9-year-old Puerto Rican girl had a red and swollen eye, and within 2 days it began to droop. Her mother diagnosed this condition as pasmo, a condition of paralysis linked to the hot-cold theory of disease. (Harwood[9] recently discussed this theory.) She began treating the condition by placing a compress soaked in camphor oil on the eye and giving the girl azufre powder sprinkled on fried eggs. When this treatment failed, she took her daughter to Puerto Rico to find the proper curative plants.

A second example concerns a young southern black woman with general weakness and skin ulcers. She visited a faith healer who gave her home remedies. No change occurred, and she sought the services of a second faith healer. Results were poor after two visits, and she then saw a third faith healer four times. She now states that she is satisfied with the treatment and is improving.

Healers and therapies in two different folk systems. One way in which an unorthodox healer validates his ability in the eyes of his patients is to tell a patient what is bothering him and what his interpersonal problems and worries are. This presents a problem for sick persons who are members of the still relatively small and tightly clustered Haitian community—they fear that the Haitian healer has heard gossip or rumors about the patient's life and problems rather than having clairvoyant ability. One of our Haitian mothers had just this concern after going to a Haitian reader.

She is now seeing a southern black healer in whom she has greater confidence.

In exception to the general pattern, a Puerto Rican espiritista with whom one of our fieldworkers has established a relationship of trust has had Cuban clients come to her to take off spells after they had consulted (unsuccessfully) Cuban espiritistas to do this job. One of the competing Cuban espiritistas even came to her for a reading, masquerading as a client, to find out how she operates.

Healers and therapies in a folk system and in the orthodox system. In addition to the folk and orthodox systems the following example illustrates the second type of behavior mentioned, the use of healers and therapies within one folk system.

A southern black woman from South Carolina, Mrs. F, drank her Geritol as usual one morning and began to have stomach pains ½ hour later. The pains continued, and 2 days later she suspected that she had been "fixed," probably by a substance added to the Geritol. She took olive oil and a few drops of turpentine on sugar cubes. Later that week she went to see a root woman, who gave her some "bush" to "work it out."

Believing that the poison was "dead," but fearing that it might have rotted away her stomach, Mrs. F went to the emergency room of a local hospital. X-rays showed that although the stomach appeared normal, "something was down there." Mrs. F again went to the root woman who then gave her a new potion to drink, which contained garlic, white onions, and mercury in addition to other ingredients. She next sought the services of a root doctor who operates a candle shop. This healer gave her powder to sprinkle in her house and candles to burn in the corners of the house; he also laid his hands on her and prayed.

After hearing from a neighbor about a sanctified woman in a farming area 20 miles south of Miami, Mrs. F began making two or three trips a week to be treated by her. The woman rubbed Mrs. F's abdomen with a red substance and prayed over her. Mrs. F subsequently reported that she felt much better. However, she continued to keep candles lighted according to her root doctor's advice, to take the garlic and mercury potion from the root woman, and to be massaged by the sanctified woman. Recently, Mrs. F went to Jackson Memorial Hospital for gastrointestinal tests to "find out what is down there." (Interestingly, Mrs. F's contacts with the orthodox system were not for curative purposes, but rather they were to check the effectiveness of the folk therapy.) Our worker first interviewed this woman approximately 8 months after the onset of her symptoms and maintained contact with her until her death a year later.

Another example concerns a Bahamian in our study who complained of abdominal and vaginal pain for months but refused to go for medical care, even if accompanied by the fieldworker and me (to insure prompt, courteous attention). She said it would be useless because her illness was caused by witchcraft, something no medical doctor could cure; the only source of help, she believed, was a root woman who she had seen several times. Ten days before her death—from an organic disease—she did visit the emergency room for treatment of a sore throat, which she defined as amenable to orthodox medical treatment, rather than for treatment of her major illness.

DISCUSSION AND CONCLUSION

Given the wide variety of healers and therapists in Miami, not only practical or obvious factors influence the choice of one over the other. Those factors which motivate an individual to accept or reject the orthodox health system, such as poor transportation or a poor "fit" between specific health beliefs and practices, provide us with only partial answers to the problem of selection. Elements which are specific to each group's health behavior add to but do not complete the picture either. We must search for deeper, more compelling motives which underlie the selection of a particular therapy or healer.

Anthropologists have proposed many hypotheses concerning motivation. Erasmas, quoted by Schwartz,[10] stated that "where medical treatment is quickly effective, dramatic and evident, it will prevail over others." Schwartz suggests that "alternative modes of curing are arranged in hierarchies of resort, with different alternatives being used as the illness progresses without cure, and according to the individual's or group's acculturative process." Another hypothesis, by Bryce-Laporte,[11] is that "when subordinate groups are only partially assimilated within a dominant culture," they tend to be bicultural in their choice of alternative beliefs and behaviors (for example, health beliefs and behaviors). Our data often indicate this simultaneous or serial use of the orthodox and traditional systems.

Still another explanation relates to etiology. Describing his health research among Mestizo communities in Peru and Chile, Simmons[12] proposes that those maladies which are assigned to "the etiological categories of severe emotional upset, ritual uncleanness, and bad air" necessitate treatment with at least one magical therapeutic technique, and a modern therapy with demonstrated value may be used in tandem.

From her study of health beliefs and practices in three Guatemalan cultures, Gonzalez[13] concluded that patients often seek relief from symptoms from a medical doctor while expecting the folk therapist to eliminate the cause of the disease. And, Egeland[14] concluded from her study of the Amish people that in the particularly crucial area of life and death, reliance on only one therapist or therapy or system of health care may be too precarious and more than one are sought.

The findings of our pilot study indicate that the scientific health care system is not sufficiently relevant to multiethnic populations in urban U.S. areas. Many persons in the ethnic groups we are studying are completely alienated from the orthodox system, and others use it serially or in tandem with folk health care systems. While we cannot disregard such considerations as language and transportation problems or the lack of cultural fit between health consumers and providers, we must be able to understand the underlying reasons for the selection of therapies and therapists. Only when we have such understanding will we be able to develop models for more appropriate health care delivery for ethnic minorities.

In the meantime, the following are some very practical measures which health personnel might find immediately helpful in providing better health care to ethnic populations:

1. Gain knowledge of the health beliefs and practices of local ethnic groups.

2. Respect the fact that these beliefs and therapies, although perhaps running counter to the scientific medical system, have survived in these populations for generations and may indeed be measurably effective. To try to change a deeply rooted health belief either by ridicule or by treating it as unscientific may not only fail but may also alienate the patient.

3. Use a treatment plan which shows understanding and respect for the patient's beliefs and which builds on these in a positive way.

Two examples illustrate the preceding points. A physician may assume that a patient from a low-income ethnic group has probably tried home remedies before coming to the orthodox system. "It is important that [he] know what the patient has been using to combat the illness—if it is harmless, it might be left in the treatment plan and the physician's own suggestions added. A harmful practice might be more readily eliminated if the physician simply suggests that since it has *not* seemed to have worked something else might be tried."[15] In developing a new treatment regimen, a physician might well integrate into it the numbers 3 and 9, for example, which are important in the folklore of Puerto Ricans and Mexican-Americans.[15]

The second example concerns the many Puerto Ricans and Haitians who subscribe to the "hot-cold" theory. This is a belief system in which illnesses are classified as hot or cold and food and medicine, also classified this way, are used to restore the natural balance in the body; a "cold" medicine would be used to counteract a "hot" disease. A Puerto Rican woman who is pregnant (considered to be a "hot" condition) will avoid iron supplements and vitamins because they are also considered to be "hot," and it is believed that they will upset the body's natural balance. The wise physician will advise the patient to take her iron supplements and vitamins with fruit juice which, because it is classified as "cool," helps to maintain the proper balance of hot and cold in the body.[9]

Another practical measure to be considered is to be able to recognize when a patient suspects that he has been hexed. He rarely would volunteer this information, but the physician should be aware that symptoms of "feeling bad," loss of weight, depression, lack of appetite, and abdominal complaints indicate possible rootwork. Often, the patient is relieved to share his fears when a concerned physician or nurse asks, Do you think something has been done to you? or Do you think you've been rooted? It is extremely important that the physician assure the patient that his symptoms are not due to rootwork and are curable with orthodox medicine, if this is true. If the physician determines the symptoms are psychogenic, he should instigate palliative, supportive therapy and also accept, without ridicule, tandem treatment by rootworkers whose job it is to neutralize or remove the spell.[16]

Many low-income ethnic groups in urban areas do not receive adequate medical care now, nor will they for many years to come. Obviously, there is no "payoff" for them to give up a health culture which has been supportive for generations in order to subscribe to the beliefs and practices of a system to which they have little access. Therefore, we can expect unorthodox health therapies to continue. Those who would try to make the scientific medical system relevant to these urban ethnic groups must first recognize the existence of other health systems and then be willing to respect and work with them. The trust and rapport thus established can form the base for a greater acceptance of the orthodox system in the future.

References

1. Weidman, H. H.; and Egeland, J. 1973. A behavioral science perspective in the comparative approach to the delivery of health care. *Soc. Sci. Med.* 7:845-860.

2. Weidman, H. H. March 8-11, 1973. *Implications of the culture-broker concept for the delivery of health care.* Paper presented at the annual meeting of the Southern Anthropological Society, Wrightsville Beach, N.C.

3. Wittkower, E. D.; and Weidman, H. H. 1967. Magic, witchcraft and sorcery in relation to mental health and mental disorder. *Top Probl. Psychiatr. Neurol.* 8:169-184.

4. Sandoval, M. 1966. *Yoruba elements in Afro-Cuban Santeria.* Madrid: University of Madrid (doctoral dissertation).

5. Herskovitz, M. J. 1971. *Life in a Haitian valley.* New York: Doubleday & Co., Inc.

6. Lauria, A. 1972. Respeto, relajo and interpersonal relations in Puerto Rico. In Cordasco, F.; and Bucchioni, E., editors. *The Puerto Rican community and its children on the mainland.* Metuchen, N.J.: The Scarecrow Press, Inc., pp. 36-48.

7. Garrison, V. Feb. 24-26, 1972. Espiritismo: Implications for provision of mental health services to Puerto Rican populations. Paper presented at the annual meeting of the Southern Anthropological Society, Columbia, Mo.

8. Suchman, E. A. 1964. Sociomedical variations among ethnic groups. *Am. J. Sociol.* 70:319-331.

9. Harwood, A. 1971. The hot-cold theory of disease. *J.A.M.A.* 216:1153-1158.

10. Schwartz, L. R. 1969. The hierarchy of resort in curative practices: The Admiralty Islands, Melanesia. *J. Health Soc. Behav.* 10:205-209.

11. Bryce-LaPort, R. S. 1970. Crisis, contraculture, and religion among West Indians in the Panama Canal Zone. In Whitten, N., Jr.; and Szwed, J., editors. *Afro-American anthropology.* New York: The Free Press.

12. Simmons, O. G. 1955. Popular and modern medicine in Mestizo

communities of coastal Peru and Chile. *J. Am. Folklore* 68:57-71.

13. Gonzalez, N. S. 1966. Human behavior in cross-cultural perspective: A Guatemalan example. *Hum. Organ.* 25:122-125.

14. Egeland, J. 1967. *Belief and behavior related to illness.* New Haven, Conn.: Yale University (doctoral dissertation).

15. Snow, L. F. 1974. Folk medical beliefs and their implications for care of patients: A review based on studies among black Americans. *Ann. Intern. Med.* 81:82-96.

16. Wintrob, R. M.; Fox, R. A., Jr.; and O'Brien, E. G. Dec. 1971. *Rootwork beliefs and psychiatric disorder among blacks in a northern United States city.* Paper presented at the Symposium on Traditional and Modern Treatments of Indigenous American People, Fifth World Congress of Psychiatry, Mexico City.

8

Relationships Between Spanish and Spanish-American Folk Medicine

George M. Foster, Ph.D.

George M. Foster, Emeritus Professor of Anthropology at the University of California, Berkeley, has had a long career of scholarship and service in the fields of medical anthropology, international health, social and economic change and development, and peasant and rural societies. He has been a consultant to Third World countries, such as India, Afghanistan, Nepal, Malaysia, Indonesia, Zambia, and various Latin American nations, on community development and health education.

Professor Foster's field research efforts extend back to his study of Yuki Indians in 1937. At present, he is engaged in a longitudinal study, begun in 1958, of socio-economic changes over time among peasants. Many of Foster's publications focus on his abiding interest in Latin American and particularly Mexican peasant society. His most recent publication is Long-term Field Research in Social Anthropology, *co-edited with T. Scudder, E. Colson, and R. V. Kemper.*

The transfer of much Spanish culture to the New World, and its subsequent assimilation with native American Indian elements to form modern Hispanic-American culture, was accomplished by both formal and informal mechanisms.

Source: Reproduced by permission of the American Folklore Society from the *Journal of American Folklore* 66:201-217, 1953.

State and Church formulated elaborate plans to guide colonial policy, particularly in government, religion, education, and social and economic forms. But also countless unplanned and informal contacts with the native peoples modified Spanish custom and belief in such areas as folklore, music, home economics, child training, and everyday family living. In medicine—particularly folk medicine—both formal and informal mechanisms have been important in the development of modern Spanish-American beliefs and practices. This paper points out a number of relationships between the two areas and raises several more general questions which are suggested by the data.

Spanish medicine at the time of the conquest of America was based largely on classical Greek and Roman practice, as modified during transmission by way of the Arab World, first through Persia and such famous doctors as Rhazes (c. 850-925) and Avincena (980-1037) and then such Hispano-Arabic physicians as Avenzoar of Sevilla (1073-1161). The systems of these men, as they influenced thought in Spain, are revealed in a series of books reprinted or published for the first time in recent years by the Real Academia Nacional de Medicina, in Madrid. Among the most interesting are Alonso Chirino's *Menor daño de la medicina,* written during the first decade of the sixteenth century but not published at that time; Francisco López de Villalobos' *Sumario de la medicina,* first published in Salamanca in 1498; Avila de Lobera's *Régimen de la salud,* 1551; and Juan Sorapán de Rieros' *Medicina española contenida en proverbios de neustra lengua,* 1616.

The Hippocratian doctrine of the four "humors"—blood, phlegm, black bile ("melancholy"), and yellow bile ("choler")—formed the basis of medical theory. Each humor had its "complexion": blood, hot and wet; phlegm, cold and wet; black bile, cold and dry; and yellow bile, hot and dry. As the three most important organs of the body—the heart, brain and liver—were thought to be respectively dry and hot, wet and cold, and hot and wet, the normal health body had an excess of heat and moisture. But this balance varied with individuals; hence the preponderantly hot, humid, cold, or dry complexion of any individual. Natural history classification was rooted in the concept that people, and even illnesses, medicines, foods, and most natural objects, had complexions. Thus, medical practice consisted largely in understanding the natural complexion of the patient, in determining the complexion of the illness or its cause, and in restoring the fundamental harmony which had been disturbed. This was accomplished by such devices as diet, internal medicines, purging, vomiting, bleeding, and cupping. For example, broth from chick peas, thought to be hot and wet, would be prescribed for epilepsy, thought to be caused by an excess of black bile, which was cold and dry. Barley, cold and dry, would be recommended for fever, caused by the hot and wet qualities of blood. An enormous pharmacopoeia, principally herbal but also including animal and inorganic substances, was drawn upon to treat illness.

Folk medicine existed side by side with formal medicine and undoubtedly overlapped it as many points. Though these beliefs and practices are not well described for that time, a fair idea of them may be deduced by subtracting the formal medicine of the sixteenth century from the folk medicine of today and by making allowance for New World influences. Sixteenth-century Spanish folk medicine represented the accretions of many centuries and many waves of invaders. It is difficult and perhaps impossible to separate these sources, but some of the more important can be named. The significance of fire and water, particularly in northwest Spain, testifies to the pre-Christian beliefs of the Celts and other early European populations. Pre-Arab Mediterranean traces appear in the continued use of votive offerings, which can be traced back to Greek and Roman temples. The universal hagiolotry and the use of religious prayers and invocations in curing practice represent Christian contributions. Moorish folk belief itself, quite apart from the classic system, has been an important source of Spanish folk medicine. Belief in the evil eye may be due to Arab contract, or it may represent an earlier Mediterranean influence.

New World Indian medicine varied from place to place, but certain general characteristics prevailed. Soul loss occasioned by fright, possession by evil spirits, and injury through witchcraft, often in the form of object intrusion, were believed to be basic causes of sickness. Probably emotional experiences which today are so commonly considered as causes of illness—shame, fear, disillusion, anger, envy, longing—have in considerable part persisted from pre-Conquest days. The shaman and medicineman used many curing techniques: herbal remedies, emetics, enemas, sucking, massage, calling upon spirits, and the like. Their understanding of the causes and cures of illness was probably not greatly inferior to that of Spanish physicians.

THE CONTACT SITUATION

Physicians were among the earliest travelers to the New World. They, and the geographier-natural historians of the time, were impressed by the different forms of flora and fauna of the newly discovered continents and classified each new discovery according to the system they knew and understood. By the end of the sixteenth century a fair part of the indigenous pharmacopoeia had been recognized and the qualities of each item described according to prevailing notions of hot, cold, wet, and dry. A chair of medicine was established at the University of Mexico in 1580, though curing had been informally taught before that at the Colegio de Santa Cruz in Tlaltelolco. The first university medical training in Peru was at the University of San Marcos in 1638. Hippocrates, Galen, Avicena, and other authorities of the Classic and Arabic periods were the basic sources of this teaching. Few changes in medical concepts and practices were apparent until the end of the eighteenth century; the isolation of Spain and the Spanish colonies from European thought and scientific progress preserved the classical theories for a century or more after they were superseded in northern Europe.

The mechanisms whereby university medical beliefs and practices filtered down to the folk level can only be surmised. In view of the relative lack of doctors, priests and other educated individuals were called upon to help the sick to a degree probably not characteristic of Spain. The same shortage of doctors stimulated the publication of guides to home curing; one of the most interesting dates from 1771 and is reproduced by Valdizán and Maldonado.[2] Among Indians and mestizos the obvious material superiority and power of the Spaniards probably placed a premium on the learning of Spanish curing practices. (The opposite also was true; the Spaniards believed the native *cuanderos* to be repositories of occult knowledge and curing magic.)

Whatever the mechanisms, a high proportion of the best medical practice of Spain at the time of the Conquest became incorporated into the folk practices of America. Simultaneously, and through informal channels, much of the contemporaneous folk medicine of the mother country was transferred to the New World. The result is a well-developed and flourishing body of folk belief about the nature of health, causes of illness, and curing techniques, made up of native American, Spanish folk, and classical medical elements.

CLASSICAL CONCEPTS IN
SPANISH-AMERICAN FOLK MEDICINE*

Spanish-American folk medicine is by no means identical in all countries, but nonetheless there is surprising homogeneity from Mexico to Chile. The same basic attitudes toward health and sickness occur, the same underlying causes of disease are believed in, a high proportion of "folk" illnesses have the same names, and much the same curing techniques and medicaments are found in all places. Much of this homogeneity stems from the nearly universal belief in the Hippocratian concept of hot and cold qualities inherent in nature and the less pronounced concept of humors associated with illness. Most herb remedies and foods are believed to be characterized by one of these two qualities, though in many places a third, "temperate," is found. Curiously, the corresponding classical concept of wet and dry seems to have entirely disappeared, as has the formal grading of degrees of intensity (from 1 to 4) of each quality. Illnesses, with perhaps less frequency, are thought to be hot or cold or to stem from hot or cold causes. The Hippocratian "principles of opposites" commonly but not always prevails in curing—for a cold illness, a hot remedy, and vice versa. Not infrequently a specific illness may have either a hot or a cold cause, and treatment will therefore vary.

In Chimbote, Peru, diarrhea may be either hot or cold in nature, depending on its cause. It is generally believed that when the body is warm, cold in the form of air, water, or food, is dangerous. One therefore avoids such things as going into the cold precipitously, bathing except under favorable circumstances, drinking iced

---

*Most of the data from the rest of this chapter is found in less detail in the two previous chapters. It is presented in detail to familiarize the reader with wide varieties of hot/cold beliefs and practices.

beverages, and eating cold foods when the stomach is hot.[3] Maintenance of health depends on a judicious combination of foods. In Lima, for example, it is popularly believed that water should not be drunk with pork because both being cold, might overtax the stomach's strength, though either can be safely taken alone. Wine, which is hot, tempers the pork and is therefore the preferred beverage with this meat. An informant from Chimbote described malaria, colds, pneumonia, other bronchial ailments, and warts as cold; he listed colic, smallpox, measles, typhoid, diarrhea, meningitis, and kidney and liver complaints as hot.

The classifications vary from country to country and place to place, and general agreement among all people even in a single town is not the rule. Nevertheless, certain general rules seem to prevail; the most marked is that (following classical theory which believed a preponderance of heat to be the normal state of the healthy body and undue cold as the condition most frequently needing remedy) a majority of medicinal herbs are classified as hot. Actually, in most of America there is a surprisingly high correspondence between the herb classification of classical authorities and those popularly ascribed today. This correspondence is somewhat less marked with respect to foods. Many people who do not classify illnesses and their causes as hot or cold nevertheless reveal the underlying presence of classical concepts in their beliefs that foods should be combined according to their hot or cold qualities or that sudden heat or cold may cause one to fall ill.

Formal concepts of humors are much less marked than those of hot and cold, though the term is often used in popular speech in discussing illness. Available data suggest that ideas are most strongly developed in Colombia. In that country "bad" humors are often associated with the blood and are believed transmissible through sexual intercourse, inhaling the breath of infected persons, or through bodily contact. Some believe that only sick people have humors, while others say that everyone has humors, either good or bad. Bad breath, fetid body oders, boils, and similar skin eruptions are among nature's ways of expelling humors from the body. Humors of adults are thought to be stronger than those of children, and children should therefore sleep apart from their parents to avoid possible sickness. Men with naturally strong humors are dangerous to wives with weak humors; through close association, particularly through sexual intercourse, such women may become thin and emaciated. Persons with strong humors are said to be especially susceptible to smallpox.

In Ecuador *mal humor*, bad humor, is reflected in boils or susceptibility to illness. In El Salvador, a man who comes in from the street perspiring or after recent sexual contact is thought to have a "strong humor." If any children are in the room he must pick them up to neutralize his humor and to prevent their falling ill of *pujo*, which in boys manifests itself in swollen testicles. In Mexico persons of irregular sex life are said to have strong humors, and their presence is thought to affect adversely sufferers from measles. Belief in humors undoubtedly was at one time much more strongly developed in Colonial America than today. A Peruvian home-remedy book of the late eighteenth century points out, for example, that caraway seeds, being hot, and dry to the third degree, drive out "cold humors," while lemon juice is good for deafness arising from them.[4]

Several other classical Spanish beliefs with American counterparts follow: Lobera[5] cautions against wearing catskin clothing or smelling catskins. Today in Colombia, Peru and doubtless other countries, cat hair is believed to cause asthma. There is also some belief in Spain that cat hair is dangerous and that sleeping in contact with cats causes scrofula.

Both Sorapán[6] and Lobera[7] warn against the danger of bad smells; Lobera specifies that latrines should for this reason be located a considerable distance from the house. Particularly in Colombia bad smells are today believed to be an important source of danger. Much resistance to sanitation programs which require the building of latrines stems from the belief that the smells which emanate produce typhoid and to a lesser extent smallpox, pneumonia, bronchitis, tumors, and other ills.

The need to maintain a clean stomach or to "clean" it, if necessary, with purges, a basic classic Spanish doctrine, is generally reflected in Spanish America today in the belief that one must periodically take a strong purge to clean out the intestinal tract. Particularly in Peru the belief in a "dirty" stomach as a cause of illness is well defined. Patent medicines known as *estomacales* (sold in all drug stores) and various combinations of herbs are taken to clean the stomach.

For wounds a classical treatment, still found in the folk medicine of Spain, is the use of spider webs to congeal blood. This appears to be general in Spanish America today; my data mention it for Chile, Peru, Ecuador, Venezuela, and Guatemala.

Cupping, known in Spanish as *la ventosa,* was basic to classical authors and was praised by Galen. *La ventosa* is widely used in Spain today for pneumonia, bruises, swelling, acute pains of all types, "cold," *paletilla* (the ailment, discussed later, caused by the displacement of organs), and other disorders. Its use in Spanish America is general for pneumonia, general pains, "air," and other ills.

Chirino[8] describes a cure for sties—rub the lids with flies. One of the most common sty cures in Spain today, it also occurs in the New World, at least in Chile and Peru.

A poultice made by opening a freshly killed small animal or bird and applying the bloody interior to the body, to treat fever or a variety of other ailments, is described by Sorapán[9] and of course goes back to classical antiquity. A poultice utilizing toads, doves, pigeons, frogs, sheep, chickens, and other living creatures is one of the most widely used folk cures in Spain today for fever, headache, wounds, meningitis, snake bite, madness, throat upsets, and other disorders. Today in Guatemala fever is treated with a poultice made of a chicken, vulture, or dog. In Colombia a pigeon is used for an illness called *mal de madre* and to ease the suffering of a dying person. In Peru a frog or a toad is used for erysipelas and for swellings and inflammations in general, and a pigeon or a vulture for meningitis. In El Salvador the meat from a freshly killed black cock is placed on the sole of the feet, under the knees, on the inner side of the armpits, and on the nape of the neck to draw out fever.

The Spaniards were intensely interested in finding new supplies of bezoar, a calcarious concretion from the stomach of certain ruminants, which they believed to be efficacious against poisonous bites and poisons in general. However, despite the world-wide fame early acquired by the bezoar of the vicuña, American deer, guanaco, and llama, surprisingly little trace of this belief remains. In Tzintzuntzan, Mexico, the *piedra de la vaca* is used against epilepsy. In Chile contact with the stone from a guanaco is thought to cure pains from *aire* and to alleviate melancholy and intestinal upsets.

The ancient belief in the therapeutic virtues of unicorn horn was twice noted. In Chile powders popularly thought to be scraping from a unicorn horn are used to treat dysentery. In Venezuela the corruption *oilcornio* is applied to archeological beads which are found in the western part of the country and are worn as a bracelet amulet against the evil eye. To be effective they must be excavated on Maundy Thursday.

Probably about half the herbs recommended by Spanish authorities of five hundred years ago are cultivated and used in Spanish America today. If frequency of use of individual herbs rather than mere presence in the pharmacopoeia is the gauge, then classical Spanish herb lore predominates today in Spanish America. As in Spain, garlic is possibly the single most important herb and figures in innumerable cures. Appearing in a wide variety of cures are other Old World herbs; among the "hot" are balm gentle (*toronjil*), alone (*sábila*), rue (*ruda*), rosemary (*romero*), oregano, pennyroyal (*poleo*), sweet marjoram (*mejorana*), mallow (*malva*), dill (*eneldo*), lavendar (*alhucema*), and artemisa (*altamisa*); among the "cold" are plantain (*llantén*), sorrel (*acedera*), and verbena. In view of the many and efficacious native American herbs, this predominance of the Spanish testifies to the force of the impact of Spanish medicine in the New World.

NONCLASSICAL RELATIONSHIPS

Many other generic relationships fall more nearly in the field of popular medicine, and the transfer of these practices and beliefs from mother to daughter countries must have been largely through informal channels. These relationships will be considered in four categories: (1) ideas of causation based on magical, supernatural or physiologically untrue, and emotional concepts; (2) specific curing techniques applicable to many different treatments; (3) specific illnesses, and (4) their special cures.

Belief in the evil eye (ojo, mal de ojo) is the most widespread of illnesses identified in terms of magical causation. Throughout Spain and Spanish America it is thought that certain individuals, sometimes voluntarily but more often involuntarily, can injure others, especially children, by looking at them. Admiring a child is particularly apt to subject him to the "eye." Unintentional eyeing can be guarded against by the cautious admirer adding "God bless you," or some such phrase, and slapping or touching the child.

The child who is thought to suffer from the evil eye normally shows rather general symptoms, such as fever, vomiting, diarrhea, crying, and loss of appetite and weight. In South America it is also often imagined that one eye becomes smaller than the other. In Andalucia and at least in Chile and Peru one explanation of what happens is that the force of the "eyeing" breaks the gall of the victim (*se revienta la hiel*).

Because the evil eye is magically induced, magical amulets help protect one. In Spain they include coral, jet (*azabache*), a small carved fist, usually of jet, with the thumb protruding between the index and middle fingers (*higa*), small booklets with a part of the books of St. John and the other apostles (*evangelios*), scapularies, a silver-mounted seed (*castaña de Indias*), and tiny bags of salt or garlic around the neck or wrist. In Spanish America amulets include coral, *evangelios*, seeds (e.g., the Mexican "deer's eye"), occasionally jet, and a bit of red color, usually in the form of a ribbon. The *higa,* the single most important charm in Spain, is common in Venezuela, but I have little information on its modern use in other Spanish-American countries. Valdizan and Maldonado quote a French source of 1732 to the effect that ladies in Lima wore an *higa* as a protective amulet,[10] and John Rowe tells me he has seen a few in Peru in recent years. It is interesting that the *higa* is ubiquitous in Brazil today.

The most widespread curing and divanatory technique in Spain for the evil eye is to drop olive oil in water. The exact method varies from place to place, but the principle is the same. The diviner places the middle finger of his or her right hand in the oil reservoir of a small lamp and allows one or more drops to fall in a glass of water. If the drops remain in the water, or if they break into smaller but distinct drops, the usual interpretation is either that the child is not suffering from the evil eye or that he is suffering but can be cured. If the oil disappears, sinks, or forms a cap over the water the child is believed to be afflicted, perhaps fatally so. Sometimes it is thought that the act of dropping the oil is therapeutic in itself. More often a curing ceremony follows. In southcentral Spain this most commonly takes the form of weighing the child in balance with an equal amount of *torvisco* (*Daphne Gnidium L.*). Then the plant is thrown on the roof, and as it dries the child recovers.

Oil divination appears to be rare in Spanish America. It is, however, briefly mentioned by Valdizán and Maldonado as occurring in the province of Tarma, department of Junín, Peru, and by Rosemberg in Argentina.[11] A second correspondence in divining occurs between Galicia and Ecuador. In the former region the distance between the outstretched hands is measured with a string, and the distance compared with that from the feet to the head. If the measures are unequal it is proof that the child suffers from the evil eye. In Esmeraldas, Ecuador, a red ribbon is used to measure the circumference of the child's thorax. It is then doubled and redoubled and used to touch several points on the child's body, while prayers are said. Always holding the measure on the ribbon, the diviner again measures the thorax, and if the distance appears to be unequal, the child is thought to have been "eyed."

Still another parallel between Spain and Spanish America is the tendency to cure the evil eye on Tuesdays and Fridays—days in both areas which are generally recognized as having superior virtues for many types of cures. The most completely described form of divining and curing the evil eye in America involves the use of a chicken egg. In Mexico, Guatemala, and Peru the egg is rubbed over the patient's nude body and then broken open for inspection. Any spots on the yolk are interpreted as "eyes," which proves the diagnosis correct. Like the Spanish divination, this is often thought to have therapeutic value—the egg draws out the "eye" from the patient. In Peru the egg is usually broken in water and beaten with the child's right hand and left foot, and often with his left hand and right foot as well, in the form of a cross. Next a cross is smeared on the victim's forehead with the mixture to complete the cure. In El Salvador the child is placed in a hammock, with a raw egg on a plate underneath. The egg is subsequently opened; if it appears "cooked" it is because the heat of the presumed evil eye has been drawn from the child, who is thereby cured. In Colombia a cure is accomplished by herbs taken internally or applied externally, accompanied by prayers. In addition, a dove egg may be broken on the back of the child's head; thereby the guilty person's offending eye loses its sight. But as the guilty person did not "eye" intentionally this is thought to be unsportsmanlike.

The origin of the egg cure in the New World is one of the mysteries of folk medicine. The only Spanish cure in any way related has to do with defective vision, for which one passes a freshly laid, warm egg across the eyes *para limpiar la vista* ("to clean one's sight"). This practice, common in El Salvador, Colombia, Ecuador, Peru, and Chile, is probably known in Mexico and Guatemala too. Because chicken eggs were absent in the New World before the Conquest, the egg cure is almost certainly Old World. Linguistic confusion is perhaps the explanation. The commonest term for evil eye in America, *mal de ojo*, means "something wrong with the eye." Because in Spain a warm egg rub is and was used for many forms of *mal de ojo*, in the clinical sense, the magical *mal de ojo* perhaps came to be cured in the same way in the New World.

"*Air*" or "*bad air*" (*aire* or *mal aire*) is perhaps the most frequent Spanish-American explanation for illness. Though mentioned in almost all descriptions of illness, its exact nature has an elusive quality which makes discussion difficult. Some forms of *aire* must certainly be pre-Conquest in origin, but other aspects of modern belief appear to stem from the Hippocratian concept of hot and cold. Thus, the most frequent explanation of the cause of the affliction is that the patient went from a closed room into fresh air or was struck by a current of air, a breeze, or wind. Other explanations, as in Mexico, are that *aire* is an evil spirit which takes possession of a person, or as in Guatemala, it is something useful in witchcraft. Though almost any illness may be ascribed to *aire,* various forms of paralysis, particularly of the face, seem to be the most common.

Air as a cause of illness has the same elusive quality in Spain as in the New World. Unfortunately, except for Galicia, it is less completely described than in America. Facial paralysis is one of the most common manifestations, but many other ailments are also ascribed to air. In Galicia air is particularly thought of as emanations from animals, individuals, corpses, occasionally places, and even heavenly bodies. Especially feared is a *gata parida* (cat which has just given birth) or a menstruating or pregnant woman who steps over a child. A menstruating woman also is dangerous to children in some, and perhaps all, Spanish-American countries. In El Salvador she should not pick up a child lest "the gall break" (*se revienta la hiel*); in Peru she may cause an umbilical hernia (*pujo*).

In many Hispanic-American countries, a coldness or illness-causing quality is believed to emanate from a corpse; therefore all persons who have contact with it must bathe or otherwise purify themselves. Children are particularly susceptible to this danger. In Guatemala, the emanation and resulting illness are called *hijillo* (from Spanish *hielo*, "ice"?), in Puerto Rico *frio de muerto* ("cold of the dead"), in Colombia *hielo de muerto* ("ice of the dead"), and in Peru *mano de la muerte,* ("the hand of death"), or *viento de la muerte* ("wind of death").

The Spanish form of this belief, *aire de los muertos* ("air of the dead"), is found particularly in Galicia, where as in the New World children are thought to be especially susceptible. As the dead person is said to have taken the life of the living to the tomb, the standard cure is to go to the graveyard to pray and urge the corpse to return life to the afflicted child. The wide distribution of this belief in the New World, the use of Spanish names to identify it, and the basic similarity with the Galician form suggest that whatever pre-Conquest ideas about the dead existed, the modern beliefs follow a Spanish pattern.

Fear of the moon is in Spain the most widely held belief in supernatural (as contrasted to magical) threats to health. Belief in the moon's power to influence men's lives and to affect the growth of plants and animals goes back to classical antiquity. Today in Spain such beliefs are still associated with agriculture, woodcutting, meat-curing, treatment of wounds, and children's health. The cold rays of moonlight are thought to exercise noxious effects on clothing or bandages left out at night. Such bandages, if not warmed by ironing, will cause wounds to fester. Swaddling clothes of children must likewise be ironed and sometimes washed as well, if the cold of the moon is not to enter the child. Moonlight may also directly enter a child. In western Spain, children sometimes wear metal moon amulets to prevent their being *alunado* ("possessed by the moon").

In the New World these exact beliefs appear not to exist, though the moon is felt to play an important part in agricultural practices and a minor part in curing. In many places, for example, cures for intestinal worms are given during the waning moon because the worms are believed to be head-up then, and the remedies more easily enter their mouths and kill them. In Colombia it is believed that hernia worsens when the moon is *brava* (apparently meaningful) and that any change of phase of the moon aggravates *erysipelas.* A parallel in Conil de la Frontera, Cadiz, is that any sore that festers during a waxing moon is called *irisipela.*

In Colombia and Ecuador the rainbow is to some extent the functional equivalent of the moon in Spain. In Colombia it is believed that the coldness inherent in the rainbow is transmitted to a child's clothing inadvertently left outside to dry and that the child will be chilled if the clothing is not ironed before being worn. Mange is the illness most frequently resulting from the rainbow's chill. In Ecuador clothing exposed to the rainbow must be disinfected by passing it over a fire. . . .

In parts of both Spain and America it is believed that illness results when real or imaginary parts of the body move from their normal positions. Restoration of the organ effects the cure. In Galicia the *espiñela* and *paletilla,* thought to be bones located respectively in the pit of the stomach and between the shoulder blades, may "fall" as a result of violent exercise or a coughing fit. The stomach also may "fall," producing a condition known as *calleiro.*

These conditions are diagnosed by palpation, by measuring the length of the patient's arms or legs, or by measuring with a string the distance from the pit of the stomach to the backbone around both sides. If the measures are unequal the suspected cause is verified. Cures are based on the principle of equalizing the measures; this is accomplished by massage and by pulling fingers, arms, and legs. Cupping and the application of poultices also are common. Fallen stomach, most common among children, is cured by holding the child upside down by its ankles and slapping the soles of its feet.

New World equivalents are "fallen *paletilla*" (*caída de la paletilla,* northern Argentina), "fallen fontanelle" (*caída de la mollera,* Mexico, Guatemala, El Salvador), "stretched veins" (*Estiramiento de las venas,* Guatemala), and a condition suggesting fallen stomach (*descuajamiento,* Colombia). These are principally childhood afflictions usually resulting from a fall or a blow. Fallen *paletilla* is diagnosed, as in Spain, by comparing the length of arms and legs. It is cured by suction (mouth, cupping), with poultices, or—in extreme cases—by placing the child in the still-warm stomach of a recently slaughtered beef. The last-named is an old Spanish cure, though it is not mentioned among common *paletilla* cures. For fallen fontanelle the patient is held upside down by the ankles, the soles are slapped, the hard palate is pressed with the thumb, and the fontanelle is sucked. For stretched veins the patient is held upside down by the ankles and the body is massaged to force the veins toward the stomach. *Descuajamiento,* diagnosed by palpation and by unequal length of the legs, is cured by holding the child by its ankles and massaging its body from bottom to top to force the stomach into place.

Strong emotional experiences that produce physiological results characterize Hispanic America much more than Spain. Fright, commonly cited in Spain as a cause of minor disturbances such as pain in the region of the appendix, fits, fainting, and boils, is particularly thought to disturb menstruation; it is not associated with soul loss. Sibling jealousy is given, but only occasionally, as the explanation of certain childhood disorders. In Navarra it is treated by surreptitiously placing a hair of the younger child in the chocolate of the older. In the New World the most important emotional experiences include fright (*susto, espanto,* in all countries, usually associated with soul loss), anger (e.g., *colerina* in Peru), shame or embarrassment (e.g., *pispelo* in El Salvador, *chucaque* in Peru), disillusion (e.g., *tiricia* in Peru), imagined rejection (in the form of sibling jealousy, e.g., *sipe* in Mexico, *peche* in El Salvador, *caisa* in Peru), desire (e.g., unsatisfied food cravings of children causing the gall to break—*se revienta la hiel*— in Chile), or sadness (e.g., *pensión* in Chile).

Several general curing techniques, used for various illnesses, are common to Spain and the New World. Some of the more important follow.

Nine-day treatment [is a general curing technique.] In Spain, treatments for disease of any gravity are usually repeated several times, usually nine times, for nine has great virtue through association with church ritual. In most of the New World many treatments are repeated nine times, or the number nine enters the formula in some other way. In Colombia, for example, to purify the blood nine piles of sarsaparilla are made. The sufferer makes a tea from each pile of succeeding days, drinks it, and keeps the herbs. Then he starts over, this time with the ninth pile, and works back through the first. . . .

In Spain many remedies are left *al sereno,* in the open air at night to gather the night's cold. This is almost equally true of the New World. In Chile carrot juice *al sereno* is used to treat jaundice, and squash seeds *al sereno* for intestinal worms. In Colombia herbs to treat conjunctivitis are left *al sereno,* as is the key rubbed over a sty in Peru. In Mexico remedies for both eyes and rheumatism are likewise *serendao.*

En Ayunas, before breakfast, is perhaps when a majority of Spanish remedies are taken. This practice, although apparently less common in the New World, is nonetheless frequent.

Silence is required in many Spanish curing acts, as is occasionally the case in the New World. *Crossroads,* particularly in Galicia, have special curative virtues; curing acts are often performed there. For example, *aire* may be cured by tying a child's feet together and taking him to a crossroads where the first passerby silently cuts the rope. In Cherán, Michoacan, Mexico, children suffering from the evil eye are taken to a crossroads by their mother, who asks all passersby to "clean" the child by ceremonially passing one of their garments over his body.

Black chicken blood or flesh figures commonly in Spanish witchcraft and curing. In Mexico the blood of a black chicken is drunk to drive out spirits due to witchcraft. In El Salvador for certain types of fever the meat poultice must come from a black fowl. In Chile sore eyes are treated with poultices made of the crests of black cocks.

Snakes, in Spain, are used for innumerable ills. The grease from fried snakes benefits almost any pain, the skins are useful for headache and toothache, and the heads are placed on snake bites. In Spanish America the snake is generally thought to be endowed with therapeutic virtues. In Mitla, Mexico, a snakeskin around the waist is thought good for rheumatism. In Ecuador snake grease is applied to boils. In Peru snake grease is used for almost any ailment.

Drying scorpions or lizards [is another general curing technique.] In Spain for some illnesses, and particularly for a lachrymal condition of the eyes known as *rijas,* a lizard, or less often a scorpion, is carried in a metal tube by the sufferer, who recovers as the animal dies and dries. The same treatment occasionally crops up in the New World. In Peru a child suffering from *irijua,* a form of sibling jealousy, wears around his neck a reed containing a scorpion, and as the insect dries the jealousy disappears. In Chile a live lizard encased in a red bag is placed over a hernia, which is cured when the lizard is dead.

Coins, which figure in a wide variety of Spanish cures, are occasionally used in the New World; in Tzintzuntzan, Mexico, they are associated with cures for diarrhea, and in Peru for nosebleed.

Cockroach broth, in Spain, is the classic treatment for a throat condition known as anginas. In Peru it is used for colic, cardiac conditions, pneumonia, and epilepsy.

Burro milk, in Galicia, is drunk for colds and jaundice; in Chile, for respiratory ailments.

Potatoes, especially in Chile and Peru, are used for such diverse things as warts, diarrhea, headache, liver conditions, erysipelas, and rheumatism. This New World medication has diffused to Spain, though its use there is less frequent. In Navarra, as in Chile, potatoes in the pocket are an amulet against rheumatism. Potato *parches,* discs of potato on the temples, are used to cure headache, especially in Galicia, as in Chile. In Spain potatoes are also used for chilblains and other illnesses.

Human and animal waste and milk [are used as cures.] The widespread use in Spain and America of human urine, human milk, and human and animal excrement doubtless represents parallel development rather than diffusion. As these remedies are worldwide they have probably been invented independently innumerable times. Human milk is used for earache and eye troubles in Spain and the New World. Snails, particularly snail mucus, are reported in Spain for the eyes, for warts, and for erysipelas; in Colombia and Peru for whooping cough, and in Chile for hernia and asthma. The lack of direct correspondence in illnesses suggests the independent invention of the use.

Hagiolotry [is] the worship of the patron saints of various illnesses and parts of the body, and of the Virgin and local images who are thought to have special powers, [and] is very important in many Spanish curing practices. Saints particularly worshiped include San Blas (throat), Santa Agueda (breasts), Santa Apolonia (teeth), Santa Lucía (eyes), San Roque (plague), San Ramón Nonato (birth), San Pantaleón, San Cosme and San Damián (physicians), and San Benito. The day of San Juan (June 24) is thought to be potent; herbs gathered this day are especially powerful, and treatments involving application of water are best done at this time. A common treatment for mange, for example, is to roll nude in the early morning dew.

Hagiolotry is poorly reported in the New World. In Chile, San Blas, Santa Lucía, and Santa Apolonia are appealed to, and it is believed that plants collected on the day of San Juan have special medicinal properties. In Peru among the saints appealed to are Santa Lucía, Santa Apolonia, and San Ramón Nonato. Medals of San Benito are common in both countries. Equally good data from the other Hispanic-American countries would probably show a similar picture. Nevertheless, hagiolotry seems much less a part of the general curing pattern in the New World than in Spain. One exception, however, has to do with votive offerings, *ex votos,* a practice apparently more widespread today in Hispanic America than in the mother country.

Prayers and spells, though commonly used on both sides of the Atlantic, are relatively more important in Spain, according to my impression. Certainly the number of recorded cases in Spain far exceeds that of the New World; the many treatments in which nothing else is done testifies to their greater importance in Spain. Nevertheless, many American prayers and spells are clearly of Spanish origin.

Folk cures in both Spain and Hispanic America play important roles. In Spain the most important class of curer is that of the *saludador,* who has a special gift, a grace (*gracia*), which characterizes individuals around whose birth special circumstances prevailed: (1) those who cried while yet unborn, provided the mother told no one; (2) those born on certain days, especially Monday, Thursday, Good Friday, and occasionally Christmas; (3) the seventh consecutive son, and less often the fifth or sixth (occasionally daughter), by the same mother. Individuals born under any of these circumstances are usually thought to have a cross on their hard palate, or less frequently a St. Catherine's wheel. Persons not born on these days, but with the distinguishing marks, also have grace. Twins generally are thought to have curing powers, particularly for stomach troubles, which they treat by the laying on of hands.

The Chilean *perspicaz* is clearly a lineal descendant of the Spanish *saludador,* for he cries in his mother's womb, he loses the power if she tells anyone before his birth, and he has a cross on his hard palate.[12] Curers with these qualifications are not known to me in the other countries under consideration. In Spanish America, as in Spain, twins are generally thought to have grace for curing. For the most part, however, New World *curanderos* have little in common with their Spanish counterparts as regards origin of knowledge or power. They are rather shamans, herb specialists, or individuals trained in some other way for their work.

A number of specific illnesses in Spain and the New World use similar or identical treatment. In most cases this appears to be due to diffusion. Throat inflammations known as *anginas* are treated in Galicia and Peru with poultices made of a frog or a toad prepared by opening the animal and applying its inner side to the sores. In at least Andalucia and Mexico toothache is explained as due to a worm inside the tooth; cloves and a child's excrement are common toothache treatments in Spain and the New World. In both areas human or animal excrement is a standard remedy for colic. The commonest treatment for erysipelas in Spain is a black cock's blood, often taken from the crest. In Peru cock's crest blood, not necessarily from a black fowl, is used. Sties in Spain, Chile, and Peru are rubbed with a key, ring, flies, or wheat grains. The commonest remedy for headaches in the New World is the plaster (*parche*) of potatoes or other substances placed on the temples. Plasters of potato, cucumber, or squash occur in Spain, though less common than other remedies. In Spain cutting the nails on Monday, and in Chile cutting them on Friday, is thought to prevent headache. In parts of Venezuela they are cut on Monday to prevent toothache. Jaundice has three principal cures in Spain: drinking water containing lice, watching flowing water, and urinating on *marrubio* herb (*Marrubium vulgare*). In Peru and Chile the louse treatment is known, and in Puru urination on verbena is listed. In Chile one urinates on bread and throws it in the street; if a dog eats the bread he catches the jaundice, curing the sufferer.

A common treatment for intestinal worms in Spain and Chile is to eat squash seeds. In Chile, Peru, and Spain dog bites, especially those of rabid dogs, are treated by burning hairs from the guilty animal and applying them to the wound. Rheumatism is treated with bee stings in Chile, with applications of human urine in Colombia, and by wearing copper wire bracelets in most American countries. All these remedies are known in Spain. Urine is a standard treatment for chilblains in both Chile and Spain.

Whooping cough remedies in Spanish America include rat broth in Colombia and the fruit of the prickly pear cactus (any one of several varieties of the genus *Opuntia*) in Peru and Chile. The former is the most widespread Spanish cure. In the Ribera del Ebro, Navarra, the juice of the leaves of the prickly pear is utilized. In Cataluña the juice or poultices of the leaves are used for bronchial ailments, including whooping cough. Nosebleed is treated in Spain and America by applying a key to the nape of the neck. Parsley nose-stoppers are reported from Peru and Madrid.

In Spain it is generally believed that pointing at stars and counting them causes warts. In Spanish America the rainbow is more frequently given as the cause, but in Chile the stars also are responsible. Peruvian and Chilean cures are obviously connected with those of Galicia and the Basque provinces. In all these places the wart is cut, causing it to bleed; grains of salt are rubbed in the blood, and then thrown on the fire. The sufferer flees, hoping to be far enough away not to hear the salt snap. In Chile and the Basque provinces the wart is rubbed with a coin which is thrown in the street. He who picks up the coin acquires the warts and thereby frees the original sufferer. The Basques rub warts with wheat which is then buried. In Chile the wheat grains are not buried but are given to dogs or chickens, who, however, do not acquire the warts. In Peru the wheat, like the salt, is thrown on the fire. Wart cures in the New World appear not to include rubbing them with garlic, the most frequent Spanish technique.

The nearly universal Spanish folk treatment for hernia in children is carried out on the mystic eve of San Juan. The child is taken to a willow thicket where two small trees are split longitudinally and tied to form an arch. A man named Juan stands on one side and a woman named Maria on the other. At the first stroke of midnight the woman passes the child through the arch to the man saying, "Juan, I give you a *niño quebrado* and want you to return him to me cured." Juan returns the child with the same words. The operation is repeated three times or until the last stroke of the clock is heard. Then the willows are bound up and if they again grow together it is a sign that the hernia will heal. Oaks and other trees may be used instead of willow.

A similar but not identical idea is found in Chile. One takes a button to a green tree and cuts a piece of bark the same size. The bark is then tied over the hernia. It is believed that as new bark grows and closes the cut on the tree the hernia will heal. In Chile and Colombia bark is otherwise associated with hernia treatment. The afflicted child's foot is placed against the tree—often a Ficus—and a piece of bark the same size and shape is cut out and hung in the smoke of the fireplace or over the door. As the bark dries the hernia heals.

CONCLUSIONS

The data suggest several tentative conclusions and raise a number of questions requiring additional study. It seems quite apparent that the medical practices of classical antiquity and Conquest Spain survive to a much greater extent in the New World than in the mother country, and are perhaps stronger than they ever were in Spanish folk medicine (as contrasted to that of the educated class). The scant traces of beliefs in humors and in the concepts of hot and cold in Spain today suggest that these ideas never were basic parts of folk belief. Superstition is so tenacious in Spain that if these ideas had been folk domain within the last several centuries they would show up in field research today. This is not the case. Intensive field questioning failed to elicit any but the most tenuous concepts of hot and cold. Leading Spanish folklorists and anthropologists (Julio Caro Baroja, Luis Hoyos Sainz, C. Cabal, José García Matos), whom I questioned, reported that such ideas were, to the best of their knowledge, completely lacking.[13] Apparently the contact situation in the New World favored widespread dissemination of much classical medical practice among the folk, a condition which never prevailed to the same extent in Spain.

A second conclusion concerns those areas in the Old and New Worlds which appear to have had greatest contact. The evidence presented here suggests that more Spanish folk medicine exists in Peru and Chile than in the other American countries considered. The remarkably complete work of Valdizán and Maldonado may contribute in part to this impression. However, other research has also led me to conclude that Peru has relatively more Spanish folklore and popular practices than, for example, Mexico; so it is not unlikely that the same would be true for folk medicine. The data also suggest that Galicia has had considerably greater contact than other parts of Spain with the New World. To American anthropologists who have been inclined to think of basic Spanish contacts as centering in Andalucía and Extremadura this may seem strange. Actually, during the past hundred and fifty years or so Galicia has been that part of Spain with most extensive contact with America; it is the only major area to which a very significant number of migrants to the New World have returned after many years of residence abroad. A special term, *Indiano,* is applied to these repatriates. They, obviously, would be important introducers of American traits, including medicine, into Spain. Lis, the most important authority on Galician folk medicine, tantalizing mentions the "great number of *curanderos* who have come from America";[14] and again, apropos of the *paletilla,* he speaks of "*curanderos* who were in America where they learned mixtures of scientific and popular (medicine)."[15] Though this is not the place for such a discussion, any consideration of the time factor in diffusion between America and Spain must place great emphasis on the part played by Galicia.

The extent to which American folk medicine has actually influenced Spain is difficult to determine. The few certain leads are through American plants and herbs. Of these, the most important is the potato, which today rather generally is recognized to have medicinal uses. Perhaps next in importance is the prickly pear cactus, which was early naturalized in Spain where it today looks as much at home as in America. Monardes[16] lists several dozen New World plants or substances of real of imagined medicinal uses which, by 1569, had reached Spain. These included copal gum (from the tree *Elaphrium jorullense*), *guayacan* (*Guaiacum sanctum*), the American sarsaparilla (*Smilax medica*), an American *cañafistula* (*Cassia fistula*), tobacco, sassafras, and the famous *jalapa* root (including a variety known as *raíz de Mechoacán*) was widely sought not only in Spain but in all western Europe for its cathartic qualities. Today these herbs appear to play little part in folk medicine. American bezoar stones, especially those from the vicuña, guanaco, llama, and deer, were mush sought during colonial times, but these also are of slight importance today in Spain. The same is true of the *uña de la Gran Bestia,* purported to be a moose hoof. Everything considered, there appears to be less American influence in the folk medicine of Spain than might reasonably be expected.

In another place I have expressed the admittedly impressionistic opinion that there are significant differences between the basic personality types of the Spaniard and the Hispano-American.[17] The Spaniard has impressed me as being an essentially stable, well-integrated individual, with few inner doubts and fears and with unlimited self-confidence. The Hispano-American, on the other hand, has struck me as resembling his North American counterpart in that an air of assurance and self confidence often masks inner doubts, uncertainties, worries, and apprehensions. Some of the data on folk medicine presented here appear to substantiate this impression. I have mentioned the relative unimportance of emotionally defined illnesses in Spain. The Spaniard falls ill because of natural and supernatural causes, because of witchcraft, or because of bad luck. But he does not tend to fall ill from psychosomatic causes, nor does his culture provide him with an easy out—in the form of emotionally based folk illnesses—whereby he can take refuge from the realities of life. This is not to say that there are no neurotic Spaniards, or that emotional unbalance does not occur. But in the popular mind life's common psychological experiences do not regularly produce adverse physiological reactions.

Contrariwise, one of the most striking characteristics of Spanish-American folk medicine is the prevalence of recognized and named illnesses or conditions which are not due to natural or supernatural causes or to witchcraft but to a series of emotional experiences which anyone can undergo and which can seriously incapacitate an individual. Anger, sorrow, sadness, shame, embarrassment, disillusion, rejection, desire, fear—all are recognized as potentially dangerous—and as leading (depending on the country) to *susto, espanto, colerina, pispelo, chucaque, tiricia, sipe, peche, caisa, pensión,* and so on.

Many of the "illnesses" are but the formal expressions of several distinct psychological phenomena. In the first place it is undeniably true that emotional experiences may be the direct causes of physiological malfunctioning, in a purely clinical sense. In other cases, however, they are manifestations of cultural definition and culturally patterned behavior. The frightened individual realizes that his fright will probably lead to illness, and he will seize upon any general and slight symptoms of discomfort which he may have had for a long time as evidence that he has indeed been frightened, and will build them up to a degree where he and his family believe that medical treatment is necessary. The mere existence of a culturally recognized condition believed to result from fright produces patients who would never be produced in a culture without such definitions and expected patterns of reactions. Finally, the functional value of emotionally defined illness as an escape mechanism is apparent. The individual who has been through an embarrassing experience, by taking refuge in a culturally acceptable illness, receives the sympathy rather than the ridicule of his fellows. Or the individual who has lost his temper may escape punishment or retribution by seeking immunity in an illness which his culture recognizes as a common result of his action.

It is impossible to say to what extent the emotional needs of the people have influenced the conceptualization of folk medicine in Hispanic America, and to what extent pre-existing cultural patterns of folk belief have influenced personality types. But it is apparent that today there is an intimate relationship between the two. Popular definition of a major category of folk disease plays an extremely important role in carrying the individual through emotionally upsetting experiences and thereby continually reinforces common aspects of personality types.

Spanish-American folk medicine appears to be marked by a strongly eclectic nature which has permitted it to pick and choose almost at random the concepts and practices which it has incorporated. In some cases entire complexes—in the sense of popular conceptualizations of causes of illnesses linked to specific symptoms and treatment—have diffused from Spain with relatively few changes. Ideas of hot and cold causes of illness and corresponding treatments, of the egg, key and fly cures for eyes, and of lice for jaundice, illustrate this type of selection. In other cases concepts of causes of disease have diffused from Spain, but not the Spanish treatments. Beliefs about the evil eye illustrate this point. And in still other cases Spanish treatments, such as a drying lizard or scorpion in a tube for sore eyes, have reached the New World but are no longer linked to those illnesses with which they are associated in the mother country. Patterning may be assumed to underlie the apparently haphazard acceptance and rejection of Spanish medical belief and practices in the New World, but available data do not permit definition of this order. Whatever the processes and reasons involved, in Spanish America native indigenous, Spanish folk, and ancient and medieval formal medical concepts have combined to form a vigorous body of folk medicine which plays a functional part in the everyday lives of the people and which will resist the inroads of modern medical science for many generations.

References

1. The Spanish data in this paper are taken from the sources given in this footnote and from my field notes from the towns of Alosno, Cerro de Andévalo, and Puebla de Guzman, in the province of Huelva; Conil de la Frontera and Vejer de la Frontera, province of Cádiz; Bujalance, province of Córdoba; Yegén, province of Granada; Villanueva del Rio Segura, province of Murcia, as well as odd notes from many other parts of the country. This field work was made possible by grants from the John Simon Guggenheim Memorial Foundation and the Wenner-Gren Foundation for Anthropological Research.

Published sources on Spain quoted or otherwise drawn upon are: Resurrección María de Azkua, *Euskaleriaren Yakintza (Literatura popular del pais vasco)*, 4 vols. (Madrid, 1947); Avila de Lobera (Luis), *El libro del régimen de la salud* (Biblioteca Clásica de la Medicina Española, Real Academia Nacional de Medicina, 5, Madrid, 1923); William George Black, *Medicina popular, un capítulo en la historia de la cultura,* trans. from the English by Antonio Machado y Alvarez, with appendices on Spanish folk medicine by Federico Rubio and Eugenio Olavarria y Huarte (Madrid, 1889); A. Castillo de Lucas, *Folklore médico-religioso. Hagiografías paramédicas* (Madrid, 1943); Alonso Chirino, *Menor daño de la medicina y espejo de Medicina* (Biblioteca Clásica de la Medicina Españols, Real Academia de Medicina, 14, Madrid, 1944); George M. Foster, "Report on an Ethnological Reconnaissance of Spain," *American Anthropologist,* 53 (1951), 311-325; Isabel Gallardo de Alvarez, "Medicina popular," *Revista del Centro de Estudios Extremeños,* 17 (Badajóz, 1943), 291-296; "Del folklore extremeño. Medicina popular y supersticiosa," *Revista de Estudios Extremeños,* no. 3 (Badajóz, 1945), 359-364; "Medicina popular y supersticiosa," *Revista de Estudios Extremeños,* no. I (Badajóz, 1946), 61-68; "Medicina popular y supersticiosa," *Revista de Estudios Extremeños,* nos. 1-2 (Badajóz, 1947), 179-196; Jose Maria Iribarren, *Retablo de Curiosidades* (Pamplona, 1948); Víctor Lis Quibén, "Medicina popular gallega," *Revista de*

Dialectología y Tradiciones Populares, I (1945), 253-331, 694-722; "Los pastequeiros de Santa Comba y San Cibran," *Revista de Dialectología y Tradiciones Pouplares,* 3 (1947), 491-523; *La medicina popular en Galicia* (Pontevedra, 1949a); "Medicina popular gallega," *Revista de Dialectología y Tradiciones Populares,* 5 (1949b), 309-332, 471-506; Francisco Lopez de Villalobos, *El sumario de la medicina, con un tratado sobre las pestiferas buvas* (Biblioteca Clasica de la Medicina, Real Academia Nacional de Medicina, 15, Madrid, 1948); Tomás Lópes-Tapia, "Contribución al estudio del folklore en España y con preferencia en Aragón," in *Sociedad Española de Etnografía y Prehistoria, Memoria* 73, pp. 247-257 (Madrid, 1929); Nicolás Monardes, *Primera y segunda y tercera partes de la historia medicinal de las cosas que se traen de nuestras Indias Occidentales que sirven en medicina,* 2nd ed (Sevilla, 1574); Ricardo Royo Villanova, "El folklore médico aragonés," *Revista Española de Medicina y Cirugía,* 19 (1936) 128-140; Juán Soropán de Rieros, *Medicina española contenida en proverbios vulgares de nuestra lengua* (Biblioteca Clásica de la Medicina Española, Real Academia Nacional de Medicina, 16, Madrid, 1949); Jesús Taboada, La medicina popular en el Valle de Monterrey (Orense)," *Revista de Dialectología y Tradiciones Populares,* 3 (1947), 31-57.

The principal Latin American countries discussed are Mexico, Guatemala, El Salvador, Colombia, Ecuador, Peru, and Chile. The data are drawn from my field notes on Mexico, El Salvador, and Chile, and from recent field research by Isabel T. Kelly (Mexico), Charles Erasmus (Colombia and Ecuador), and Ozzie Simmons (Peru and Chile), anthropologists of the Institute of Socila Anthropology. Greta Mostny contributed data from Chile, José Cruxent has supplied information on Venezuela and Cataluña, and the Servicio de Investigaciones del Folklore Nacional of the Venezuelan Ministry of Education has given data on Venezuela.

Published sources on Latin America quoted or otherwise drawn upon are: Richard N. Adams, *Un análisis de las enfermedades y sus curaciones en una población indigena de Guatemala* (Instituto de Nutrición de Centro América y Panama, Guatemala City, 1951); Ralph L. Beals, *Cherán: A Sierra Tarascan Village* (Smithsonian Institution, Institute of Social Anthropology, Publication 2, Washington, 1946); George M. Foster, *Empire's Children: The People of Tzintzuntzan* (Smithsonian Institution, Institute of Social Anthropology, Publication 6, Mexico City, 1948); John Gillin, *The Culture of Security in San Carlos* (The Tulane University of Louisiana, Middle American Research Institute, Publication 16, New Orleans, 1951); John Gillin, *Moche: A Peruvian Coastal Village* (Smithsonian Institution, Institute of Social Anthropology, Publication 3, Washington, 1947); Elsie Clews Parsons, *Mitla: Town of the Souls* (University of Chicago, Ethnological Series, Chicago, 1936); Elsie Clews Parsons, *Peguche: A Study of Andean Indians* (University of Chicago, Ethnological Series, Chicago, 1945); Hermilio Valdizán and Angel Maldonado, *La medicina popular peruana,* 3 vols. (Lima, 1922); Julio Vicuña Cifuentes, *Mitos y supersticiones: estudios del folk-lore chileno recogidos de la tradición oral* 3rd ed. (Santiago, 1947); Charles Wisdom, *The Chorti Indians of Guatemala* (University of Chicago, Ethnological Series, Chicago, 1940).

2. Validizán and Maldonado, 1922, III, 109-316.

3. Unless otherwise indicated the words "hot" and "cold" as applied to illness, remedies, medicines, and food are used in the Hippocratian sense of qualities, and do not refer to actual temperature.

4. Valdizán and Maldonado, *op. cit.*, 485, 455.

5. Lobera, 1923, 68.

6. Sorapán, 1949, 1956.

7. Lobera, *op. cit.*, 58.

8. Chirino, 1944, 285.

9. Sorapán, *op. cit.*, 214.

10. Valdizán and Maldonado, *op. cit.*, 114.

11. *Ibid.*, 112.

12. Vicuña, 1947, 91.

13. José Cruxent, however, remembers that in his childhood in Cataluña certain foods were thought to be hot and others cold. Iribarren (1948), writing of the Ribera del Ebro, Navarra, says: "with respect to chilling, the folk follow the Hippocratian doctrine which speaks of wetness, dryness, of heat, cold and temperatures" (p. 77). In his rather complete discussion of folk medicine he does not elaborate this point.

14. Lis, 1949a, 16.

15. *Ibid.*, 168.

16. Monardes, 1576.

17. Foster, 1951, 315, 324.

9

American Indian Medicine

Virgil J. Vogel, Ph.D.

This chapter was taken from American Indian Medicine, *which is an expanded version of Virgil J. Vogel's dissertation, "American Indian Medicine and its Influence on White Medicine and Pharmacology" (University of Chicago, 1966). Dr. Vogel's long interest in the American Indians and their cultural influence has taken him to over sixty Indian reservations and communities. He was professor of history at Truman College, City Colleges of Chicago, until his retirement in 1980. His other publications include "American Indian Foods Used as Medicine," in* American Folk Medicine, *edited by Wayland C. Hand (Berkeley, 1976), and* This Country Was Ours: A Documentary History of the American Indian *(New York, 1973).*

The central figure in Indian healing is the medicine man, often called, by ethnologists, by the Asian term *shaman,* and by the early observers, juggler, conjurer, sorcerer, quack, priest, and even physician. Ackerknecht took sharp issue with the last designation, arguing that medicine men and modern physicians are antagonists and not colleagues; all they have in common is that both treat diseases. The medicine man, he wrote, "is rather the ancestor of the priest, the antagonist of

Source: From Vogel, V. J. 1970. *American Indian medicine.* Norman, Okla.: University of Oklahoma Press, pp. 22-35. Copyright 1970 by the University of Oklahoma Press, Publishing Division of the University.

the physician for centuries. If there is any ancestor or colleague of the physician in primitive society, it is the lay healer, usually a woman, the midwife."[1]

The medicine man is indeed many things. He is, wrote Roland Dixon, "in the lower stages of culture, at once healer, sorcerer, seer, educator, and priest; but while often the single shaman sums up in himself thus all or most of these functions, there is frequently specialization, as a result of which each of these activities is exercised by a different person."[2] In some tribes, several classes of medical practitioners are distinguished. Among the Ojibwas, Hoffman described four: highest in rank were the priests of the *Midewiwin,* or medicine society, to which membership was gained by initiation and the payment of gifts. Next in rank were the *Wabenos,* "dawn men," practicers of medical magic, hunting medicine, love powders, etc.; third were the *Jessakid,* seers and prophets, revealers of hidden truths, possessors of a gift of clairvoyance received from the thunder god. Last were those whom most modern opinions have held to be the most useful of the lot, *Mashki-kike-winini,* or herbalists, who were generally denominated medicine men, as their name implied.

> Their calling [wrote Hoffman] is a simple one, and consists in knowing the mysterious properties of a variety of plants, herbs, roots and berries, which are revealed upon application for a fee. ... Although these herbalists are aware that certain plants or roots will produce a specified effect upon the human system, they attribute the benefit to the fact that such remedies are distasteful and injurious to the demons who are present in the system and to whom the disease is attributed. Many of these herbalists are found among women, also; and these, too, are generally members of the Midē-wiwin.[3]

Hoffman also noted that the Mide societies were the main opposition to the introduction of the Christianity, due to the fact that "the traditions of Indian genesis and cosmogony and the ritual of initiation into the Society of the Mide constitutes what is to them a religion, even more powerful and impressive than the Christian religion is to the average civilized man." He saw the purpose of the society as the preservation of Indian traditions and as giving "a certain class of ambitious men and women sufficient influence through their acknowledged power of exorcism and necromancy to lead a comfortable life at the expense of the credulous."[4]

Hoffman's view that the medicine men were insincere exploiters of their people was not shared by all who studied them. Hrdlicka believed that many of them, at least, were sincere,[5] while Dr. Brooks declared that:

> ... the removal of the foreign body on the part of the priest has precisely the same significance as the very similar ceremonies practiced by our shamen. The attempt to deceive and willful faking is not in the mind of the respectable practitioner any more than it is in the mind of our psychiatrists when they do practically the same thing in their practice.[6]

Dr. Stone relates the impression of Washington Mathews that the performers of the Navaho mountain chant (a curing ritual) so thoroughly believed in "the supernatural powers of their own deceptions that even during the practice before the performance he has seen the men trembling with fear and awe and looking as pale as an Indian could look, from sheer emotion."[7]

Medicine societies are found in a number of tribes besides the Ojibwas and Menominees as reported by Hoffman. Arthur C. Parker described thirteen such organizations still functioning among the Senecas early in the present century,[8] and in recent years the well-known writer Edmund Wilson described the "Little water ceremony" of the Senecas (also mentioned earlier by Parker), which he was privileged to attend.[9] Some of the rituals of Seneca medicine societies, such as the sprinkling of water to banish disease, and the chanting in unison of certain songs in language unintelligible even to the participants,[10] are suggestive of certain practices of some of the Christian churches.

Leslie White described in detail the functioning of thirteen medicine fraternities among the Zũnis, each of which was charged with the treatment of a different disease or complex of diseases, or conjuring exercises, such as prayers for rain.[11] Ralph Linton has told of a number of medicine societies that once existed among the Pawnees.[12]

INDIAN DEFINITION OF MEDICINE

The meaning of the term *medicine* to an Indian was quite different from that which is ordinarily held in white society. To most Indians, medicine signified an array of ideas and concepts rather than remedies and treatment alone. George Bird Grinnell, who was intimately associated with northern Plains tribes, has written:

> All these things which we speak of as medicine the Indian calls mysterious, and when he calls them mysterious this only means that they are beyond his power to account for. ... We say that the Indian calls whisky "medicine water." He really calls it mysterious water—that is, water which acts in a way that he cannot understand. ... In the same way some tribes call the horse "medicine dog," and gun "medicine iron," meaning mysterious dog and mysterious iron. He whom we call a medicine man may be a doctor, a healer of diseases; or if he is a juggler, a worker of magic, he is a mystery man. All Indian languages have words which are the equivalent of our word medicine, sometimes with curative properties; but the Indian's translation of "medicine," used in the sense of magical or supernatural, would be mysterious, inexplicable, unaccountable.[13]

John James Audubon, the painter, thought it notable that Missouri valley Indians called the steamboat "great medicine."[14] Even a glance at the map reveals the varied applications of the term "medicine" by the Indians: Medicine Bow, Wyoming; Medicine Hat, Alberta; Medicine Lake, Montana; Medicine Lodge,

Kansas; Medicine Mound, Texas; and Medicine Park, Oklahoma. There are also, in Indian parlance, such things as medicine stick, big medicine, bad medicine, good medicine, medicine dance, medicine pipe, medicine drum, and war medicine. "Whereas we think in terms of drugs, ointments, or cathartics which will benefit the body in a predictable fashion," wrote Robert F. Greenlee, "the Seminole thinks of benefits which one can produce only through the office of the medicine man." This functionary believes that he can surely cure if he can recite the prescribed medicinal formulas, perform the necessary rites, and blow on the brewed medicine in a certain way. His medical theory arises from the reasoning that "he can control the forces of nature and hence make disease yield to his personal efforts."[15] Consequently, curative agents are indeed "medicine," but only one kind of medicine, and that only in association with prescribed rites. Greenlee further remarked that the Seminole concept of medicine covers diagnosis, the curing of bodily ills, and mysterious mental ailments. The medicine man is entrusted with ceremonies connected with birth and death, magical ceremonies, and the perpetuation of tribal lore. He further served as the spokesman of the group in Indian-white relations.

Maddox has stated that savage medicine includes "clairvoyance, ecstasism, spiritism, divination, demonology, prophesy, necromancy, and all things incomprehensible. Hence the medicine man is not only the primitive doctor, but he is the diviner, the rain-maker, the soothsayer, the prophet, the priest, and in some instances, the chief or king."[16] Indeed, some of the better-known Indian "chiefs" were in fact medicine men: Corn Planter, Gall, Sitting Bull, Joseph, Geronomo, Cochise, and others.[17]

Medicine power is often attributed to a fetish or charm adopted to typify a tutelary demon, or mystery guardian, and the superior performance on one "juggler" over another is often attributed to the fact that his "medicine" is the stronger. Medicine is also associated with magic numbers, as it sometimes is among whites ("lucky seven," "unlucky thirteen"). The usual sacred number among Indians is four, signifying the cardinal directions, but sometimes six, adding the up and down directions. Medical prescriptions will sometimes specify, for this reason, a certain number of remedies, or the administration of the remedies for so many days, or that they be gathered in so many places.

Omens were watched for by Indian doctors to determine the probable results of treatment, or to foretell future events. This practice was well developed in Middle and South America[18] but also persists among North American tribes, as it does among white people. Ruth Landes reported that when her Kansas Potawatomi informant left the reservation for war industry and marriage, "he found that his white associates also observed omens everywhere, divined by cards, ghosts, and dreams, and solicited Indian shamans for love medicine."[19]

EQUIPMENT OF THE MEDICINE MAN

The medicine man was equipped with paraphernalia and equipment appropriate to his calling. These might include special costume, such as animal skins as shown in

George Catlin's famous painting of the Mandan medicine man, a medicine bundle that contains charms and fetishes, medicine sticks serving as an offering, a warning, or an invitation,[20] and sometimes a bag of herbs. The function of providing the herbs was sometimes relegated to an assistant, or "apothecary." The medicine man might also have a drum, rattle, a scarification instrument—in former times made of flint, obsidian, or snake fangs—a hollow bone for sucking, a mortar and pestle for mixing medicines, and, in many places, a syringe for injecting medicine into wounds or administering an enema.

From the religious viewpoint, which was uppermost to the Indian, the medicine bundle was perhaps the most important. In the thirties the medicine bundle cult still survived among the Kansas Potawatomis, along with the more recent "religion" or drum dance, and the peyote religion, as one of the three curing cults still extant.[21] The medicine bundle was usually made of an animal skin, often from a totemic animal, and included such fetishes as deer tails, dried fingers, and often the maw stone of a buffalo.[22] These bags were handed down from father to son, or to newly initiated medicine men by the instructor. La Potherie has described a seventeenth-century Miami medicine bag:

> In the cabin of the great chief of the Miamis an altar had been erected, on which he had caused to be placed a Pindikosan. This is a warrior's pouch, filled with medicinal herbs wrapped in the skins of animals, the rarest that they can find; it usually contains all that inspires their dreams.[23]

The charms in the medicine bag, to ward off evil, were often more important than the curative agents, which they might or might not contain. Benjamin Hawkins reported that the Creeks carried in their shot bags "a charm, a protection against all ills, called the war physic, composed of . . . bones of the snake and lion."[24]

The use of charms or fetishes is old in human history. While the French Jesuits ridicules the Indian charms, they soberly wrote of miraculous cures performed by swallowing in water or in broth a little dust from the tomb of Kateri Tekakwitha, the saintly Iroquois Christian girl who died in 1680.[25] Several cures attributed to baptism are recounted in the *Jesuit Relations,* including "instant" recovery of an Indian child so ill with "consumptive fever" that he was "reduced to a mere skeleton."[26] One account from Virginia related the cure of an Indian boy through baptism performed according to the liturgy of the Church of England.[27] Cure by relics is claimed in an account written in Illinois in 1700 by Father Jacques Gravier:

> I have found an excellent remedy for curing our French of their fever. I promised God, jointly with Pierre de bonne,—who had a violent tertian fever for a long time,—to recite for 9 days some prayers in honor of Father Francois Regis, whose relics I have. These I applied to him at his Strongest paroxysm, which suddenly ceased, and he has had none since.[28]

Father Gravier reported four other cures accomplished in the same way. "A small piece of Father Francois Regis's hat, which one of his servants gave me," he wrote, "is the most infallible remedy that I know of for curing all kinds of fever." In an earlier instance, Pierre Biard in 1612 cautiously suggested that he may have cured the son of an Indian chief of a dangerous illness, after the French apothecary had failed, by "putting upon the sufferer a bone taken from the precious relics of the glorified Saint Lawrence . . . at the same time offering our vows to him, and then he improved."[29]

According to John G. Bourke, the South Texas Mexicans put a string of coral beads around the neck to stop nosebleed,[30] a practice similar to the Penobscot custom of preventing bleeding by wearing a necklace made of bloodroot.[31] Bernard Romans, who would have no truck with Indian "superstitions," reported that Spaniards in the Gulf region wore "the nest of the great travelling spider sowed in a rag about their neck as a sure way to assuage a hecktick fever, and I think with great success."[32]

Charm remedies and sympathetic magic are reported among the Pennsylvania Germans and numerous other American subcultures. In eighteenth-century Pennsylvania, Joseph Doddridge relates, "charms and incantations were in use for the cure of many diseases. I learned, when young, the incantation in German, for the cure of burns, stopping blood, for the toothache, and the charm against bullets in battle."[33] These parallels in the practices of the two races are cited as examples of their universality and do not indicate that either race learned them from the other.

INDIAN METHODS OF TREATMENT

There were variations in healing procedure from tribe to tribe, and in different culture areas. However, there were some methods which were nearly universal. A survey of all of them is quite outside the scope of this study, but much of the procedure common to eastern Woodland tribes can be seen in the description provided by Pierre de Liette for the Illinois-Miami tribes of the late seventeenth century. He reported that most of the old men were healers, and that when a person was sick, his relatives would hang in the cabin certain gifts for the medicine man, such as a kettle, guns, or blankets. The healer was summoned, and would question the patient about the nature and extent of his illness. The healer would then leave, and return with his bag of medicines, and his *chichicoya,* or gourd rattle. The rattle was shaken, while the healer intoned in a loud voice that certain animal spirits had revealed to him the proper remedies, which were certain to cure. He next called for warm water, and, taking some of it in his *micoine* (spoon), he mixed his remedies, and the medicine was swallowed by the patient. The healer would also take some of the medicine in his own mouth, spout it upon the seat of pain, and bandage it. He returned twice a day and sang incantations, followed by violent sucking of the ailing parts of the body. He then revealed an object said to have been drawn from the body, such as an eagle claw or cougar's hair, which was called the cause of the ailment. Then in a long song:

> He thanks his manitou with his *chichicoya* for making it possible for him frequently to obtain merchandise through his favor. He takes his patient out for a bath, or washes him in the cabin, according to the season. He takes what had been hung up for him in the cabin and carries it off without saying anything. The relatives rise and pass their hands over his head and his legs, a sign of profound gratitude. Generally they do not cure the sick, although assuredly they have excellent drugs, because they are ignorant of internal maladies.[34]

While De Liette believed that their treatment of internal diseases was ineffective, he praised their treatment of wounds and thought that the sucking process was a good device to remove infection.

Indian medical treatment is here seen as a combination of rational and religious practices, differing from the usual white practice in that *both are performed by the same functionary* among the Indians. In our own society there are some religious sects which combine treatment with supernatural appeals and some which eschew medical treatment altogether. Comparing the two, Dr. Harlow Brooks commented: "I fail to find in the service of our modern faiths anything more dignified, beautiful, and worshipful than some of the chants or 'dances' of the red man, conducted for the benefit of the sick, or for the purpose of imploring the assistance of their divine being in the welfare of their people."[35]

Tribal differences, however, should not be overlooked. It was one scholar's opinion that "the New England Indians apparently had nothing like those formal, elaborately organized priesthoods of the West and South which dominate most discussions of Indian cults and superstitutions."[36] Similar claims to a separation of medical practice from ritual have been made for the Catawbas.[37] Some classes of practitioners, such as midwives and herbalists, minimized or dispensed with ritual, and it was not commonly employed in the treatment of external injuries for which the cause was obvious.

Among the Winnebagos, the medicine man scattered tobacco, feathers, or some such substance to exorcise the spirit causing the disease, meanwhile repeating prayers, often in ancient, unintelligible dialect. Sometimes a dog was sacrificed to prevent an illness from attacking other members of the family.[38] Tobacco is also used among the Seminoles,[39] and other tribes to ward off evil influences, not only of disease, but of such natural phenomena as storms and lightning. It was used by the Virginia Indians, wrote John Smith, to "offer the water in passing fowle weather."[40]

The use of rattles or drums seems to be universal. "To cure the sick," Smith wrote, "a man, with a Rattle, and extreame howling, showting, singing and such violent gestures and Anticke actions over the patient, will sucke out blood and flegme from the patient, out of the unable stomacke, or any diseased place."[41]

Maximilian reported among the Blackfeet: "In all cases they have recourse to the drum and rattle, and have great confidence in the intolerable noise caused by those instruments."[42]

Herbs employed by the medicine men were believed to derive their strength from ceremonies performed to make them powerful. Among the Onondagas, wrote the Jesuit priest Jean de Quen, "all the village Sorcerers and Jugglers, the Physicians of the Country, assemble, to give strength to their drugs, and by the ceremony performed, to impart to them a virtue entirely distinct from that derived from the soil."[42] The same procedure is reported among the Miamis by Charlevoix:

> The whole town being assembled, one of these quacks declares he is going to communicate to the roots and plants, of which he takes care to provide good store, the virtue of healing all sorts of wounds, and even of restoring the dead to life. He falls immediately to singing; the other quacks make responses to him, and it is believed that during the concert, which would not appear to your ear very melodious, and which is accompanied with many grimaces on the part of the actors, the medicinal quality is communicated to the plants.[44]

The doctrine of signatures played an important role in Indian medicine, as it once did in European medicine. "Like cures like" was the essence of this belief; thus, yellow plants were good for jaundice; red ones were good for the blood. Some part of the plant might resemble the organ of the body it was designed to cure, according to this belief. Reminders of the former prevalence of such conceptions among Europeans are indicated by plant names such as hepatica, formerly believed to be useful in liver complaints, and lungwort, once believed valuable in pulmonary infections.[45] Speck called this belief "sympathetic influence" and gave several examples of it among Indians. The form and the Indian name of ginseng (*Panax quinquefolius* L.), a noted panacea, indicated its value to the Penobscots for promoting female fertility. The use of wormroot (*Apocynum cannabinum*) for worms, and snakeroot (*Aristolochia serpentaria*) for fits or "contortions" were determined from their appearance. Elm bark was used in this tribe for bleeding lungs because of its slippery quality, and bloodroot was used to prevent bleeding because of the red juice contained in it.[46]

The Indians also commonly believed that certain roots or plants were beneficial to the system because they were distasteful and injurious to the demons present in the body which were causing the disease.[47] Consequently, foul-tasting medicines, emetics, and purges, were often used.

THE RESULTS OF SHAMANISTIC TREATMENT

The shaman was often successful, not only in the treatment of Indians, but also whites. Most writers have attributed this success at least in part to psychological factors not recognized in earlier times but given much attention today. Many curative measures, Rivers has indicated, "owe their success to the faith they inspire, or to the more mysterious property we call suggestion."[48] James Mooney recognized this when he wrote that:

> The faith of the patient has much to do with his recovery, for the Indian has the same implicit confidence in the shaman that a child has in a more intelligent physician. The ceremonies and prayers are well calculated to inspire this feeling, and the effect thus produced upon the mind of the sick man undoubtedly reacts favorably upon his physical organization.[49]

Josiah Gregg, writing of the Comanches in the 1830's, remarked that "they have great faith in their 'medicine men,' who pretend to cure the sick with conjurations and charms; and the Comanche and many others often keep up an irksome, monotonous singing over the diseased person, to frighten away the evil spirit which is supposed to torment him; all of which, from its effect upon the imagination, often tends, no doubt, to hasten recovery."[50] Such views have been finding increasing corroboration among modern anthropologists, physicians, and others. Dr. Ackerknecht has written that "the participation of the community in the healing rites, and the strong connection between these rites and the whole religion and tradition of the tribe, produce certain psychotherapeutic advantages for the medicine man which the modern physician lacks."[51]

THE MEDICINE MAN AND WHITE SOCIETY

The Indian medicine man, being also a priest and highly respected tribal leader, was long recognized by the whites as a principal barrier to the eradication of Indian culture. John Bourke saw in the medicine man "an influence antagonistic to the rapid absorption of new ideas and the adoption of new customs." He believed that only "after we have thoroughly routed the medicine men from their intrenchments and made them an object of ridicule" could whites "hope to bend and train the mind of our Indian wards in the direction of civilization."[52] More recently, Huron H. Smith reported that "the government takes cognizance of the Indian medicine man and is trying to wean the Indians away from his dominance."[53]

The hostility of the Christian missionaries to the medicine men is revealed in many of their accounts. Thus, all of the principal forces of European erosion of Indian society have been brought to bear in the assault against the medicine man. To the extent that his influence was weakened, white influence was able to penetrate. The campaign has made great headway, and yet the old ways, sometimes driven underground, continue to flourish in many ways. Even though Indians are coming to depend more upon white doctors and hospitals, provided to them free if they are on reservations, they sometimes resort to their medicine men if a quick cure is not forthcoming.[54] If the Indian medicine man eventually disappears, he will nevertheless have left to mankind an important store of remedies and curing methods, which, however irrational his notions about them, have often proved useful to the conquerors and will stand as his enduring monument.

References

1. Ackerknecht, E. H. 1942. Problems of primitive medicine. *Bull. Hist. Med.* 11:508-509.

2. Dixon, R. 1908. Some aspects of the American shaman. *J. Am. Folklore* 31:7.

3. Hoffman, W. J. 1891. *The Midēwiwin or "grand medicine society" of the Ojibwa.* Seventh Annual Report, Bureau of American Ethnology, 1885-1886. Washington, D.C.: U.S. Government Printing Office, p. 159.

4. Hoffman, W. J. 1891. *The Midēwiwin or "grand medicine society" of the Ojibwa.* Seventh Annual Report, Bureau of American Ethnology, 1885-1886. Washington, D.C.: U.S. Government Printing Office, p. 159.

5. Hrdlicka, A. 1908. *Physiological and medical observations among the Indians of southwestern United States and Northern Mexico.* Washington, D.C.: U.S. Government Printing Office, p. 223.

6. Brooks, H. 1933. The medicine of the American Indian. *J. Lab. Clin. Med.* 19:16.

7. Stone, E. 1962. *Medicine among the American Indians.* New York: Hafner Press, p. 92.

8. Parker, A. C. 1909. Secret medicine societies of the Seneca. *Am. Anthropologist* 11:161-185.

9. Wilson, E. 1960. *Apologies to the Iroquois.* New York: Farr, Straus & Cudahy, Ch. 9.

10. Parker, A. C. 1909. Secret medicine societies of the Seneca. *Am. Anthropologist* 11:161-185.

11. White, L. 1927. *Medicine societies of the Southwest.* Chicago: Department of Anthropology, University of Chicago (doctoral dissertation).

12. Linton, R. 1923. *Annual ceremony of the Pawnee medicine men.* Chicago: Field Museum of Natural History.

13. Grinnell, G. B. 1935. *The story of the Indian.* New York: D. Appleton-Century-Crofts, pp. 180-181.

14. Audubon, J. J. 1960. *Audubon and his journals,* vol. 2 (M. R. Audubon, editor). New York: Dover Publications, Inc., p. 19.

15. Greenlee, R. F. 1944. Medicine and curing practices of the modern Florida Seminoles. *Am. Anthropologist* 46:317-319.

16. Maddox, J. L. 1923. *The medicine man: A sociological study of the character and evolution of shamanism.* New York: Macmillan, Inc., p. 25.

17. Verrill, A. H. 1943. *The American Indian: North, South and Central America.* New York: New Home Library, p. 124.

18. Brinton, D. G. 1876. *The myths of the New World,* 2nd ed. rev. New York: Henry Holt, pp. 106, 297.

19. Landes, R. 1963. Potowatomi medicine. *Trans. Kans. Acad. Sci.* 76:572.

20. Verrill, A. H. 1943. *The American Indian: North, South, and Central America.* New York: New Home Library, p. 125.

21. Landes, R. 1963. Potowatomi medicine. *Trans. Kans. Acad. Sci.* 76:588.

22. Linton, R. 1923. *Annual ceremony of the Pawnee medicine men.* Chicago: Field Museum of Natural History.

23. Kellogg, L. P., editor. 1917. *Early narratives of the Northwest, 1634-1699.* New York: Charles Scribner's Sons, p. 87.

24. Hawkins, B. 1848. *A sketch of the Creek country in the years 1798 and 1799.* Savannah: Georgia Historical Society. p. 79.

25. Thwaites, R. G., editor. 1789. *The Jesuit relations and allied documents: Travels and explorations of the Jesuit missionaries in New France, 1610-1791,* vol. 45. Cleveland: Burrows, p. 79.

26. Thwaites, R. G., editor. 1789. *The Jesuit relations and allied documents: Travels and explorations of the Jesuit missionaries in New France, 1610-1791,* vol. 42. Cleveland: Burrows, pp. 145-147.

27. Force, P. 1838. *Tracts and other papers, relating principally to the origin, settlement, and progress of the colonies in North America.* Canton, Ohio: Smith & Bevin, p. 9.

28. Thwaites, R. G., editor. 1789. *The Jesuit relations and allied documents: Travels and explorations of the Jesuit missionaries in New France, 1610-1791,* vol. 45. Cleveland: Burrows, pp. 107-109.

29. Thwaites, R. G., editor. 1789. *The Jesuit relations and allied documents: Travels and explorations of the Jesuit missionaries in New France, 1610-1791,* vol. 19. Cleveland: Burrows, p. 19.

30. Rourke, J. G. 1894. Popular medicine, customs, and superstitions of the Rio Grande. *J. Am. Folklore* 7:137.

31. Speck, F. G. 1915. *Medicine practices of the Northeastern Algonquians.* Proceedings of the Nineteenth International Congress of Americanists. Washington, D.C., p. 311.

32. Romans, B. 1962. *A concise natural history of East and West Florida.* Gretna, La.: Pelican Publishing Co., Inc., p. 168.

33. Doddridge, J. 1876. *Notes on the settlement and Indian wars of the western parts of Virginia and Pennsylvania.* Albany, N.Y.: Joel Munsell, p. 172.

34. Quaife, M. M., editor. 1962. *The western country in the seventeenth century: The memoirs of Antoine Lamothe Cadillac and Pierre Liette.* Secaucus, N.J.: Citadel Press, pp. 144-145.

35. Brooks, H. 1933. The medicine of the American Indian. *J. Lab. Clin. Med.* 19:13.

36. Bradley, W. T. 1936. Medical practices of the New England aborigines. *J. Am. Pharm. Assoc.* 25:142.

37. Speck, F. 1944. Catawba herbals and curing practices. *J. Am. Folklore* 57:38-39.

38. Bergen, F. D. 1896. Some customs and beliefs of the Winnebago Indians. *J. Am. Folklore* 9:53-55.

39. Greenlee, R. F. 1944. Medicine and curing practices of the modern Florida Seminoles. *Am. Anthropologist* 46:323.

40. Tyler, L. G., editor. 1959. *Narratives of early Virginia, 1606-1625.* New York: Barnes & Noble Books, p. 51.

41. Tyler, L. G., editor. 1959. *Narratives of early Virginia, 1606-1625.* New York: Barnes & Noble Books, p. 51.

42. Thwaites, R. G., editor. 1904. *Early Western travels, 1748-1846,* vol. 23. Glendale, Calif.: Arthur H. Clark Co., p. 120.

43. Thwaites, R. G., editor. 1789. *The Jesuit relations and allied documents: Travels and explorations of the Jesuit missionaries in New France, 1610-1791,* vol. 42. Cleveland: Burrows, p. 173.

44. de Charlevoix, P. F. X. 1923. *Journal of a voyage to North America,* vol. 1 (L. P. Kellogg, editor). Chicago: Caxton Club, pp. 316-317.

45. True, R. H. 1901. Folk materia medica. *J. Am. Folklore* 14:106.

46. Speck, F. 1944. Catawba herbals and curing practices. *J. Am. Folklore* 57:306.

47. Hoffman, W. J. 1891. *The Midēwiwin or "grande medicine society" of the Ojibwa.* Seventh Annual Report, Bureau of American Ethnology, 1885-1886. Washington, D. C.: U.S. Government Printing office, p. 159.

48. Rivers, W. H. R. 1924. *Medicine, magic, and religion.* New York: Harcourt Brace Jovanovich, Inc., p. 122.

49. Mooney, J. 1891. *The sacred formulas of the Cherokees,* Seventh Annual Report of the Bureau of American Ethnology, 1885-1886. Washington, D.C.: U.S. Government Printing Office, p. 323.

50. Gregg, J. 1904. Commerce of the prairies, or the journal of a Santa Fe trader. In Thwaites, R. G., editor. *Early western travels, 1748-1846,* vol. 23. Glendale, Calif.: Arthur H. Clark Co., pp. 334-335.

51. Ackerknecht, E. H. July 1946. Primitive medicine: A contrast with modern practice. *Merck report,* p. 8.

52. Bourke, J. G. 1892. *The medicine-men of the Apache,* Ninth Annual Report of the Bureau of American Ethnology, 1887-1888, Washington, D.C.: U.S. Government Printing Office, pp. 451, 594.

53. Smith, H. H. 1923. *Ethnobotany of the Menomini Indians.* Milwaukee: Milwaukee Public Museum, p. 20.

54. Ritzenthaler, R. E. 1953. *Chippewa preoccupation with health.* Milwaukee: Milwaukee Public Museum, p. 202.

10

Bisayan Filipino and Malayan Folk Medicine

Donn V. Hart, Ph.D.

Donn V. Hart is Professor of Anthropology and Director of the Center for Southeast Asian Studies at Northern Illinois University. He spent 1979 in the Philippines where he investigated the social control role of ethnomedicine among Bisayan Filipinos. A member of many professional organizations, Dr. Hart has taught in the Philippines as well as in various American universities, including Yale and Syracuse University, and has lectured for the Peace Corps. His latest book is Compadrinazgo: Ritual Kinship in the Philippines.

Bisayan Filipinos support at least two, often competing, medical systems. When ill, they may consult both the indigenous curer and the western trained physician. Certain illnesses are assigned to such natural causes as overeating, poor diet, excessive drinking, physical abuse of the body, infections, and accidents. Such ordinary ailments normally are treated with home remedies. Other illnesses are believed caused by supernatural agents. There are the invisible spirits "who replicate the life of the peasants but possess supernatural powers denied most humans."[1] Sickness and death may also result from the actions of angered ancestral spirits,

Source: From Hart, D. V. 1969. *Bisayan Filipino and Malayan humoral pathologies and folk medicine and ethnohistory in Southeast Asia.* Ithica, N.Y.: Cornell University, Southeast Asia Program, pp. 14-18, 29-31, 35-43.

witches, persons with the evil eye, or the lethal bite or powers of preternatural animals.

If the patient either does not recover or worsens, he seeks the advice of the various folk medical specialists. Depending upon the individual, his financial resources, and the illness, modern western drugs may be sought, including hospitalization in the provincial capitals. These two medical systems are not totally separated. Some physicians in Dumaguete accept aspects of the hot-cold syndrome, whereas traditional curers are not beyond recommending aspirin or giving their patients injections.[2]

A variety of traditional curers, including shamans, both diagnose and treat the sick. Some part-time specialists limit their practice to specific types of afflictions, e.g., boils, fractures, bones or food lodged in the windpipe, sickness caused by fright, by supernaturals, etc. Although the etiology of an illness may be supernatural, herbal remedies can be used. Other forms of treatment are massage, dry cupping, "fumigating" the patient with incense, prayers at both the household altar and the church, magical incantations, amulets, food offerings to the spirits and ancestral souls, and a few modern drugs.

Curers often diagnose sickness by feeling the patient's pulse. According to a Cebu City curer, "The pulse is the best spot to tell the illness of the patient because it is an outlet, a "substation," of the heart. If the pulse lies, then the heart lies."[3] A Lalawigan curer said an ill person's pulse may be hot or cold, depending on the type of sickness. A healthy person has stabilized his unique balance of hot, cold, and air elements in the body. When the body becomes too hot (or too cold), the velocity of the blood's circulation is increased (or decreased). Loss of appetite and general malaise occurs, lowering the normal defenses against illness. The healer most respected by Caticuganers claimed he could diagnose the sickness of a villager by feeling the pulse of the messenger who came to fetch him to the patient. The messenger's pulse duplicated the abnormal beating of the sick person's pulse, although he did not contract the latter's illness.

Latin American and Philippine folk medical complexes assert that exposure to excessive real heat or cold is harmful. The following paragraph, written about Tzintzuntzan, Mexico, is largely true in Caticugan and Lalawigan.

> Heat may attack the body following exposure to high temperatures such as the rays of the midday sun, a hot bath, and radiation from a cooking fire or pottery kiln. "Heat" may also attack the body as a consequence of strong emotional experiences such as anger, fright, envy, or joy (which are classified as "hot" experiences, from injudicious ingestion of hot foods and drinks, and from the emanations believed to be given off by a corpse).[4]

In Lalawigan, however, great fright or joy are regarded as cold not hot experiences.

A woman in Caticugan reportedly became blind because she constantly baked rice cakes in an outdoor oven, and failed to protect her eyes from the fire. In

Caticugan illness may occur if a female irons clothing (using a charcoal iron) and immediately afterwards washes her hands in cool water. Sudden changes in the weather, "strong winds and vagrant breezes," vapors that rise from the ground when the sun appears after a lengthy rain, simultaneously eating or drinking certain hot and cold foods, or exposure to the night air are alleged causes for illness in Caticugan and among other Christian Filipino groups.[5]

In Malitbog, a predominantly Protestant village in Panay, the residents believe that over-exposure to the sun or heat from the kitchen cooking fire turns a mother's milk rancid; as a result her nursing infant may become ill with a stomach-ache or loose bowels.[6] In summary, both metaphysical and real hot and cold temperatures, when absorbed by the body in excessive amounts, result in sickness.

One feature of the "complexion" of the humors, in the classical sense, was their quality of air or vapor. Both Latin Americans and Filipinos accept the possible baneful effect on their health of air or wind (Sp. *aire* or *mal aire*). Among Filipinos air (Ceb. and Sam. *hangin,* also meaning wind) may produce illness in two basic ways. First, exposure to a normal draft or breeze may bring illness, e.g., a cold. If one absorbs excessive amounts of hot or cold air, the balance of these principal elements in the body may be disturbed. The Caticugan mother wraps the navel of her infant with a cloth to prevent air from entering its body through this alleged aperture. Coconut oil in which *pauli* roots have soaked is rubbed on the skin to keep "the wind from penetrating one's pores." Air circulates in the veins. Dr. Jocano writes that the barriofolk of Malitbog believe that if hot air is absorbed through the pores and carried by the blood to the brain cavity, mental illness may occur in which the victim becomes extremely hostile.

A second association of air, or wind, with illness is that it may be the means by which the spirits (Ceb. *ingkanto*) propel thorns, pebbles, bones, or other foreign objects to penetrate magically the body. Many aches and pains in Caticugan and Lalawigan are the result of the spirits' "missiles" "shot" by air into one's legs and arm joints.[8] The Balangingi Samals have the same troubles with their *jin.*

Jocano reports that "All diseases, for the farmers of Maltibog, are caused by either supernatural beings or by the unbalanced relationship of elements inside the body due to the imbalance of the elements in the body by air or the overconsumption of cold or hot foods."[9] The relationships between excessive exposure to hot and cold air and disease concepts among Bisayan Filipinos are more complicated than this short summary indicates. For example, a Cebu City *mananambal* (traditional curer) told Lieban that a person who has eaten spoiled food becomes vulnerable "to a wind containing both hot and cold elements."[10]

Filipinos in Tuburan, Santolan, Caticugan and Lalawigan also associate hotness with the supernatural. These villagers usually erect their dwellings only on cold sites. Building a residence on a hot location would bring sickness and bad luck to the occupants. There are numerous techniques to select a proper location. In Tuburan, a carabao (water buffalo) is staked on a prospective site. The new building is constructed only on the spot where the animal finally lies down to rest since this area is regarded as cold (*mahamog*).[11]

One of several ways Caticuganers determine if the environmental spirits approve a new housesite is to bury a green coconut in which the fluid inside cannot be heard when the nut is shaken. The next morning the nut is unearthed and shaken. If the liquid inside is heard, the area is regarded as hot, i.e., the spirits disapprove its use as a housesite.[12]

INDIGENOUS SOUTHEAST ASIAN HOT-COLD SYNDROME

Sources on various Bornean groups were searched to determine the possible presence of an indigenous hot-cold dichotomy or humoral pathology features of their traditional medicine. Most of these societies have been largely isolated from the main streams of Indian, Arab, Chinese, and Spanish influence in Southeast Asia. For those societies where this dichotomy occurs, no convincing evidence exists to date that the concepts were borrowed from these external cultural traditions.

No Bornean society was located, in the sources examined, that systematically classifies foods, medicines, and diseases on a hot-cold basis. Bornean folk medicine does not appear to have any pronounced humoral qualities. When the hot-cold concept occurs, it is related primarily to the structure of the universe. For example, humans who disturb the world's hot-cold balance suffer sickness and other misfortunes. The Kelabit believe the universe is controlled by a hot-cold balance that began with a struggle between fire and water during the origin of the human world.[13] They assert that humans, their domestic (but not wild) animals, dwellings, and personal possessions may petrify from intense cold if certain customs are violated.[14]

Williams reports that

> The people [Dusun] of Sensuron [Sabah] feel that the state of the universe as well as omens of personal fortune are responsible for sickness. The condition of a "hot universe" . . . is feared greatly since at such a time the "fever of sickness" affects man, plants, and animals. When the universe is . . . "cool," then it is believed personal fortunes would be good and men can expect to be in good health and live to the limits of their fate.[15]

The Dusun also fear precipitation that occurs when the sun is shining. Such "hot rain" not only causes fatal fevers and jaundice but the "evil spirits are much in evidence and particularly virulent during showers of the kind."[16]

The Rungus Dusun of Sabah (North Borneo) believe that illicit sexual intercourse creates heat that spreads in "an ever-widening circle involving the couple, their kin, and the community, so that illness and death increase, humans and animals fail to produce, crops wither and die, and the world itself becomes increasingly dry and hot."[17] A major wedding ritual is the sacrifice of a pig to "cool" the marriage; a similar ritual with the same purpose has been reported for other Dusun-speaking groups. Apparently the hot-cold dichotomy among the Dusuns and Kelabit is activated only by illicit sexual relations and the violation of various other mores that causes an abnormal heating or cooling of the universe.

Publications on various primitive Philippine cultural minorities in northern Luzon and Mindanao do not report a hot-cold dichotomy or humoral pathology as part of their concepts of the universe or traditional medicine.[18] Since these societies often retain features once typical of lowland Christian Filipinos, a wide-spread occurrence of these beliefs would have strongly suggested their preHispanic presence in the lowland. In summary, and on the basis of this survey, none of the Southeast Asian nonliterate societies examined in Borneo or the Philippines has a well-developed humoral pathology. Although a hot-cold dichotomy appears among some Bornean groups, no similar complex was found for groups in northern Luzon or Mindanao.

THE HUMORAL PATHOLOGY OF
THE BURMESE AND THAI

The Ayurvedic medical system diffused to Tibet, Mongolia, China, Japan, and Southeast Asia. At the start of this century, this Indian medical system spread from Mongolia to Russia where it is called "Tibetan" since its concepts first reached the Mongols through the Tibetans.[19] Of special concern to this study is the humoral pathology, primarily derived from the Ayurveda, of the Theravada Buddhist Burmese and Thai. Although no thorough study has been made of Burmese humoral pathology, its main contours can be sketched.

Burma

Forchhammer's claim that all Burman science, including medicine, was derived from India has been judged "exaggerated."[20] However, a recent and careful enquiry into folk medicine states that many Burmese medical books are based on translations of the Ayurvedic sumhitās of Susruta and Charaka.[21] The following material indicates that the Burmese humoral pathology absorbed many basic Ayurvedic principles.

Most Burmese believe that the 32 component parts of the body are grouped under five elements (dat): earth (pahtawi), water (abo, apaw or arbaw), fire (teizaw), air or oxygen (wayaw), and ether (agatha).[22] These elements, arranged on the opposite sides of the body, are also patterned differently for males and females. There are three humors (dawthas): wind (lay), bile (thechi), and mucus or phlegm (thalait). One humor may predominate or several may combine to produce disease; each humor may be excessive, retained, scanty, exhausted, or decomposed. Their exact status is determined by the age of the patient, symptoms of the disease, climate, day of the week, etc.[23]

For the Burmese, "Illness comes from throwing the locus and the amount of the elements out of proper combination. ... It is the proper balance of the elementals that is 'health' and disturbances of the balance that are 'ill health,' and medicine is a series of techniques to restore harmony and balance."[24] When the earth *dat* (forming the bones, muscles, etc.) is disturbed, loss of strength, emaciation, and diarrhea results. If the *teizaw* element, or bodily heat, is upset, fever or loss of appetite occurs. Various sicknesses are associated with the days of the week. If one becomes sick on Sunday, the cause is an excessive amount of the earth *dat* that creates an unhealthy state of the fire *dat*.[25]

Various "cold-and-hot-caused diseases" require "balance-restoring" foods and medicines. Traditionally, there are 96 ailments that may result when the body's humoral balance is upset.[26] As a result, most foods eaten in Nondwin and elsewhere in Upper Burma fall into one of four classes. These classes are: (1) *pu, sat,* and *hka* (different kinds of heat); (2) *cho, chin,* and *a* or *e* (different kinds of cold); (3) *sein,* bland taste; and (4) *ngan* and *hpan,* neutral foods.[27] Some foods are classified as both hot (cold) and bland. As in Latin America and the Philippines, a food's category is not necessarily dependent on its physical taste, form, or texture.

Scott described two categories of traditional Burmese curers. One type is *datsayas* (*hsaya,* expert or master), or dietists, who trust solely to regulating the patient's diet for restoration of the humoral equilibrium. The *beindawsayas,* the more numerous of the two, rely upon various drugs for treatment. Sometimes a *hsaya* combines both types of treatments.[28]

Thailand

The *Handbook on Thailand* notes that the Thai supposedly lack a single, consistent theory of the cause of sickness. It is quite possible that the absence of a unitary focus may be a function of our limited knowledge of this aspect of Thai traditional culture. For

> behind much of the diagnosis, explanation and cure of disease is the idea, not always clearly articulated, that the body [and all nature] is composed of the four elements—wind, water, fire and earth—and that sickness results from or is a symptom of imbalance in the proportions or arrangements of these elements. Imbalance of the body's wind is the explanation for fainting; earth in the joints, it is believed, results in rheumatism. Such imbalance may occur through magical or natural causes.[29]

Thai folk medicine, borrowing heavily from the Ayurveda, also has absorbed Chinese elements, but the latter are difficult to document.[30]

There are two sets of Thai terms for the four elements.[31]

1. Air   *Ākāt*
   (wind)   *Lōm*   *Wayo*

2.	Earth	*Din, Thīdin*	*Patawee*
3.	Water	*Nam*	*Ahpo*
4.	Fire	*Fai*	*Dech'o* or *Dach'o*

Patawee is the Sanskrit/*pratiwill* and *wayo* the Sanskrit/*vayul.* The *thī* of *thidīn* comes from Chinese and is the basic term for earth used in Chinese religions. Since Thai words of Indian origin usually begin with the prefix *ah* or *a* (long *a*), *apho* may be a derivative. *Dech'o,* or *dach'o* (Thai, heat, fire, might, or power) is also suspected to be of Sanskrit origin.[32]

Both the Thai and Burmese believe that there are exactly 96 humoral ailments; these disabilities "are the inevitable result of any excess in the amount of any one of the primary elements."[33] Actually, a deficiency of an element may also produce an abnormal equilibrium, resulting in sickness.[34] If fire (or any of the other three elements) penetrates an individual, the excess deranges the healthy balance of the body. The victim becomes ill with fever, measles, smallpox or other ailments. Internal disturbances may also upset the balance of the elements; for example, apoplexy results when the wind element, blowing from all parts of the body, concentrates on the heart.

Illnesses that are difficult to diagnose usually are blamed on the abnormal accumulation or deficiency of wind (or air) in the body.[35] A common expression for sickness among the Thai is: "It is the wind."[36] Thai medication "whether of mineral, vegetable, or animal origin, aims at adding to or taking away from the constitutive elements what they lack or what they have in excess."[37] The four major categories of medicine (with numerous subdivisions) are those associated with fire, water, earth, and wind.[38]

Ayurvedic, Burmese, and Thai traditional medicine accept a causal relationship between the etiology of disease and the seasons, including each month. Each element is associated with certain months; during this period the element's influence predominates. Ailments blamed on excessive heat are more prevalent during the hot (dry) season, whereas those caused by water occur more frequently during the rainy part of the year.

Burmese, Thai, and Malaysians have synthesized with Ayurvedic and Hippocratic concepts the belief that the environmental and other spirits control the four elements of the body, and hence may cause illness by disturbing their balance. These preternatural beings also control the external elements that are directed, for cause, into the victim's body resulting in sickness or death.[40]

> As spirits have control over elements of the world, they may control the elements of the body too. A spirit may cause a disproportion of some bodily element and bring on sickness. When this happens, the thing to do is to exorcise the spirits and expel them by incantation and the sprinkling of holy water which has been blessed by the monk.[41]

In summary, it is obvious that Burmese and Thai humoral pathology borrowed extensively from Ayurvedic doctrine. Available information on these two traditional medical systems is so meager that the probability of Chinese influence can merely be suggested. Sources that assert Chinese influence never offer any documentation. Until detailed field studies are made of Burmese and Thai folk medicine, more precise statements concerning possible relationships with external sources are inappropriate.

It is beyond the scope of this chapter to discuss extensively the agents and techniques by which Indian culture diffused to Southeast Asia, a subject of current dispute among scholars of this region.[42] Preceding sections of this study, however, have indicated (or implied) that in Latin America and parts of Southeast Asia, humoral pathology and Ayurvedic medical concepts were brought to these areas by bearers of the Great Tradition. Yet today these intrusive cultural elements are aspects of the Little Traditions of the rural population.

The spread of Hinduism-Brahmanism into Southeast Asia was basically ". . . an aristocratic process, [whereas] Buddhism involved cultural transfer at the popular levels."[43] Early Brahman immigrants often gained the favor of Southeast Asian nobility with knowledge of their Great Tradition—mythology, law, royal genealogies, ritual, folklore, Sanskrit, etc. They were also involved in the "treatment of illnesses" and the "distribution of curative medicines."[44]

Most aspects of the Great Tradition of India could not have been transmitted to Southeast Asia by the uneducated Dravidians involved in the trading activities between the two regions. However, Ayurvedic medicine probably was, as it is today, widely known in village India—unlike the situation in rural Spain. These Indian sailors and traders, therefore, could have introduced basic Ayurvedic concepts to port city Southeast Asians. However, mastery of the esoteric doctrines of Ayurveda required extensive specialized training and knowledge of the literature; these features of the medical complex must have been brought to Southeast Asia by other agents.

If the Brahmans exposed Southeast Asian nobility to Auyrvedic practices, this elite probably encouraged Ayurvedic specialists to come to their courts as resident physicians. The "Indianization" of Southeast Asia was partly the result of the initiative of Southeast Asians. Furthermore, ". . . Indian medicine could incorporate indigenous anatomical and physiological speculations and each country's recipes for cures [more easily than could] mathematics and other sciences of a universal nature [that] did not lend themselves to local variation."[45]

Ayurvedic knowledge could also have reached members of the Southeast Asian elite through translations of Indian texts. Indian medicine, for example, is traditionally believed to have been introduced into Thailand by Thai translations of the medical treatises of Khomarabhacca who lived during the time of Buddha.[46] If this hypothetical reconstruction of the major modes of transmission of Ayurvedic medicine is valid, the next question is how these concepts diffused outward from the elite and the court circles to the Little Tradition of the villagers.

It is believed that one group of mediators between the Great and Little Traditions in Burma and Thailand were the Buddhist monks. They have always acted, as they do today, as medical therapists. Unlike the aristocratic, pollution-haunted Brahmans, they had intimate contacts not only among local court circles but with the peasants. In addition, Buddhism's introduction to Southeast Asia was mainly "... by South-East Asians, notably Mon monks, who went to Ceylon to study, to collect canonical texts, and to receive orthodox ordination."[47] While in Ceylon they could have been exposed to Ayurvedic specialists and texts whose knowledge they later propagated among the faithful in their homelands.

In summary, it is possible that the religious in both regions, the Buddhist monks in Southeast Asia and the Catholic priests in Latin America, and perhaps also the Philippines, played a crucial role in linking these intrusive elements of the Great Traditions with the Little Traditions of the indigenous populace of the countryside.

References

1. Hart, D. V. 1966. The Filipino villager and his spirits. *Solidarity* 1:66.

2. Hart, D. V.; Rajadhon, P. A.; and Coughlin, R. J. 1965. *Southeast Asian birth customs: Three studies in human reproduction.* New Haven, Conn.: Human Relations Area Files, p. 21.

3. Lieban, R. W. 1967. *Cebuano sorcery: Malign magic in the Philippines.* Berkeley: University of California Press, p. 82.

4. Foster, G. M. 1967. *Tzintzuntzan: Mexican peasants in a changing world.* Boston: Little, Brown & Co., p. 88. Among the items used in the posthole ceremony for new Caticugan residence are small *lag-it* (Ceb. hard and sharp) stones. These stones, always under water in the river, are believed to guarantee that future occupants of the dwelling will have a "watery, cold mind," i.e., will not be quick to anger. Hart, D. V. 1959. *The Cebuan Filipino dwelling in Caticugan: Its construction and cultural aspects.* New Haven, Conn.: Cultural Report Series, Southeast Asia Studies, Yale University, p. 35.

5. Guthrie, G. M.; and Jacobs, P. J. 1966. *Child rearing and personality in the Philippines.* University Park: Pennsylvania State University Press, pp. 130, 132; Hart, D. V.; Rajadhon, P. A.; and Coughlin, R. J. 1965. *Southeast Asian birth customs: Three studies in human reproduction.* New Haven, Conn.: Human Relations Area Files, p. 13; Lieban, R. W. 1967. *Cebuano sorcery: Malign magic in the Philippines.* Berkeley: University of California Press, p. 81; Nurge, E. 1958. Etiology of illness in Guinhangdan. *Am. Anthropologist* 60:1161-1162. In Cagicugan and Lalawigan, a person may become ill when exposed to heat and then subjected to cold, a condition called *pasma.* In Lalawigan air, or wind blowing from the forest, is considered cold, whereas wind coming from the sea is hot.

6. Jocano, F. L. 1969. *Growing up in a Philippine barrio.* New York: Holt, Rinehart & Winston, p. 35.

7. Gillin, J. 1951. *The culture of security in San Carlos: A study of a Guatemalan community of Indians and Ladinos.* New Orleans: Middle American Research Institute, Tulane University, p. 107. Many middle American Indians believe that *aire* may be self-activating or used by the spirits as a vector. Adams, R. N.; and Rubel, A. J. 1967. *Sickness and social relations.* Austin: Institute of Latin American Studies, University of Texas, p. 338. Among Mexican-Americans, good health "... is the result of perfect equilibrium between these internal humors and *aires,* as well as between man and his family, and between man and God." Kiev, A. 1968. *Curanderismo: The Mexican-American folk psychiatry.* New York: The Free Press, pp. 43, 46, 131.

8. Jocano, F. L. 1968. Cultural perception of food and its implication for technological change: A case study. Paper delivered at the seminar on Production of Protein-Rich Foods from Local Sources, Manila.

9. Personal communication from Dr. F. Landa Jocano.

10. Personal communication from Dr. Richard Lieban.

11. Jocano, F. L. 1968. Cultural perception of food and its implication for technological change: A case study. Paper delivered at the seminar on Production of Protein-Rich Foods from Local Sources, Manila, p. 9.

12. Hart, D. V. 1959. *The Cebuan Filipino dwelling in Caticugan: Its construction and cultural aspects.* New Haven, Conn.: Cultural Report Series, Southeast Asia Studies, Yale University, p. 31.

13. Some information on Kelabit was obtained from Professor Harrison through personal correspondence.

14. Harrison, T. 1959. *World within: A Borneo story.* London: Cresset Press, pp. 114-116.

15. Williams, T. 1965. *The Dusun: A North Borneo society.* New York: Holt, Rinehart & Winston, p. 34. If a kite, a red-colored bird (*Haliastur indus*), lights on an unfinished Dusun dwelling, the house is doomed supernaturally to destruction by the " 'red-hot' ... quality inherent and conducted by the bird." Harrison, T. 1960. Birds and men in Borneo. In Smythies, B. E. *The birds of Borneo.* Edinburgh: Oliver & Boyd, p. 23.

16. Evans, I. H. N. 1923. *Studies in religion, folk-lore and custom in British North Borneo and the Malay Peninsula.* Cambridge, Mass.: Cambridge University Press, p. 175. The Negritos and Semai of Malaya share this belief. Williams-Hunt, P. D. R. 1952. *An introduction to Malayan Aborigines.* Kuala Lumpur: Government Printing House, pp. 64, 72; and Dentan, R. K. 1968. *The Semai: A nonviolent people of Malaya.* New York: Holt, Rinehart & Winston, pp. 20-21. Dentan thinks the Semai concept of "hot rain" may be of Malayan origin. Also see Appell, G. N. 1968. A survey of the social and medical anthropology of Sabah: Retrospect and prospect. *Behav. Sci. Notes* 3:1-54.

17. Appell, G. N.; and Harrison, R. 1969. The ethnographic classification of Dusun-speaking peoples of North Borneo. *Ethnology* 8:222. In a personal communication, Professor Appell added that if the people of a village suffer from an unusual number of colds, others may jokingly remark that the village is hot; if there is little sickness in the community, it is said to be cool. Alien traditions with the strongest impact on the Dusun-speaking people are, in order, Chinese, coastal Islam, and Western. No archeological evidence has been found of Indian influence. Appell, G. N.; and Harrison, R. 1969. The ethnographic classification of Dusun-speaking peoples of North Borneo. *Ethnology* 8:213.

18. Of special assistance in this research for the Philippines was Saito, S. 1967. *A preliminary bibliography of Philippine ethnography.* Manila: Ateneo de Manila (mimeographed). Also see Villegas, A. 1923. Primitive medicine in the Philippines. *Ann. Med. Hist.* 5:229-241. Professor Eggan reported these concepts were unknown among primitive groups he studied in north-central Luzon. Also see Guthrie, G. M. 1964. *Impressions of Ifuago health and social activities.* University Park: Pennsylvania State University (mimeographed).

19. Filliozat, J. 1946. *The classical doctrine of Indian medicine: Its origins and its Greek parallels* (trans. from French by Dev Raj Chanana). Delhi, India: Munshiram Manoharlal, p. 30.

20. Forchhammer, E. 1885. *An essay on the sources and the development of Burmese law.* Rangoon: Government Printing, p. 21; and Spiro, M. F. 1967. *Burmese supernaturalism: A study in the explanation and reduction of suffering.* Englewood Cliffs, N.J.: Prentice-Hall, Inc., p. 148. Although the Persians and Arabs had direct, if limited, commercial contacts with Lower Burma as early as the 9th century, it appears unlikely they contributed any of their medical knowledge to the Burmese. Khan, M. S. 1936. Muslim intercourse with Burma: From the earliest times to the British conquest. *Islamic Culture* 10:409-427.

21. *Report of the Committee on Enquiry into the indigeneous system of medicine.* 1951. Rangoon: Government Printing & Stationery, p. 5.

22. Nash, M. 1965. *The golden road to modernity: Village life in comtemporary Burma.* New York: John Wiley & Sons, Inc., p. 193. Scott lists the same elements but adds that ether was usually disregarded by traditional curers. Scott, J. (Shway Joe). 1910. *The Burman: His life and notions.* London: Macmillan, Inc., p. 418. Another source states a fifth *dat,* as *ākāśa,* or the organs of the senses, e.g., eyes, ears, nose, etc. *Report of the Committee of Enquiry into the indigeneous system of medicine.* 1951. Rangoon: Government Printing & Stationery, p. 16. This term is identical with the Sanskrit term for space or emptiness (*akāśa* or *antariksa*), known in Burmese as *agatha.* Filliozat, J. 1946. *The classical doctrine of Indian medicine: Its origins and its Greek parallels* (trans. from French by Dev Raj Chanana). Dehli, India: Munshiram Manoharlal, p. 26. The Sanskrit term for wind or air is *vāyu*; fire, *tejas*; water, *ap*; and earth, *prthvī.*

23. *Report of the Committee of Enquiry into the indigeneous system of medicine.* 1951. Rangoon: Government Printing & Stationery, p. 17. Scott adds

that "... it is important to know in what proportion the *dat* should be present." Scott, J. (Shway Joe). 1910. *The Burman: His life and notions.* London: Macmillan, Inc., p. 418.

24. Nash, M. 1965. *The golden road to modernity: Village life in contemporary Burma.* New York: John Wiley & Sons, Inc., p. 194. Also see Hart, E. 1897. *Picturesque Burma: Past and present.* London: J. M. Dent, p. 180. It appears that traditional Laotian medicine also is based on a humoral pathology basis for their concept of disease includes the idea analogous "to the humors of European physicians a few centuries ago." Laotians believe the body is composed of such basic elements as air, water, and fire. Stomach ache is diagnosed as trouble with the air element, whereas fever occurs "because the fire element is too strong." Halpern, J. M. *Laotian health problems.* Los Angeles: University of California, Department of Anthropology (Paper No. 19), nid., p. 20.

25. MacDonald, K. N. 1878. *The practice of medicine among the Burmese translated from original manuscripts, with an historical sketch on the progress of medicine, from earliest times.* Edinburgh: MacLachlan & Stewart, p. 22.

26. Hart, E. 1897. *Picturesque Burma: Past and present.* London: J. M. Dent, p. 180.

27. Nash, M. 1965. *The golden road to modernity: Village life in contemporary Burma.* New York: John Wiley & Sons, Inc., p. 195. Nash lists the classification of more than 50 Burmese foods. The Judson Burmese-English dictionary gives somewhat modified definitions of some of these terms. *Pu* and *sat* are hot, but the former is hot, in the sense of warmth, whereas the latter is hot, in taste or pungency. *Hka,* defined as bitter, could be associated with hot. Nash states *cho, chin* and *a* (or *e*) are different kinds of cold; the dictionary defines *cho* as sweet, *chin* as sour and *a* (or *e*) as cold. Nash defines *sein* as a bland taste, the dictionary gives raw. Although *ngan* and *hpan* are listed as neutral foods, their dictionary definitions are salty and astringent (slight sour). Adoniram Judson, A. 1921. *The Judson Burmese-English dictionary* (rev. and ed. by Robert C. Stevenson, rev. and ed. by F. H. Eveleth). Rangoon: American Baptist Missionary Press, pp. 644, 355, 371, 299, 287, 158, 375, 322, and 684.

28. Scott, J. (Shway Joe). 1910. *The Burman: His life and notions.* London: Macmillan, Inc., p. 418; *Report of the Committee of Enquiry into the indigeneous system of medicine.* 1951. Rangoon: Government Printing & Stationery, p. 16.

29. Sharp, L., editor. 1956. *Handbook on Thailand.* New Haven, Conn.: HRAF, p. 489; Young, E. 1900. *The kingdom of the yellow robe: Being sketches of the domestic and religious rites and ceremonies of the Siamese.* Westminster: Archibald Constable, p. 122; Bradley, D. B. 1967. Siamese theory and practice of medicine. *Sangkhomsat Parithat* 5:103 (reprinted from *Bangkok calendar,* 1865).

30. Landon, K. R. 1939. *Thailand in transition: A brief survey of cultural trends in the five years since the revolution of 1932.* Chicago: University of Chicago Press (distributor), pp. 139-140.

31. The Thai terms in the second column are honorific words, whereas those

in the first column are ordinary Thai. Bradley, D. B. 1967. Siamese theory and practice of medicine. *Sangkhomsat Parithat* 5:104 (reprinted from *Bangkok Calendar,* 1865).

32. Cabaton, A. Siam. In Hastings, J., editor. 1921. *Encyclopedia of religion and ethics.* New York: Charles Scribner's Sons, pp. 11, 484.

33. Young, E. 1900. *The kingdom of the yellow robe: Being sketches of the domestic and religious rites and ceremonies of the Siamese.* Westminster: Archbald Constable, p. 122.

34. Bradley, D. B. 1967. Siamese theory and practice of medicine. *Sangkhomsat Parithat* 5:104.

35. Young, E. 1900. *The kingdom of the yellow robe: Being sketches of the domestic and religious rites and ceremonies of the Siamese.* Westminster: Archbald Constable, p. 122; Bradley, D. B. 1967. Siamese theory and practices of medicine. *Sangkhomsat Parithat* 5:104.

36. Langdon, K. R. 1939. *Thailand in transition: A brief survey of cultural trends in the five years since the revolution of 1932.* Chicago: University of Chicago Press (distributor), p. 140.

37. Cabaton, A. Siam. In Hastings, J., editor, 1921. *Encyclopedia of religion and ethics.* New York: Charles Scribner's Sons, p. 484.

38. Bradley, D. B. 1967. Siamese theory and practice of medicine. *Sangkhomsat Parithat* 5:105.

39. Hofauer, R. 1943. A medical retrospect of Thailand. *J. Thailand Res. Soc.* 34:193ff; Bradley, D. B. 1967. Siamese theory and practice of medicine. *Sangkhomsat Parithat* 5:103.

40. Bradley, D. B. 1967. Siamese theory and practice of medicine. *Sangkhomsat Parithat* 5:104-105; Harris, G. L., et al. 1966. *Area handbook for Thailand.* Washington, D.C.: U.S. Government Printing Office, p. 259.

41. Landon, K. R. 1949. *Southeast Asia: Crossroad of religions.* Chicago: University of Chicago Press, p. 27. The Thai "attribute the non-equilibrium of the four elements and hence their illnesses to spirits, and consult the sourcerer rather than the doctor; besides the sorcerer often the ordinary doctor." Cabaton, A. Siam. In Hastings, J., editor. 1921. *Encyclopedia of religion and ethics.* New York: Charles Scribner's Sons, p. 484.

42. Hall, D. G. E. 1964. *A history of South-East Asia.* London: Macmillan, Inc., pp. 17-18; Hall, D. G. E. 1966-1967. Recent tendencies in the study of the early history of South-East Asia. *Pacific Affairs* 39:339-348; Cody, J. F. 1964. *Southeast Asia: Its historical development.* New York: McGraw-Hill Book Co., pp. 41-44; Coedès, G. 1967. *The making of South East Asia* (trans. by H. M. Wright). Berkeley: University of California Press, pp. 54-55.

43. Cody, J. F. 1964. Southeast Asia: Its historical development. New York: McGraw-Hill Book Co., p. 43.

44. Ferrard, G. 1919. Le K'oven-louen, et les anciennes navigations inter-oceaniques dans les mers du Sud. *J. Asiatique.* Cited by Coèdes, G. 1968. *The*

Indianized states of Southeast Asia (ed. by W. F. Vella; trans. by Susan Brown Cowing). Honolulu: East-West Center Press, p. 22.

45. Coèdes, G. 1967. *Making of South East Asia.* (trans. by H. M. Wright). Berkeley: University of California Press, p. 226.

46. Cabaton, A. Siam. In Hastings, J., editor. 1921. *Encyclopedia of religion and ethics.* New York: Charles Scribner's Sons, p. 484. Khomarabhacca wrote under the name Rokhanithan.

47. Hall, D. G. E. 1964. *A History of South-East Asia.* London: Macmillan, Inc. p. 22. Also see Leslie, C. 1967. Professional and popular health cultures in South Asia: Needed research in medical sociology and anthropology. In Morehouse, W., editor. *Understanding science and technology in India and Pakistan.* Albany: Foreign Area Materials Center, University of the State of New York, pp. 27-42.

11

Health Care of the Chinese in America

Teresa Campbell, M.S.
Betty Chang, R.N., D.N.S.

Teresa Campbell is a Professor of Nursing at San Francisco State University. She has taught community health nursing in an urban setting for eighteen years. Her research and publications have focused on transcultural health care, as well as a variety of other topics. From 1959 to 1960, she served as a nurse on the S.S. Hope *in Indonesia and Vietnam.*

Betty L. Chang is an Assistant Professor in the School of Nursing, University of California, Los Angeles, where she teaches in the graduate medical-surgical clinical specialist program. Her research and published work have dealt with the relationships between Asian-American ethnicity and health care, and various aspects of health care of the elderly, particularly the evaluation of health care from the clients' perspective. Her clinical practice has involved patient care in a variety of settings, including coronary care units, acute medical-surgical units, pediatrics, rehabilitation, and skilled nursing facilities.

Source: From Campbell, T.; and Chang, B. Health care of the Chinese in America. *Nurs. Outlook* 21:245-249. Copyright © 1973, American Journal of Nursing Company. Reproduced with permission, from *Nursing Outlook.* April, 1973, Vol. 21, No. 4.

Chinese people in America prefer to work in restaurants, laundries, and sewing shops; they have a low rate of juvenile delinquency; they always take care of their own; they are "inscrutable." These stereotypes are about as far as most non-Asians go in thinking about the Chinese who live in this country. Their superficial ideas result from limited personal contact and from a paucity of literature on this group.

The stereotypes are rooted, in fact, in the history of the Chinese people's adjustment to an alien society. During the settlement in America, as an example, the Chinese handled racial hostility by developing businesses and seeking employment where there was little competition from the white population. Today, many new immigrants, although better educated than their predecessors, are limited by language and continue to seek menial jobs in the restaurants, laundries, and sewing shops of Chinatown. This does not mean, however, that such occupations are part of their "culture."

Similarly, the fact that for many years the Chinese enclaves in American cities were populated by men fostered the myth of a low juvenile delinquency rate. (The Exclusion Act of 1924 prevented the entry of Chinese women into this country.) However, the arrival of Chinese wives starting in 1965 changed the composition of Chinese families and increased the number of Chinese youths in the United States. Today, the delinquency among the young in Chinese communities is a serious problem.

In China before the revolution, the lineage and clan, as well as numerous specialized associations, were the means for fulfilling the social needs of the individual in the village. When Chinese first entered this country over 100 years ago, they established the same type of formal groups they had known at home—the family name associations, tongs, and benevolent associations—to meet their social welfare needs. However, their increasing social and health problems now demonstrate that without help the Chinese can no longer "take care of their own." Among their health problems are a high incidence of visual problems, immunization deficiencies, and dental caries; in San Francisco the tuberculosis rate among Chinese is three to four times that of the city as a whole.[1] In addition, the environmental conditions in San Francisco are particularly poor, with a very high population density—often whole families living in two rooms and sharing a community toilet facility and kitchen with other families.

The legend of "inscrutability" may derive from different orientations to body language. An observer of one nationality, for instance, may see things in body language that are completely missed by someone of a different nationality.[2]

Because of this and other differences in cultural orientation, health professionals would ideally belong to the same ethnic group as the population they serve. If this is not feasible, a knowledge of customs and culture will help any health worker serve more effectively. Certainly a knowledge of Chinese folk medicine and health practices, attitudes, and beliefs as they are manifested by the Chinese in America is very important.

The number of Chinese people in this country is relatively small—a little over

435,000, according to the 1970 census. Most of them live in the urban central city, mainly in the western states, although the largest Chinese-American community (over 69,000) is in New York City. San Francisco runs a close second.

Population statistics, however, should be of little concern to the nurse caring for a Chinese-American patient or family; no matter how few members of this ethnic group she sees, she needs the health-related information.

THREE MAIN GROUPS

The Chinese people in this country fall into three main groups: (1) individuals who were born in China and immigrated from rural villages 40 to 50 years ago—they are the strongest believers in Chinese folk medicine and continue to influence the health practices of their immediate families; (2) new immigrants who have arrived over the past 20 years from a number of Asian countries and Hong Kong; and (3) first- and second-generation American born Chinese. Members of this last group, while oriented to Western medicine, bow to the pressures of their elders in practices of folk medicine. One young pregnant Chinese woman who was a registered nurse, for instance, routinely followed her obstetrician's orders, but at the same time, under pressure from her mother and mother-in-law, ate special foods and herbs to insure birth of a healthy baby.

Chinese folk medicine evolved from an Eastern philosophy which holds that the elemental forces controlling the universe pervade all aspects of human endeavor. The universe is thought of as a vast entity, each organism in it conceived as an open system that interacts and is affected by others in the universe. The energy for regulating the universe is composed of two opposing forces, the Yin and the Yang.

YIN AND YANG

The Yin represents the female, negative force: darkness, cold and emptiness. The Yang represents the male and positive force, producing light, warmth, and fullness. All things or beings in the universe consist of a Yin and a Yang, and if peace and harmony in society and health in the mind and body are to be maintained, the two energy forces must be in perfect balance. An imbalance is thought to cause catastrophe and illness.

The Yin and Yang energy forces are embodied in the autonomic nervous system as elsewhere in the body. Thus, the sympathetic system responds to stress by mobilizing the body for defensive action, much as the Yang is said to protect the body from outside infiltrations. An excess of Yang causes fever, dehydration, irritability, and tenseness.

In contrast, the parasympathetic system is generally concerned with restoring and conserving body energy and controlling the digestive process, and Yin is thought to store the vital strength of life. A person with too much Yin catches cold easily, is nervous, apprehensive, and predisposed to gastric disorders. Further, various parts of the body correspond to principles of Yin and Yang. For example, the body surface is Yang; inside is Yin. Some organs are Yang; others are Yin.

When a Chinese person is ill, he may go to a Western doctor or to a practitioner of Chinese medicine. Or he may see both. The Chinese specialist will be an acupuncturist, an herb pharmacist, or an herbalist, whose treatments often overlap and duplicate each other.

The herbalist diagnoses by interrogating, observing color, tongue, and perspiration, listening to sounds of the body and taking the pulse. He will then formulate a prescription of herbs that either he will fill directly or that can be filled by the herb pharmacist. A patient may also go directly to the herb pharmacist, tell him his symptoms or what he wants, and receive a prescription.

An acupuncturist will use basically the same procedure as the herbalist for making a diagnosis. He then treats the patient by inserting fine needles into a number of the 365 body points where channels or ducts called meridians extend internally. Acupuncture is gaining in popularity in San Francisco and was recently included as acceptable treatment by Teamster Local 856 for medical insurance coverage.

CHINESE VS WESTERN MEDICINE

Some persons believe that Western medicine is for Westerners and Chinese medicine is for Chinese. Others think that Western medicine is best for some diseases, like tuberculosis, but that Chinese medicine is more effective for skin diseases and blood disorders. Still others believe that a combination of both provides the best treatment. Therefore, the professional health worker should encourage a Chinese patient to let his Western doctor know what medication he is receiving from his herbalist. Herb prescriptions may contain the same chamical ingredients as Western medicine and might result in an overdose or adverse reaction in the patient. For instance, Ma Huang, or Chinese ephedra, a major source of ephedrine, is an herb used in the treatment of pulmonary disease. Ginseng, one of the most commonly used herbs, is viewed in Chinese folk medicine as a panacea. However, it is classified by many Western physicians as a tonic-stimulant and its use is contraindicated in hypertension.[3]

Chinese patients frequently switch doctors and herbalists and may see two or three during the same period. This shopping around for doctors is an attempt to find the most promising cure. It is important for the health professional to know what medication the patient is receiving from each doctor, and the patient must give this information to his doctors. But a Chinese patient is often reluctant to tell his doctor directly that he is seeing another one for fear that the doctor will "lose face."

The professional in such a situation can obtain the patient's permission to let him tell the doctor, and it is important to have the permission. Irreversible distrust developed in one family toward a community health worker who, without the family's knowledge, told the doctor that his patient was seeing another doctor as well.

One conflict between Chinese folk medicine and Western medical practice is medication. Increasingly, Chinese people are recognizing the value of Western drugs, but they continue to use herbs for certain ailments as they see fit. And the health worker cannot always justify one type of medicine over the other. A diabetic woman, for instance, refused to continue taking her oral hypoglycemic agent and, instead, started taking a medicine prescribed by an herbalist. On later home visits, the health worker found that the patient's urine tested negative on the Clinitest, her arthritic pain had diminished, and she seemed to be progressing without any apparent problems related to her diabetes.

SOME DIFFERENCES

An important difference between Western medicine and Chinese folk medicine is the administration of medication. When a patient receives one dose of a prescription from an herbalist for instance, he is told to return if he doesn't feel better—one dose of any correct medication should cure him. And so the patient has difficulty comprehending why Western doctors give so many pills to be taken over a long period. The health professional working with a Chinese patient must help him understand that there is a difference between Western medicine and Chinese medicine. Concrete illustrations help. If the patient's blood pressure has stabilized, for instance, the health worker can explain how the medicine he is taking has helped.

Another difference is the form of the medication. A Chinese person boils the herbs he has received from the herb pharmacist in the amount of water and for the time prescribed to get the right concentration of broth. Liquid medications cleanse the intestines, stimulate the circulation, and restore the balance between Yin and Yang. Why is Western medicine dispensed in pills or capsules and with few directions?

The health professional again must explain that Western medicine is different from Chinese medicine—that it comes in different forms and must be taken over a longer time. He can also explain that just as herb broth comes in child and adult doses, so, too, does Western medicine. If one pill is for the treatment of a child, then two pills may be necessary to treat an adult.

CHECKING THE MEDICATIONS

Some Chinese keep all the medicine they have received and take it at their own discretion at various times for numerous ailments. They also tend to borrow and loan medications at will. The health worker visiting in the home should ask to see all the medications the patient has and learn which ones he is taking. Although he can try to persuade the patient to dispose of all old medications or let the professional destroy them, he is usually not successful. As an alternative, he should have the patient take the medications to the doctor.

It is clear from these examples that extensive health teaching and supervision is necessary to help Chinese believers of folk medicine understand the correct use of Western medicine.

FOOD AND DISEASE

Food is thought to play a part in the cause and treatment of diseases. In Chinese philosophy, *chi* (literally, "air," "breath," or "wind") is an energy present in all living organisms. Food, when metabolized, is transformed into *chi* and becomes either a cold Yin energy force or a hot Yang energy force. Illnesses caused by Yin excesses are treated by hot foods; those caused by Yang excesses are treated by cold foods. The symbol of Yin and Yang is [shown in Fig. 11-1].

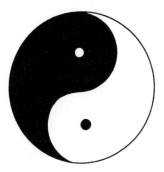

Figure 11-1. Yin and Yang symbol.

This theory is demonstrated in the following instances. Cancer is viewed as a cold disease. When a Chinese child in a large San Francisco hospital was diagnosed as having leukemia, the mother immediately asked the Chinese student nurse whether it resulted from improper eating—possibly too many cold foods in the diet. In another situation, a Chinese patient suffering from an ear infection, a hot disease, refused scrambled eggs, a hot food, because a hot illness needs to be treated with cold foods such as wintermelon. The common ginger root is believed to be a hot food and is used to strengthen the heart (Yang organ) and to prevent and treat nausea and dyspepsia (Yin excess disorders).

The knowledge of hot and cold foods is passed down in the family by tradition and practice. At present, there is no complete listing of hot and cold foods. A health professional in an institution might encourage family members to bring in Chinese dishes which support the Yin and Yang beliefs if the foods are not contraindicated.

FOOD HABITS AND NUTRITION

Like those in any other ethnic group, Chinese have definite food preferences based on cultural eating patterns. A health professional needs to be alert to food patterns so that a therapeutic diet compatible with the patient's beliefs and preferences can be selected. Some older Chinese, for instance, believe that drinking ice water shocks the system and is harmful to health. Also, because of a history of inadequate sanitation in China, Chinese have habitually boiled their drinking water.

As a result, many Chinese prefer to drink hot water, which is often brought to the hospital in a Thermos by their families. If there is no family to bring a Thermos to a patient, the professional might inquire if the patient would like hot drinking water.

Similar unsanitary conditions have made raw vegetables generally unacceptable to Chinese from overseas, where organic fertilizer was used. Uncooked vegetables caused illnesses, and, as a result, eating them has not been a regular part of the dietary pattern.

Then, too, milk and milk products have been scarce in the Far Eastern countries, and people's taste for them may not have developed. Thus, they tend to dislike foods containing milk or milk products—particularly in dishes like cheese and creamed foods where the milk or cream flavors is not disguised. In diets that call for a higher intake of calcium, health professionals can suggest modifications or substitutes: custards are usually well-liked, and milk with Ovaltine, or simply warm milk with sugar added. Green leafy vegetables also contribute a large part of the total calcium in the diet.

Another example is rare beef, which may not be acceptable, since in most Chinese foods beef is cooked until the blood is no longer apparent. The health professional can list for the dietition all the various food likes and dislikes of the patient, so that meals can be as appetizing as possible.

It is common knowledge that the preparation of Chinese food requires soy sauce. Its high sodium content makes it a problem in restricted-sodium diets, for experience has shown that it is useless to instruct the patient to eliminate soy sauce. Greater success has been attained by having the patient measure and limit the amount of soy sauce for cooking. He should also avoid dried, salted, or preserved foods. The San Francisco Heart Association has diet instructions and sample menus printed in Chinese and English for Chinese patients on restricted-sodium diets.

FOOD SUBSTITUTIONS

Although health professionals are knowledgeable about the "basic four" in nutrition, they need to know about using food substitutions for a Chinese diet. One such is the versatile tofu, a soybean curd made by precipitating protein of soybean milk by the use of calcium or magnesium salts. Tofu is a commonly used food in the Chinese diet that is a good source of protein, relatively high in iron, and if made with calcium salts can contribute a considerable amount of calcium, which is often deficient in the Chinese diet. A 2-inch cube portion of tofu can substitute for a protein equivalency of two to three ounces of hamburger, or two eggs.

Half a cup of rice or *mein* (Chinese noodles) can be substituted for one slice of bread or a serving of potatoes. In a diabetic diet, Oriental foods can take the place of Western foods, which may not be familiar to the patient. Emphasis should be placed on approximate portions of meats and starches rather than exact measurements. There are relatively few concentrated sweets in the Chinese diet, so eliminating them is not a problem for most Chinese persons with diabetes.

CARE DURING PREGNANCY

Folk medicine practices during the childbearing periods are assiduously enforced in many Chinese families. Practices vary from family to family. For instance, some Chinese women avoid excessive use of soy sauce during pregnancy so that the baby will not be too dark. Shellfish during the first trimester may be shunned in the belief that the baby will thus be prevented from developing allergies later in life. Some young women refuse to take iron supplements because they think that the iron will harden the bones and make delivery difficult. During the seventh and eighth months of pregnancy, ginseng is sometimes taken as a general tonic to strengthen the expectant mother.

The health professional supervising the care of a Chinese family may acknowledge that these are indeed the family's practices and help by suggesting some scientifically based health measures that are not in conflict with folk medicine beliefs. Eating foods from the family's usual diet that are high in calcium and iron can be stressed.

Major conflict with Western medicine occurs during the postpartum period when the health professionals' recommendations are incompatible with principles of Yin and Yang. The traditional postpartum convalescence consists of a one-month period during which the new mother's dietary and health practices are directed toward decreasing the Yin energy forces or cold air in the body. The pores are believed to remain open for 30 days postpartum, during which time cold air can enter the body.

As a result, a new Chinese mother is forbidden to go outdoors or to take a shower or tub bath. The health professional can demonstrate an understanding of the Chinese mother's beliefs and support her in continuing with sponge baths, emphasizing pericare, breast care, and other activities contributing to her total comfort and well-being.

The classical Chinese postpartum diet is high in hot foods. Most fruits and vegetables, considered cold, are avoided. Basic mainstay of a postpartum and lactating diet generally consists of rice and eggs and a chicken soup containing pig knuckles, vinegar ginger, rice wine, and sometimes peanuts. Because the vinegar in the soup helps to transfer tricalcium phosphate from the bone of pig knuckles into solution, the traditional soup may supply some of the calcium essential in the diets of postpartum and lactating women. The alcohol in the rice wine may stimulate bleeding, and its addition should be postponed for at least two weeks postpartum.

The health professional can be supportive to the new mother who eats this soup but should encourage her to supplement her diet with other foods that are culturally acceptable as well as nutritious, such as eggs, meat or liver.

IN THE HOSPITAL

Members of the Chinese community are most reluctant to be admitted to hospitals. They feel: (1) hospitals are unclean and individuals die there; (2) there will be no one to translate for them; (3) surgery, considered very mutilating, may occur; (4) a patient's spirit may get lost and be unable to find its way home; and (5) Chinese food will not be served. Ideally, Chinese patients would be admitted to hospitals staffed by Chinese-speaking professionals, but this is seldom possible. Bilingual family members, however, can be encouraged to remain with the non-English-speaking patient.

The importance of having an interpreter at hand was made clear when one young Chinese woman who attempted suicide was admitted to the emergency room of a large hospital. The non-Asian doctors examined her and sutured her lacerated wrists, but because of the language barrier, they did not discover until later that she had also swallowed poison.

When a Chinese person is admitted to a hospital, his family usually leaves some valuable jewelry on him for status, and some jade for good luck. To avoid loss, family members should be encouraged to take all jewelry with them.

Elderly Chinese patients may have large amounts of money hidden in the linings of their clothing. The nurse should see that some member of the family removes most clothing until the day the patient is to be discharged. If a patient dies in the hospital, the family may then be reluctant to accept his clothing, for it is considered to contain evil spirits. Or the family may return later and request all or part of the deceased person's clothing. The health professional should therefore itemize the clothing of the deceased and keep it in a safe place.

UNDERSTANDING EACH OTHER

Health professionals frequently label the practitioners of Chinese folk medicine ignorant and superstitious. In turn, the practitioners of Chinese folk medicine frequently reject Western medicine because it is alien to their basic philosophy and beliefs. Better understanding of Chinese folk medicine by health professionals will contribute to the acceptance of health care by a portion of our community which is still for the most part not reached.

References

1. Chinatown U.S.A. 1970. *Calif. Health* 2:27-28.
2. Fast, J. 1971. *Body language*. New York: Pocket Books, p. 157.
3. Zacharoff, L. Feb. 2, 1972. A new look at ginseng. *San Francisco Examiner Chronicle*, p. 5.

Part II Review

SUMMARY

The growing debate between health care providers who support folk healers and those who support scientific practitioners is not unlike the old rural-urban debate in sociology. It may be helpful to review that argument as a means of placing folk and orthodox medicine in a proper transcultural perspective.

Rural-Urban Dichotomies

Romantic conceptualizations assign different values to rural (folk) and urban (scientific) communities. Some individuals maintain idyllic images of rural life. "Rural" conjures up the smell of freshly mown fields, herds of cattle or sheep, fields of crops, a country store, and farmers in blue jeans. From this perspective the Third World indigenous curer is the prototype of the sturdy, independent person in a natural, unspoiled environment. Conversely, urban life is viewed as unnatural and, indeed, bad.

On the other hand, there are those who view the city as the center of civilization, the epitome of progress and the good life. From this perspective, the urban dweller is the prototype of a truly civilized person. Unlike Rousseau, who viewed rural people as "noble savages," critics of rural life label rural people as "country bumpkins" who do not share in the richness of culture found in urban areas. Even the urban Third World curer is viewed as someone slightly removed from the Neanderthal man.

Somewhere between these two extremes is a more accurate picture of rural and urban life. In terms of life styles, there is much similarity between urban-oriented and rural-oriented people. Both share and are influenced by the products of urbanization. Both have been enculturated in a country that has strong folk cultures, but folk cultures do not yield willingly to technology. Before the introduction of rapid transportation, mass communication, and other intrusions of urban culture into rural communities, villages and small towns were isolated very much like Washington Irving's Sleepy Hollow. There was an overriding sense of independence, on the one hand, and ethnic solidarity, on the other. The range of interaction was restricted primarily to the rural community. This set of circumstances resulted in community efforts to retain folk beliefs and practices while fueling prejudice against outsiders and new medical beliefs and practices. Contact with the outside was intermittent and slow coming, but once contact was established through explorers, exploiters, and churches, folk beliefs and practices were altered forever.

New Forms of Medical Care

It is erroneous to cling to the stereotype of the traditional curer who, according to George Foster and Barbara Anderson:

> Is known to us all: a wise and skilled person who knows not only the patient but also the family, who is aware of the social and personal tensions of the patient's life, who sees relief from interpersonal stress as essential to relief from physical symptoms. The stereotypic curer is, in short, a social pathologist, able and willing to spend unlimited time with a single patient, little concerned with payment.[1]

A few of these types still exist in both indigenous and scientific health care systems, but most care givers are very much concerned with remuneration for their services. For example, Irwin Press notes that urban *curanderos* in Bogotá use techniques identified with both traditional folk and modern medical sources.[2] Many of the curers that Press observed scheduled as many as 70 patients a day, and each visit lasted less than 15 minutes. With few exceptions, the Bogotá curers charged fees—some of them quite high.

The behavior of Third World patients is also changing. Many of them utilize the services of curers in two or more medical systems. Sometimes this is done simultaneously. The reason for this behavior is simple; they want a wide and, hopefully, sound variety of opinions and advice to select from. It is not uncommon for persons in all ethnic groups—Third World and non-Third World—to try one curer after another to secure effective treatment. Nor is this sampling process limited to indigenous curers. Western health personnel also are consulted about problems in which they are believed to have expertise.

The process of shopping around for curers and patronizing indigenous curers and modern medical personnel is occurring throughout the world. For example, this behavior has been documented in several Third World communities, including Taipei, Kota, Hong Kong, Bankok, Bono, and Pustunich.[3-8] Closer to home, Robert Edgerton and coauthors studied *curanderismo* in East Los Angeles and concluded that in spite of a long tradition, "its importance has diminished greatly. Both ethnographic observations and formal interviews indicate that for Mexican-Americans in East Los Angeles, the preferred treatment resource for mental illness is the general physician, not the curandero."[9] From these data we can surmise that when effective medical treatment is available in Western systems, is delivered by empathic persons at a price Third World people can afford and at convenient times and places, it will be the first choice for many and perhaps most persons.[10]

Aware of these trends, a growing number of traditional curers are engaging in a process that David Landy called "role adaptation"–the process of updating traditional therapies by incorporating elements of scientific medicine.[11] Role adaptation involves a wide range of behavior. Some curers convert almost completely to a Western system of behavior; others select only those elements that will preserve their status while at the same time minimally altering their behavior. In any case, the pattern of the interrelationship between traditional medicine and modern medicine appears to be universal and irreversible. Thus, all health care systems must meet the needs of Third World and Western people.

Integration or Pluralism

Whether or not to integrate into Western society is a question that most Third World people ponder. This is an especially sensitive issue for indigenous curers. The dilemma is somewhat similar to that of the early European immigrants to the United States. When they initially came to this country during the nineteenth century, the Poles, Greeks, Germans, Italians, and other groups clustered together in their own ethnic enclaves. Gradually, either they or their children moved out of their ethnic neighborhoods into the larger community. Along with this change came a merging of languages, customs, habits, dietary patterns, and medical practices.

While the European ethnic groups were assimilating into a nebulous American melting pot, Third World people present at that time were not assimilated. Some Third World activists argue that pluralism, not assimilation, is the most viable goal for Third World people. Switzerland is an example of pluralism that may be the most acceptable to Third World and non-Third World people:

> The standard example of cultural pluralism is Switzerland, a country that maintains a high degree of national unity although it has no national language and is religiously divided. In Switzerland, Protestants and Catholics have been able to live agreeably under the same government, while speaking either German, French, or Italian. Since the Swiss citizen does not feel that either his religious loyalty or his ethnic identification is threatened by other Swiss, he is free to give complete allegiance to the Swiss nation as a common government that allows for the tolerance of distinctly different cultural groups. Canada, with a division between the French and the English, and Belgium, with a division between the French and the Flemish-speaking populace, are other examples of cultural pluralism. The different groups that make up a pluralistic society in these nations frequently engage in a struggle for influence, but the essential ideal is that national patriotism does not require cultural uniformity and that differences of nationality, language, or even race do not preclude loyalty to a common government.[12]

Within a similar framework it would be possible for Third World people to adopt Western medicine without losing other aspects of their ethnicity. If this is not possible, what happens to individuals who, against strong community injunctions, maintain their traditional medical beliefs and practices?

The intracommunity health care conflicts have left many Third World people, especially curers, feeling marginal. According to Robert E. Park, the marginal person is one whom fate has condemned to live in two societies and in two, not merely different but, antagonistic cultures.[13] Although Park used the term "fate" in his definition, we consider marginality to be the result of a complex social system. As such, marginality is not the result of accidental phenomena but predictable occurrences within a social framework. One may or may not feel "condemned." Or, as Milton M. Goldberg observed, if:

> (1) The so-called "marginal" individual is conditioned to his existence on the borders of two cultures from birth, if (2) he shares this existence and conditioning process with a large number of individuals in his primary groups, if (3) his years of early growth, maturation and even adulthood find him participating in institutional activities manned largely by other "marginal" individuals like himself, and finally, if (4) his marginal position results in no major blockages or frustrations of his learned expectations and desires, then he is not a true "marginal" individual in the defined sense, but a participant member of a *marginal culture,* every bit as real and complete to him as the non-marginal culture to the nonmarginal man.[14]

Medical marginality, therefore, is characterized by the following conditions. First, there must be a situation that places two medical systems in lasting contact. Second, one system must be dominant in terms of legal and political power. This is the nonmarginal of the two systems. Its members are not particularly influenced by or attracted to the marginal system. Third, the boundaries between the two systems are sufficiently defined for the members of the marginal system to internalize the patterns of the dominant system and not be satisfied with their socially prescribed inferior status.

At one time or another, adolescents, career women, migrants, chiropractors, bilingual persons, monks, the physically handicapped, middle-income groups, Catholics, factory foremen, druggists, emancipated men, and sociologists of knowledge have all been defined as being situationally marginal. Thus, indigenous curers join a long and distinguished group of persons. Most persons in marginal environments, including curers, are well-adjusted, nonmarginal group participants.

Health Beliefs

We cannot fully appreciate the present without understanding the past. Ethnic group health practices are derived from basic needs and fears. Insecurity is a result of failure to cope with minority-group status. Although folk medicine may be defined as primitive by outsiders, it is functional for the persons within a culture.

Cultural differences are not merely barriers that keep people out; they also keep ethnic people in.

Health beliefs and behavior may be viewed as crucial dimensions of societal institutions. It is important to start where the client or patient is in terms of health care beliefs and practices. The scientific method is not always best for health care investigation. Whichever method is used, the patients' beliefs should be respected. In fact, in all situations, respect, trust, and unconditional positive regard are needed for effective health care to occur.

Values are based on needs that may have little basis in environmental realities. Social scientists have not been able to clearly separate interrelated variables such as politics, religion, and education. Most attitudes are learned, and few attitudes are based on logical, rational analyses. Once group attitudes are learned, they are reinforced in a variety of behaviors.

Religious beliefs and traditions are usually integral aspects of folk medicine. The semantics of a culture are seen in their definitions of life, illness, and death. Even within religion there is a healer class or ranking system. An individual's concept of the spiritual universe shapes his or her behavior. Consequently, religion is an important factor shaping this definition of life and appropriate behavior. In all societies, cultural transfer is a result of political and economic progression.

Questions for Further Study

1. When does the health care provider have the right to contradict a patient's cultural beliefs?

2. Why should low-income ethnic people utilize scientific medical systems that have not been supportive to them?

3. How can the health care provider communicate acceptance?

4. Is more knowledge rather than increased technology needed by ethnic persons in the lower socioeconomic classes?

5. How can the health care provider resolve conflicts between scientific medicine and folk medicine?

6. To what extent should the health care provider work within the patient's medical belief system?

7. How can the hot-cold dichotomy be useful in modern medicine?

References

1. Foster, G. M.; and Anderson, B. G. 1978. *Medical anthropology.* New York: John Wiley & Sons, Inc., p. 249.

2. Press, I. 1971. The urban curandero. *Am. Anthropologist* 73:741-756.

3. Unschuld, P. U. 1976. The social organization and ecology of medical practice in Taiwan. In Leslie, C., editor. *Asian medical systems.* Berkeley: University of California Press, pp. 300-316.

4. Carstairs, G. M.; and Kapur, R. L. 1976. *The great universe of Kota: Stress, change and mental disorder in an Indian village.* Berkeley: University of California Press, p. 66.

5. Lee, R. P. L. 1975. Toward a convergence of modern and traditional medical services in Hong Kong. In Ingman, S. R.; and Thomas, A. E., editors. 1975. *Topias and utopias in health: Policy studies.* The Hague: Mouton, p. 400.

6. Boesch, E. E. 1972. *Communication between doctors and patients in Thailand,* I. Saarbrucken: University of the Saar, Socio-Psychological Research Centre on Development Planning, p. 34.

7. Warren, D. M. 1974-1975. Bono traditional healers. *Rural Africa* 26:33-34.

8. Press, I. 1975. *Tradition adaptation: Life in a modern Yucatan Maya village.* Westport, Conn.: Greenwood Press, Inc., p. 196.

9. Edgerton, R. B.; Karno, M.; and Fernandez, I. 1970. Curanderismo in the metropolis. *Am. J. Psychotherapy* 24:133.

10. Foster, G. M.; and Anderson, B. G. 1978. *Medical anthropology.* New York: John Wiley & Sons, Inc., p. 253.

11. Landy, D. 1974. Role adaptation: Traditional curers under the impact of Western medicine. *Am. Ethnologist* 1:103-127.

12. Horton, P. B. 1965. *Sociology and the health sciences.* New York: McGraw-Hill Book Co., pp. 310-311.

13. Park, R. E. 1928. Human migration and the marginal man. *Am. J. Soc.* 33:881-893.

14. Goldberg, M. M. 1941. A qualification of the marginal man theory. *Am. Soc. Review* 6:53. Used by permission of the American Sociological Association.

EXERCISES

Exercise 1: Substitute

A Puerto Rican patient in considerable pain rings for assistance. You are filling in for the nurse assigned to the patient's floor. When you enter the room and offer to help, the patient cries out, "You're not *my* nurse. He understands me. No woman can help me. I want my nurse, not you."

1. How do you feel about the patient's comments?
2. How will you respond to him?
3. What are some cultural factors that may be relevant to understanding the patient?

Exercise 2: Rejection

You have been hired by the Bureau of Indian Affairs to be a public health practitioner with responsibility for residents of an Indian reservation. Despite being well trained, you are having difficulty gaining the trust of the Indians.

1. What are some cultural factors contributing to your rejection by the American Indians?

2. What personal and professional qualities do you have that may be (a) helpful to establishing rapport and (b) detrimental to establishing rapport?

3. How will you try to gain community acceptance?

Exercise 3: Behavior

This questionnaire is designed to measure your human relations style. There are no right or wrong answers. For the results to be meaningful, you must answer each question truthfully.

After each statement are three possible behaviors. Place a number "3" beside the behavior you would *most likely* make, a "2" beside the behavior you would next likely make, and a "1" beside the behavior you would *least likely* make.

1. When leading a team meeting, I would:

_____ (1) Keep focused on the agenda.

_____ (2) Focus on each team member's feelings and help each person to express his or her emotional reactions to the issues.

_____ (3) Focus on the different positions team members take and how they deal with each other.

2. A major objective of a health practitioner is:

_____ (4) To maintain an organizational climate in which health care can take place.

_____ (5) To promote the efficient operation of her or his job.

_____ (6) To help patients/clients to better understand themselves.

3. When a strong disagreement occurs between me and a colleague of another ethnic group about work to be done, I would:

_____ (7) Listen to the person and try to understand his or her point of view.

_____ (8) Ask other persons familiar with the work to mediate the dispute.

_____ (9) Support my colleague for asking his or her question about the work.

4. In evaluating ethnic team members' performance, I would:

_____ (10) Involve all team members in setting goals and evaluating individual performance.

_____ (11) Try to objectively assess each person's accomplishments by using standardized instruments.

_____ (12) Allow each ethnic group person to determine her or his own goals and performance standards.

5. When two patients from different ethnic groups get into an argument, I would:

_____ (13) Help them deal with their feelings as a conflict resolution strategy.

_____ (14) Encourage other practitioners to help resolve the argument.

_____ (15) Allow both persons to express their views but keep the focus on institutional regulations.

6. The best way to motivate patients/clients who are not following their health plan is to:

_____ (16) Point out to them the importance of the plan and their responsibilities.

_____ (17) Try to get to know the patients better so that I can motivate them.

_____ (18) Show them how their lack of cooperation is adversely affecting themselves and their loved ones.

7. The most important element in judging my professional performance is:

_____ (19) My technical skills and ability.

_____ (20) How I get along with my colleagues and help them to get work done.

_____ (21) Success in accomplishing goals that I set for myself.

8. In dealing with minority group issues, I:

_____ (22) Deal with such issues only when they disturb the health care atmosphere.

_____ (23) Encourage all of my colleagues to understand the history and cultural conditioning of ethnic minorities.

_____ (24) Help my colleagues to understand their own personal attitudes toward ethnic minority groups.

9. My foremost goal as a health care professional is to:

_____ (25) Make sure that all of my patients/clients have clear knowledge of their health plan.

_____ (26) Help patients/clients to work effectively in groups and to use this relationship to achieve better health.

_____ (27) Help each patient/client become responsible for his or her own health care.

10. The difficulty with being a professional is that:

_____ (28) It is hard for me to handle all the job-related details.

_____ (29) I do not have enough time to really get to know my patients/ clients as individuals.

_____ (30) It is hard for me to keep in touch with my colleagues.

**Do not turn to the next page until you have
answered all of the preceding questions.**

SCORING SHEET AND INSTRUCTIONS

1. Transfer your answers to the scoring columns, placing a 1, 2, or 3 beside each question number.

A	B	C
(1) _____	(2) _____	(3) _____
(4) _____	(5) _____	(6) _____
(7) _____	(8) _____	(9) _____
(10) _____	(11) _____	(12) _____
(13) _____	(14) _____	(15) _____
(16) _____	(17) _____	(18) _____
(19) _____	(20) _____	(21) _____
(22) _____	(23) _____	(24) _____
(25) _____	(26) _____	(27) _____
(28) _____	(29) _____	(30) _____
Total _____	Total _____	Total _____

2. Add up your totals for each column. The three totals combined should equal 60.

3. Mark your score for each column on the bar graph below. Fill in each bar.

A. Organizational

B. Individual

C. Group

0   5   10   15   20   25   30

INTERPRETATION

The longest bar represents your foremost concern in work-related situations. For example, some practitioners are more concerned with their own individual growth and integrity than that of their colleagues or institution (employer). The shortest bar indicates the area you may tend to overlook. Practitioners who are least concerned with group relationships may have difficulty effectively working with ethnic minority and poor patients/clients.

PART III
Patient Care

The chapters in Part III are designed to provide practical suggestions for effective patient care. Although the chapters focus on specific ethnic groups, the suggestions in each are based on sound nursing practices and good human relations. Consequently, many of the suggestions are applicable to all ethnic groups. It is our intention to use these pages to bridge the formidable gap between academic theories and health care. All of the authors bring their many years of experience to bear on the topic. We hope you will think of other ways to provide better care to Third World patients.

12

Religious Beliefs and Healing

George Henderson, Ph.D.
Martha Primeaux, R.N., M.S.N.

Countless persons in extreme physical pain have refused a cure or medical help because it was not consonant with their religious beliefs. Some individuals, such as Christian Scientists who refuse blood transfusions, have died as a result. Health care practitioners should understand a patient/client's illness in terms of his or her religious beliefs. More than any other institution, religion attempts to lift humans above pain, illness, and death.

THE ULTIMATE QUEST

The collective efforts of the human race to understand its various illnesses is a classical study in folk medical beliefs and practices. Throughout history, human beings have tried continually to understand their present health conditions by extracting significance from their past and even by adopting folk medicine for their present health care in an attempt to be healthier in the future. The health of an individual, as well as of the human race, reflects a direct relationship between folk medicine and scientific medicine.

All ethnic groups are concerned with the need for structuring their health values. In this regard, perhaps the oldest source of values is religion, which addresses "man's concern for his ultimate value and how to attain it, preserve it, and enjoy it."[1] Despite differences, despite elaborate schemes for determining and systematizing health values, history attests to the ever-present impact of religious beliefs, rituals, and practices on scientific medicine.

It is certainly understandable that attempts to define and relate practically to our existence are difficult. More likely than not, our confrontations with the universe arouse complex emotions within us. That is, most people are puzzled by the cyclic patterns of the seasons, the unerring polarities of days and nights, the conflict between their own reason and emotion, the glorious process of birth, and the inevitable call of death. They are mentally shaken when they consider the idea of infinite time and compare it with their limited life spans. Indeed, most people are terrified when they realize their susceptibility to disease and illness. In short, life seems to have a meaning beyond our power of comprehension.

Historically, religion is one of the foremost institutions humans have turned to in an attempt to work out the meaning of illness and health. Thus, religion is both a catalyst to understanding basic elements of health and a philosophic border within which to give at least a semblance of order to these conditions. Because the varieties of religious beliefs and practices are almost unlimited, we are faced in this text with the tremendous problem of selecting representative denominations and sects that will do justice to the topic and at the same time provide insights into their contribution to health care. Given the magnitude of the task, we have elected to focus mainly on the religious contributions of Christian cultures.

BASIC FOUNDATIONS

Religions contribute to understanding health care because they offer what is perhaps our most comprehensive beliefs about the basic nature of human beings—beliefs that have significantly affected theories and practices of medical care. This observation is borne out in a brief glance at the religious-medical practices of primitive peoples. The word "primitive" is used here in the sense of "lineally ancestral," not with the negative or culturally prejudiced connotations it has acquired over the years.

The religious beliefs and practices of primitive societies were animistic and reflected preoccupation with *mana,* a term adopted by anthropologists to designate the force or forces that primitive people believed to pervade the world.[2] Mana encapsulated belief in a powerful, invisible, all-pervading force at work in the universe. The primitive influence on modern consciousness is obvious; today, most people still believe in invisible electrons, that is, in invisible powers.

Mana also encompassed the ancient belief in one total, universal Energy; however, primitive people felt little need to give consistent answers regarding the number of manas. This attitude is deeply embedded in modern temperament: "We still do not know whether existing power is all one or whether it is distributed among dispersed parts."[3] The implications of mana were far reaching in terms of ancient life styles; "from it developed polytheisms, pantheons interrelating gods . . . trinities, duotheisms, hierarchial systems of gods of their incarnations, as well as varieties of monotheisms, pantheisms and panentheisms."[3]

Since mana's effect on us may be good or bad, we, like primitive people, are constantly experimenting with ways to control it. Manas that manifest themselves in the wind, sun, thunder, and time generally are beyond our power. Other manas, such as those in rocks, animals, and persons, frequently are within our power.

In Egypt and Mesopotamia, animism influenced a complex polytheism that in turn gave way to a belief in one supreme God, Yahweh.[4] From Yahweh, Moses eventually received the Ten Commandments, a covenant or contract under which Yahweh would protect the Hebrews. In return, the Hebrews were to serve Yahweh forever by living out the terms of the contract. Two contributions to health care beliefs are apparent: (1) monotheism, a theological reference point that not only articulates our relationship to the question of ultimacy but also offers the ideal conditions of human behavior and health; and (2) the existence of a contract that spells out our responsibilities.

In early civilizations, health care practitioners were both religious leaders and healers. For example, in 3000-4000 B.C., many Middle Eastern cultures treated disease by casting out evil spirits through incantations. Herbs and healing magic were integral aspects of Greek and Roman medicine. The belief in healing magic was even more widespread outside the Greco-Roman world.

> For instance, the Persians recognized three forms of physicians whose respective tools were the knife, the drug and the spell, and considered the last the best: in the Far East therapy had to take into account the work of gods, demons and ill-wishers; and in the Judaic scriptures paranormal cures such as Abraham's prayer against barrenness, the banishment of a boil by Isaiah (who, however, treated an ulcer with a preparation of figs) and the cures of leprosy by Moses and Elisha take their place beside miracles of prediction.[5]

Among some cultures, the sick were believed to be possessed by evil spirits. Such a belief is found in both the Old and New Testaments. For the sick to get well, someone had to banish (exorcise) the evil spirits. Until they were cured, the sick were outsiders; they did not belong in the larger society.

The advent of Greek medicine did much to reduce the importance of the demonic theory of suffering. Hippocrates, the founder of modern medicine, viewed disease as the result of natural rather than supernatural causes, and from this perspective, sick persons should not be rejected from society.

In the Greek's relationship to their gods we see the first nationwide attempts to free people from the paralyzing fear of the omnipotent, omnipresent Unknown. Magic, a powerful force in the world before this period, was seriously challenged. It is true that often the Greek gods were only slight improvements on their worshippers and that there were beast gods, but the rationality of Greek mythology is astonishing.

There are threads of Greek and Roman thought running throughout Hebraic writings, and the impact of primitive Greek religions on Western society is seen in our nation's philosophic, rational, and scientific characteristics. Edith Hamilton observed that the Greeks' religious beliefs and practices make us aware that most Americans are their intellectual, artistic, and political descendants. "Nothing we learn about them," she wrote, "is alien to ourselves."[6] With the advent of Homer's Greece about 1000 B.C., humankind became the center of the universe, the most important thing in it. A Western ethnocentric view holds that it was in Greece that humankind first systematically pondered what it was to be alive and well.

The most obvious contributions of Christianity to health care center on the teachings of Jesus. Although 2000 years of conflicting interpretations leave most investigators unsure of their views, some interpretations have greatly influenced health care. For example, to believe that an individual's illness is "the will of God" has profound implications. Christians who follow this belief behave differently than those who do not. Although there is little disagreement among religious scholars about Jesus' concern for the sick, there is considerable disagreement about the causes of sickness and the most effective cures.

In the New Testament, the attention Jesus gave to the sick is closely tied to his ministry of forviging sins. A residual effect of such thinking still exists in modern times; it is demonstrated when religious bodies sit in judgment and attach the label "sickness" to much that they assess as immoral. Some other religious groups adopt a scientific posture that does not associate sickness with moral guilt. The scientific approach has no room for either moral judgment or forgiveness—both of which are cornerstones of Christian beliefs.

MINISTERS AND PRIESTS

It is helpful to understand the functions performed by Protestant ministers and Roman Catholic priests in health care settings, especially hospitals. In addition to talking with patients, ministers may read from the Bible or pray with patients; Roman Catholic priests may hear confessions and distribute communion. Compared with the Protestant minister:

> The work of a Roman Catholic priest is different in form, though it is essentially about the same things. ... One difference which immediately catches the eye is that the work of the Roman Catholic priest is marked less by words than by actions. The minister is called a servant of the word of God (*verbi divini minister*), while the most characteristic task of the priest is the administration of sacraments. Of course, the priest also talks with the sick—a great deal of emphasis is placed on this—and, of course, the minister is entitled not only to proclaim the word but to administer the sacraments of baptism and the last supper (the two sacraments, sacred acts, which Protestants and Roman Catholics have in common). But the emphasis is different, more on the word with one, on the sacrament with the other.[7]

Protestant and Roman Catholic words and sacraments are basically the same in that they are meant to help the patient. This is true whether we are talking about washing away sin through baptism, lighting a candle to make visible the burning up of life, or feeding with bread in the eucharist as a means of strengthening life.

When dealing with dying patients, ministers and priests focus on three aspects of the experience. First, there is a visible reaction in the dying person. During this phase the religious emphasis is on the faith in God. Second, after experiencing an initial reaction to dying, the patient may feel a fear of dying, which may give way to the fear of judgment. During this phase, religious leaders try to help patients to get their lives in order. The third phase is the desire for death. The religious emphasis is on returning to God. In ancient Judaic terms, dying is being gathered to one's fathers.

Both the minister and the priest try to

> help the patient to understand how he sees life, what faith means for him, what significance it brings to his life and how that significance may grow deeper. One could perhaps say that the priest as much as the minister tries to accompany the patient to the point where the sacrament can convey its saving power most fully and bring the sick in touch with Christ.[8]

Faith Healers

Faith or miracle healing has existed in every society from the earliest times in history to the present day.[9] During the past century, modern medicine has accepted the premise that many diseases are psychogenic in origin and may be helped by faith healing. Diseases in this category include gastric ulcers, high blood pressure, coronary thrombosis, diabetes, vasomotor rhinitis, rheumatoid arthritis, and asthma. The Roman Catholic Church has a set of four rigid criteria for validating miracle cures. First, the cure must be noteworthy, edifying, and reasonable. Second, it usually must be instantaneous, although some miracles develop over a period of time. Third, it must be lasting in its effect. Fourth, there must be an overwhelming weight of evidence that the event did in fact occur and that it cannot be explained by any natural explanation. St. John Vianney, St. Francis Cabrioni, and St. John Bosco are three of the more famous Roman Catholic saints. Protestants do not have an agreed-upon set of criteria for validating miracle cures.

One verse in every seven of the Gospels and one in 14 of the Acts provide biblical references to therapeutic activities that suggest faith healing. Of the scores of miracle events ascribed to Christ, approximately three dozen fit the description of faith healing: lepers, the blind, and the crippled were cured. Christ's techniques—praying and commanding the sick to be well, laying on hands, and instructing the afflicted person to pursue a specific course of action—have been adopted by modern evangelists.

Four principles of Protestantism lend themselves to faith healing: (1) a resolution to live by faith; (2) freedom to initiate a new life; (3) openness to truth, which is revealed in both scientific and nonscientific experiences; and (4) the call to a vocation in the world, such as caring for the poor, sick, and orphans. Evangelical conservative Christians relate their healing activities to belief in authentic and authoritative Holy Scriptures; in the life, teachings and sacrificial death and resurrection of Jesus Christ; and in an eternal life.[10]

Evangelists reject the notion that healing occurs by God in only some situations. Evangelists believe that it is God who heals in all situations, although through different persons, modalities, and techniques. Many Americans are ministered to by deliverance evangelists—itinerant male and female preachers who claim the Holy Ghost has given them the gift of divine healing. On a broader scale, Pentecostalism is composed of many fundamentalist or evangelical denominations, sects and cults concerned primarily with holiness (a state of moral and spiritual purity), literal interpretation of the Bible, and a renewal of the Pentecostal experience. Most Pentecostals believe in divine healing, prophecy, speaking in tongues (ecstatic speech induced by religious emotion), and working miracles. However, there are distinct differences among faith healers.

Some faith healers believe that all disease is the work of the devil and that the only cure is to place our trust in the Lord. Others believe that both disease and medicine (including herbs) are the work of the devil. Yet other faith healers believe in divine healing but not to the exclusion of scientific medical cures. Several non-Pentecostal groups believe in elements of faith healing. Mormons utilize "holy handkerchiefs," which are part of a healing tradition dating back to Joseph Smith in the nineteenth century. Baptists, Congregationalists, Methodists, Lutherans, and Unitarians are part of a long list of other religious groups that have a history of faith healing.

SELECTED DENOMINATIONS

The egalitarian nature of Pentecostal faith healing services is especially appealing to ethnic minorities, women, and poor people. This is not to deny the appeal of traditional religious denominations and sects. However, the balance of this chapter briefly reviews a few of the religious denominations whose beliefs often conflict with those of health practitioners. Additional information can be obtained from the references cited.*

Jewish Congregations

Jewish religion is not a synonym for Judaism, which encompasses the total Jewish culture, history, religion, and philosophy of life.[11] Judaism emphasizes our

---

*See Mead, F. S. 1975. *Handbook of denominations in the United States,* 6th edition, Nashville: Abingdon.

responsibility for proper decisions and behavior, and it encourages self-reliance and independence. Consequently, Jewish theology mandates fulfillment of our duties and obligations to God through our relationships in human society, especially with members of our family.

Judaistic principles of freedom of will, justice, love, righteousness, thanksgiving, hope, purity, repentance, prayer, and resurrection of the dead are found in the Torah and Talmud. All of these principles lead to an enlightened oneness with God. There is no original sin in this doctrine, and humans are believed to be inherently good. Nor is there a need for a mediator between humans and God; thus immortality can be attained without Christ or other religious mediators.

All three divisions of American Judaism—Orthodox, Reform, and Conservative—place great faith in science in general and scientific medicine in particular. Jewish patients tend to be concerned with the meaning of pain and its significance in relation to the health and welfare of their families. Thus Jewish patients, fearing habit formation, are often reluctant to accept drugs. Even after taking drugs and being relieved of pain, they worry about its recurrence. In these and other ways, Jewish patients exercise a commitment to health that is intellectual, free of mystical components.

Seventh-Day Adventist Church

The Seventh-Day Adventist Church has a unique set of beliefs that affect the health practices of its followers.[12] Two prominent beliefs are that Christ's return to earth (Second Coming or Advent) is imminent and that Saturday, the seventh day of the week, is the Sabbath rather than Sunday, the first day of the week. Good health for the Adventist depends on an orderly life. If we could live by the Ten Commandments, Adventists believe, a good life would be assured. The Seventh-Day Adventist Church emphasizes the hosistic nature of human beings and the belief that the body, mind, and spirit are part of the greater whole. The body, then, is the temple of the Holy Spirit. This view supports active involvement in health, nutrition, and education—all considered integral aspects of the Gospel.

Adventists abstain from the use of alcoholic beverages, tobacco, and nonmedically prescribed drugs. These abstentions are complemented by concern for helpful diet, exercise, and frame of mind. In many ways, the Seventh-Day Adventist patient is an ideal person for rehabilitation routines.

Church of Christ Scientist

Christian Science presents a metaphysical approach to religion, sickness, and healing.[13] The ultimate human reality, Christian Science asserts, is mental or spiritual, not material or physical. Therefore because sickness, whether of mind or body, is of a mental origin, it can be cured through proper mental processes. Consequently there is no mind-body dilemma for the Christian Scientist.

The body is its own laboratory.

Christian Science treatment consists of prayer and counsel with the sick person; however, there are no clergy in Christian Science. Instead, healing is facilitated by certified practitioners who employ three dimensions of therapeutic treatment. The first dimension focuses on "affirmation and denial" or "argument," that is, the practitioner tries to destroy the sick person's belief in suffering. The second dimension of treatment consists of "absolute consciousness of good"— convincing the individual that he or she is well and knows it. The third dimension, "impersonal treatment," is carried out alone by the practitioner, who focuses on his or her own thoughts to free the inflicted person of belief in sickness.

Christian Science therapy is not like other forms of spiritual healing. There are no prayers that involve emotional, ritualistic appeals to God. Rather, healing is private, abstract, and highly intellectual. Nor do Christian Science practitioners lay on hands as do some practitioners in other religious sects. Drugless healing as found in osteopathic and chiropractic medicine are accepted by Christian Scientists; so, too, are natural methods of healing—dietary regulation and manipulation of the body.

Native American Church

The Native American Church has more Native American members than any other church in America.[14] It is a Christian church whose rituals and beliefs represent almost every North American Indian tribe. The most controversial healing practice is the use of the peyote cactus; thus the designation of its members as Peyotists.

Members of the Native American Church believe in both the Great Spirit of Indian religions and the Christian Trinity—the Father, the Son, and the Holy Ghost. Peyotists believe that: (1) through prayer and communion with God our sins are forgiven and we can be cured of illness; (2) the earth is our mother and she must not be abused or treated disrespectfully; (3) all people are brothers and sisters; and (4) the universe is an harmonious creation and each of us must fit into it with love, peace, charity and humility. Peyotists also believe in abstinence from alcohol.

The peyote service is a total audience participation activity. All members participate equally in the praying, drumming, singing, and speaking. Following Indian tradition, tobacco is part of the service. By consuming peyote the members believe that they are able to establish a closer contact with God. The entire peyote ritual is performed under the guidance of a road chief. The attraction of the Native American Church is clear when we recount the insensitive deeds of early missionaries.

Missionaries looked at the feats of medicine men and proclaimed them to be works of the devil. They overlooked the fact that the medicine men were able to do marvelous things. Above all, they overlooked the fact that what the Indian medicine men did *worked*. Most missionary activity centered on teaching and preaching. The thrust was to get the Indians to memorize the Large Catechism, the Small Catechism, the Apostles Creed, the Nicene Creed, the Ten Commandments, and other magic rites and formulas dear to Christianity. Salvation became a matter of regurgitation of creeds. In a very real sense, then, Christianity replaced living religions with magic.[15]

The religions of Native Americans are religions of the land. To understand this, we must understand the nature of sacred mountains, sacred hills, sacred rivers, sacred burial places, and other sacred geographical features. The Native American Church incorporates these concepts into its doctrines. Finally, it is important to note that Peyotists also believe that scientific medicine can be used to supplement peyote services.

Eastern Orthodox Church

Christian churches are divided into three major sections: (1) Roman Catholic, (2) Eastern Orthodox, and (3) Protestant. The Eastern Orthodox (Greek) Church claims to be the "direct heir and conservator" of the original Christian (primitive) church.[16] Historically, the Eastern Orthodox Church has been divided into independent ethnic churches—Albanian, Bulgarian, Georgian, Greek, Romanian, Russian, Serbian, and Syrian.

The Eastern Orthodox Church does not believe that God created humans in His image; however, we have the potential to become like God in terms of His goodness. Nor does the Orthodox doctrine subscribe to the original sin of Adam; rather, each of us is guilty if in our freedom we elect to imitate Adam. In the Eastern Orthodox Church salvation is a community, not an individual, activity. Thus, we are not saved *from* the world but *with* the world. In essence, salvation is achieved through reconcilation with God, ourselves, our neighbors, and nature.

The Eastern Church believes that humans need the Spirit of God for healing to occur. Caring for the sick has a special place in the church. For example, if a man is sick, the priest visits him to pray over him. If the man is gravely ill, the priest will administer the sacrament of Holy Unction. Since this latter activity consists of seven lessons about the miracles of Jesus, it is preferable, but not mandatory, that seven priests be present, each to read a lesson and to anoint different parts of the body with oil. Furthermore, members of the family and the congregation are present during the Holy Unction. Eastern Christians, like other Christians, are encouraged to pray for and visit sick persons. Persons "possessed" with spirits are exorcised by priests with special healing powers.

In addition to religious healing services, Orthodoxy encourages the sick to seek out scientific medical cures. Basil the Greek, a fourth century Eastern priest, established hospitals for the sick, asylums for the poor, and hospices for travelers.

Church of Jesus Christ of Latter-Day Saints

Latter-Day Saints are better known as Mormons. Based on the Bible and Joseph
Smith's *The Book of Mormon,* the religious doctrines are similar to those of many
conservative Protestant churches.[17] However, unlike conservative Protestants,
Mormons believe that two personages of God—the Father and the Son—have bodies
of flesh and bones, whereas the Holy Ghost does not. Salvation for humans will
come through the atonement of Christ and by obedience to the laws of the gospel.
Explicit in the Mormon's faith is belief in baptism by immersion in water.

Healing takes on an aspect of faith healing discussed earlier: laying on of hands.
Mormons also believe in speaking in tongues, visions, and prophecy. Mormons will
also seek scientific relief for illness and poverty. Mormons have established
worldwide missions to spread their gospel at home and abroad.

SUMMARY

Although no attention has been given to black religions, it is important to note the
manner in which Africans and later black Americans were able to reshape white
religions to meet their needs. This phenomenon is certainly evident in Protestant
and Roman Catholic splinter churches.

> For all its deficiencies and excesses, the religion that the slave practiced was
> his own. It was unmistakably the religion of an oppressed and segregated
> people. It had, of course, common features with Protestantism and in the
> French and Spanish areas, with Roman Catholicism. But it was forged not in
> the drawing rooms of the southern mansions, nor in the segregated balconies
> of the northern churches. It was born in Blackness. Its most direct
> antecedents were the quasi-religious, quasi-secular meetings which took
> place on the plantations, unimpeded by white supervision and under the
> inspired leadership of the first generation of black priests taken in slavery. It
> was soon suppressed and dominated by the Society for the Propagation of
> the Gospel in Foreign Parts and the colonial churches—especially the
> Baptists and Methodists. But the faith that evolved from the coming
> together of diverse religious influences was *tertium quid,* distinctly different
> from its two major contributors.[18]

A similar observation can be made for ethnic minority churches in nontraditional denominations. Most churches, regardless of ethnic composition, adhere
to the basic religious beliefs and healing practices of the surrogate church. Only by
becoming aware of the similarities and differences will health care personnel be
optimally effective in involving all sick persons in their rehabilitation.

References

1. Bahm, A. J. 1964. *The world's living religions.* New York: Dell Publishing
Co., Inc., p. 16.

2. Bahm, A. J. 1964. *The world's living religions.* New York: Dell Publishing Co., Inc., p. 36.

3. Bahm, A. J. 1964. *The world's living religions.* New York: Dell Publishing Co., Inc., p. 40.

4. Smith, H. W. 1932. *Man and his gods.* New York: The Viking Press, p. 15.

5. Rose, L. 1968. *Faith healing.* London: Victor Gallancz, pp. 25-26.

6. Hamilton, E. 1942. *Mythology.* Boston: Little, Brown & Co., p. 7.

7. Faber, H. 1971. *Pastoral care in the modern hospital.* Philadelphia: The Westminster Press, p. 79.

8. Faber, H. 1971. *Pastoral care in the modern hospital.* Philadelphia: The Westminster Press, p. 80.

9. Simson, E. 1977. *The faith healers: Deliverance evangelism in North America.* St. Louis: Concordia Publishing House, p. 14.

10. Vayhinger, J. M. 1973. Protestantism: Conservative-evangelical and the therapist. In Cox, R. H., editor. *Religious systems and psychotherapy.* Springfield, Ill.: Charles C Thomas, Publisher, p. 58.

11. Donin, Rabbi H. H. 1973. *To be a Jew.* New York: Basic Books, Inc., Publishers.

12. Evans, H. S. 1973. The Seventh-Day Adventist faith and psychotherapy. In Cox, R. H., editor. *Religious systems and psychotherapy.* Springfield, Ill.: Charles C Thomas.

13. DeWitt, J. 1971. *The Christian Science way of life.* Boston: Christian Science Publishing Society.

14. Bergman, R. L. 1971. Navajo peyote use—its apparent safety. *Am. J. Psychiatry* 128:695-699.

15. Deloria, V. Jr. 1969. *Custer died for your sins: An Indian manifesto.* New York: Macmillan, Inc., pp. 108-109.

16. Constantelos, D. 1967. *The Greek Orthodox church.* New York: The Seabury Press.

17. Smith, J. 1971. *The book of Mormon.* Salt Lake City: Deseret Book.

18. Wilmore, G. S. 1972. *Black religion and black radicalism.* New York: Doubleday & Co., Inc., p. 18.

13

Cross-cultural
Patient Care

George Henderson, Ph.D.
Martha Primeaux, R.N., M.S.N.

As illustrated earlier, nursing is a process that revolves around interaction between two or more persons with the explicit end goal of better preventive and remedial health services. Clearly, this process works best when the nurse and the patient know and respect each other. By now it should be evident that the nurse-patient relationship has interpersonal as well as physiological dimensions. The more effective nurse is in tune with conditions that promote a patient's physical and emotional well-being.

CULTURALLY DIFFERENT PATIENTS

Total patient care will remain an ideal and not a reality until those responsible for patients are trained in both the scientific and the human relations dimensions of health care. Because medical schools and schools of nursing have been slow to incorporate behavioral science knowledge into an experiential educational component, the average physician or nurse lacks the necessary skills to be optimally effective care providers.

    Since it is the nurse who works most closely with patients, her or his lack of sensitivity to Third World people and poor patients can be disastrous. In short, whether she or he is working in a public or private hospital, public health agency, physician's office, or industry, whether she or he is in an urban or rural setting, or among reservation Indians, patients represent diverse ethnic, social class, age, sex, and religious backgrounds. Indeed, when we get beyond a patient's welfare, social security or hospitalization number, the social dimensions of human existence are extremely complex. These dimensions play a critical role in patients' reactions to their own illness, hospitalization, treatment, and rehabilitation. Nor should we overlook the importance of sociocultural factors in determining the quality of interaction between the nurse and the patient.

Students exposed to concepts found in introductory psychology and sociology courses are well aware of the communication barriers fostered by poverty, racism, sexism, agism, and elitism. For example, a white person who has been taught to dislike black Americans is likely to react to black patients with hostility. Conversely, black Americans who have been taught to dislike whites are likely to be uncommunicative or hostile when with a white nurse.

The more effective nurses are skilled in working with patients of varying backgrounds. Knowledge of sociocultural factors are the foundations on which they build their interpersonal and intergroup behaviors. Even more basic to this process is the realization that the nurse is the primary person in picking up significant clues that bear on response to treatment. Such clues relate to the patient's readiness to follow a prescribed diet or exercise or his or her confusion about the physician's behavior. People who are in pain, confined to a bed, and feeling helpless are dependent on physicians and nurses—too few of whom are sensitive, caring persons. In some subcultures a hospital is where people go to die, in other cultures birth and death are thought of together—the same people who bring children into the world gather to bathe and bury the dead.

It is not uncommon for patients to be unable or too terrified to communicate verbally their innermost feelings. Thus, the ability to read nonverbal cues is quite helpful to nurses. Feelings are communicated not only through words but also through the eyes, skins, and gestures. Learning how to see and feel with patients is just as important as learning how to listen to their words.

The presence of patients from multicultural and multiethnic backgrounds is a source of potential problems. These problems center on language and cultural differences. Much of this grows out of *ethnocentrism,* the belief that one's own group is superior to others. Nurses bring their ethnocentrism with them to their jobs. These sets of attitudes, beliefs, and values also characterize social classes. The effects of group conditioning can be seen in the way people express emotions. For example, depending on our cultural conditioning, fear may be experienced in the back of the neck, in the pit of the stomach, in the head, or in the buttocks. Furthermore, an individual's initial concern for hygiene, nutrition, and privacy are culturally determined.

Cultural understanding does not mean being culture free or indifferent. Nurses not only do but should adopt beliefs, values, and attitudes that are consonant with their subgroup identities. Patients and nurses are different. But it is more basic than this—people are different.

Since people are different, considering people as being different is not "prejudice." The prejudiced are not those who insist that people are different in various respects and by various reasons, but those who deny it. Insisting that people who are different are not different means making propaganda for misunderstanding each other. Since we are different, we can only understand each other if we admit and are aware in what respects and why we are different. Prejudice comes in only if we misinterpret the existing differences in terms of inferiority and the like.[1]

It is counterproductive to "treat all patients alike." For example, black Americans are not Polish Americans; Catholics are not Protestants; women are not men; and physically handicapped are not physically able. There are some human characteristics that all people share (for example, physical needs for food and shelter), there are some characteristics that some people share with certain other people (for example, cultural languages and relations), and there are some characteristics that people share with no other groups (for example, unique racial or ethnic historical conditions, such as slavery). The secret to effective nursing is knowing the similarities and differences between groups. Lectures alone are seldom enough to teach this kind of social perception. Interaction with people of different backgrounds is also required. At the same time, care must be taken to avoid creating ethnic stereotypes and generalizations that do not leave room for individual differences. For example, education and social class can be great equalizers, causing ethnic minorities to behave similar to their Anglo peers.

Most patients, especially ethnic minority patients, need help to understand and optimally utilize services that health professionals offer. The nurse can assist a patient by explaining the services. Like it or not, nurses are expected by most patients to interpret what is happening in the medical setting. To be optimally helpful, a nurse must understand how a patient feels about himself or herself as well as how a patient feels about what is happening (or going to happen) to him or her.

Marie Foster Branch and Phyllis Perry Paxton list the following behavioral objectives for cross-cultural nursing:

1. Delivery of holistic patient care that emphasizes the integral relationship between the psychosocial-spiritual-environmental aspects of the person.

2. Facilitation of the nurse-patient relationship through the development of special resources (such as Spanish proficiency and the inclusion of bilingual-bicultural nursing personnel).

3. Establishment of family involvement in the healing process.

4. Obtainment of knowledge of nontraditional community resources (Latino stores, and so forth).

5. Assessment of signs of illness and referral to appropriate folk health practitioners.

6. Enlistment of the help of folk health practitioners for culture specific conditions.

7. Enlistment of in-service programs in places of employment that would further explain health practices specific to that locale.

8. Promotion of the concept of cultural pluralism in the education of nurses. This type of nursing education would prepare practitioners to assist persons with different cultural backgrounds, values, beliefs, and practices regarding health care maintenance.[2]

POVERTY-STRICKEN PATIENTS

According to Abraham Maslow, all human beings strive to satisfy five basic needs: physiological, safety, belongingness and love, esteem, and self-actualization.[3] The location of a patient on the physiological/self-actualization continuum determines how and to what extent he or she is motivated to satisfy other needs. Physiological needs are the first to be satisfied by every patient, and the need for self-actualization is the last to be fulfilled. According to this theory, the basic physiological needs do not contradict the need for self-actualization but, instead, complement it.

All patients need food and shelter as well as safety and love, but once satisfied, these needs give way to the development of the inner being. Simply stated, once the basic needs are met, we no longer are content to *have* something significant but rather desire to *be* something significant. The satisfaction of a need for food is a motivator only when a patient is hungry.

Once basic physiological needs have been filled, a patient's actions are controlled by the need for safety. Therefore physically safe hospitals, clinics, and homes are important for patient care, too. After the first two needs (physiological and safety) are fulfilled, the patient will feel, as he or she has never felt before, the absence of a close personal relationship. It is during this period when patients develop emotional attachments to nurses, who become substitute parents, lovers, and friends. Thus, emotional hunger takes the place of physiological hunger in each patient's consciousness. If this hunger is displaced to a nurse of a different ethnic background, the patient may experience guilt, shame, and even anger. An inexperienced nurse is often confused by love-hate emotions acted out by patients seeking belongingness and love.

Once the belongingness need is satisfied, the patient is likely to be concerned with achieving a stable, firmly grounded, high evaluation of self. Esteem needs can be divided into two parts: self's view of self and other's view of self. At this stage, a patient's query "How do I look?" is more than idle conversation. If nurses cling to monocultural concepts of beauty, it will be impossible for them to accept physical features that deviate from their subcultural normative standards.

Effects of Poverty

Most patient-centered health care plans are designed to enhance self-actualization in patients. The self-actualized patient strives to do what he or she, as a unique person, is able to do. For a variety of reasons, a few ethnic minority and poverty-stricken patients are self-actualized individuals.

Some nurses fail to realize that poverty-stricken patients are people who have feelings similar to their own. Most low-income patients are sensitive, concerned, and easily embarrassed. An old proverb states that poverty does not destroy virtue, nor wealth bestow it. Oblivious to this fact, many nurses respond to poverty-stricken patients in patronizing and humiliating ways. If a nurse considers herself to be the expert on patient care, she frequently rules out a peer relationship with nonprofessional people, especially low-income persons. "I don't tell them how to run their homes," these paragons of medical excellence say, "so why should they try to tell me how to do my job?" Frequently, nurses who assume this posture are afraid of poverty-stricken patients.

Before nurses can interact successfully with poverty-stricken patients, they must be educated about the physical and social environments of low-income neighborhoods and communities. This includes an awareness of what poverty-stricken homes are like. More than anything, it is necessary to understand the basic factors of survival within subcultures of poverty.

Physical Environment. Physical appearance is one of the most revealing characteristics of most low-income neighborhoods. Neglect and disorder are common. Buildings are in a state of deterioration, highlighting structural neglect and social decline. Slum neighborhoods are overcrowded with buildings, and buildings are overcrowded with people. The population consists mainly of people who are not welcome in other areas or who cannot afford to live elsewhere. Slums have unusually low standards of sanitation, and garbage-strewn streets and alleys are overrun by rats. Infant and maternal mortality rates are high, as are unemployment and underemployment. Vice is rampant in the slums, although it is by no means confined to this area. Slums are the habitat of occupationally marginal men and women and the hiding place of fugitives.[4]

Home Environment. With this kind of community to live in, it is not hard to see the problems low-income people face. Recreational facilities are almost nonexistent, and therefore children play in the streets and alleys. Parents who can must usually work long hours to earn barely enough for subsistence. When at home, low-income parents are often too tired or busy worrying about where their next meal will come from or how they are going to pay this month's rent to listen or pay attention to their children. This is not to say that the children are neglected and unloved. Parental frustration tolerance levels are low, and the way low-income parents generally discipline their children is with a "good whipping."[5]

There usually are few books in the home. If books are present, lighting may be so inadequate that it is difficult for children to read, if they know how. Some poverty-stricken parents believe it is more important for their children to get out and work than to go to school. Most low-income homes are way stations, places to catch a meal and get some rest before moving on to another destination. (Many affluent homes are way stations, too.) Parents tend to exercise little jurisdiction over preschool children, who come and go as they please. Other siblings—mainly older sisters and brothers—become mammas and papas for the younger ones.[6]

Many poverty-stricken families, especially black American families, are mother dominated. Historically, it has been difficult for nonwhite men to obtain work, whereas it has always been easy for nonwhite women to get menial jobs. In some cases, the low-income male's resentment of the female's domination is exhibited in various behavior patterns, such as sleeping during the day, staying out all night, drinking, or beating his wife and children.[7] (Middle-class males behave in this manner, too.)

Typical Low-Income Patients

Most of the poor patients receiving health care are not chronic recipients of welfare. The typical low-income patients have less than an eighth-grade education and, if employed, work as unskilled and service workers. The family's income per person is less than the minimum wage. They do not get their names in the news as outstanding representatives of their race or ethnic group, nor do they show up on welfare rolls or in crime statistics.

Few patients from low-income families—welfare and nonwelfare—enter health care facilities with a predisposition to be uncooperative, but we must remember that these facilities form drastic contrasts to low-income homes. Health facilities are relatively clean, whereas most low-income homes are dirty. Health facilities are sanctuaries of silence; slums are noisy. Health facilities are organized around schedules and regulations, whereas slum interaction is based on strict but informal codes of conduct. Nurses are well-educated, most adults in slums are poorly educated. It is little wonder then that a health facility brings culture shock to the newly admitted, poverty-stricken person. A final word of caution is in order: poverty does not respect race or ethnic background; no one is safe from it. Finally, it is important to know that most low-income people do not have regular preventive medical checkups because they cannot afford them. Few individuals of any income group would not, if given the opportunity, avoid an illness.

PROVIDING EQUAL TREATMENT

The newborn baby is frequently referred to as the best representative of democracy that our nation is able to produce. Every baby is born free of prejudice. Unfortunately, this condition is only temporary, because every baby quickly learns the prejudices that are part of his or her environment. Thus, although every individual comes into this world free of prejudice, most are socialized by extremely prejudiced people.[8]

Many of a nurse's personal preferences are prejudgments—decisions made on the basis of inadequate information. However, being against someone or something is not necessarily a *prejudice*. When based on facts, an attitude opposing (or supporting) someone or something is a *bias* that does not violate democratic principles. For example, a nurse is not behaving prejudicially if she concludes after interacting with nasty, uncooperative patients that she does not like them, but few people collect enough facts to allow them to make objective judgments.

Prejudices tend to multiply and spread to areas unrelated to the initial object of concern. Whites prejudiced against nonwhites find it relatively easy to reject disadvantaged whites also, especially the physically handicapped, welfare recipients, and poorly educated individuals. The bigot blames others for various social misfortunes: inflation, recession, high taxes, and, interestingly, racism.

It is also important to note that not all prejudices are harmful or negative. Some, such as clothing preferences, are both harmless and a source of amusement to others. Prejudicial behavior can support a group rather than oppose it. Black, brown, red, and yellow power advocates, for instance, state that they are for their people and not against other groups.

The most insidious prejudices are those negative attitudes directed toward groups, especially racial, ethnic minority, and sexual groups. These prejudices take on the form of assumptions or generalizations about all or most members of a particular group ("You know how *those* people are!"). Such *in-group* versus *out-group* hostility can threaten the foundation of any health care plan. We are born, educated, married, employed, and buried within the perspective of one factor: group affiliation. The behavior, customs, and habits of out-group patients frequently are labeled "strange" and "inferior."

It is both amazing and frightening to observe health care professionals rejecting patients without knowing whom or what they are rejecting. When such rejection occurs, health professionals are hating on the blind faith that they are right and that individuals advocating tolerance and acceptance are wrong. *Ignorance,* therefore, is one of the primary causes of prejudice. Without understanding the historical and cultural backgrounds of other people, we cannot fully appreciate their cultural backgrounds and contributions. The most negative aspect of ignorance is that people afflicted with this social disease are also socially blind.

Ignorance leads members of one ethnic group to assume that theirs is superior to all others and is characterized by high morality and intelligence, whereas members of other groups are of generally low morality and intelligence. Nurses engaging in such assumptions have not learned that (1) all people are of the same genus and species, (2) there are more differences within ethnic groups than among them, and (3) apparent group differences are largely due to environmental and cultural conditions.

Ignorance is not the only cause of prejudice. Institutions of higher learning have their share of well-educated but extremely prejudiced persons. Their prejudices, especially ethnic and racial prejudices, are deeply rooted in emotions. Scientific studies have shown that prejudice is based on fear of the unknown, and fear is based on insecurity. For example, many whites are fearful that if nonwhites ever achieve positions of power, they will imitate racist whites and become hostile and oppressive. Thus *hostility* growing out of frustration and insecurity is another cause of prejudice. The irrational hatred of some nurse educators makes it clear that education is not a guaranteed deterrent to prejudice.

Group prejudices are expressed in terms of *stereotypes*—false images of out-groups. Stereotypes are given verbal expression: "Jews are pushy," "black Americans are lazy," "Indians are drunks," "Mexicans are smelly," "poor whites are trashy." Clearly these images are false, but they trigger the premature social, economic, and physical deaths of groups so labeled. Of course, we can find individuals to fit the stereotypes, but we can find many more who do not. It is likely that the prejudiced person will dismiss the minority persons who do not fit the stereotype as being "different," "exceptional," or "not like the others."

Because we are creatures of culture, our attitudes, feelings, and values make objective thinking difficult. In any case, *it is behavior, not attitudes, that comprise the major human relations problems confronting nurses.* There are many laws against discriminatory behavior, but there are none against prejudicial attitudes. A nurse does not have to like a patient to give him or her good care. Ideally, effective health care is the result of all health care personnel accepting and respecting the differences of others—patients and nonpatients.

NURSES WHO CARE

Sister Madeleine Clemence Vaillot described the nurse who cares:

> The nurse does not make decisions on the patient's behalf, no matter how much wiser she may be than he in matters of health; she does not substitute her strength for the patient's weakness, not even to spare him suffering at all cost. The role of the nurse is to help the patient become an authentic person and to use his situation and illness for doing so. ... The nurse helps the patient to be; to be self-accepting, with insight, capable of bearing all the consequences of his actions without excuses or alibis, open to love, open to life with all its richness and diversity but also to its concomitant suffering.[9]

Dr. Francis Peabody of Harvard University, one of the founders of medicine in America, stated that the secret of the care *of* the patient is the care *for* the patient.[10] Ethnic minority and poor persons who have been subjected to nonmedical depersonalizing conditions and suddenly find themselves confined to a hospital bed are not likely to feel cared for; they are given wrist bands, expected to divulge intimate secrets about their health and feelings, deny their sexuality, and repress such natural responses as fear, anger, and impatience.

To the average nurse, what constitutes a "good" patient? Undeniably, the good patient is the patient who does not give us "any trouble." The good

patient is cooperative, readily submitting to Rx. The good patient
cooperatively gags on the Levin tube as it passes his uvula; he patiently
extends his arm for the intravenous therapy; he obediently exposes an
already over-perforated upper outer quadrant; he may grouse, but he
submissively partakes of the prescribed 200 mg. salt luncheon, as though it
has not lost its savor. This then is the good patient—he cooperates.[11]

Nurses who care do not try to make patients conform to a rigid set of
dehumanizing behaviors. Furthermore, they are sensitive to the patients' needs and
by being so are less likely to respond insensitively.

Cultural insensitivity can be seen in the belief that no matter how many times
nonwhite patients are bathed, they are always dirty. The "dirt" usually is dead skin
that sheds in the water. Whites shed dead skin too, but because of its light
pigmentation, it is difficult to see in the water. Hair care or the lack of it is another
area of insensitivity. Because a patient's feeling of well-being is often related to how
she imagines others view her, it is necessary that nurses be able to assist all patients
in caring for their hair. Contrary to popular belief, the hair of black patients is not
difficult to take care of.

To provide effective special diets, nurses must be knowledgeable of cultural
foods. Ignorance of cultural tastes has resulted in many patients electing not to eat
prescribed meals. In hospitals, unmet food preferences often result in patients
asking relatives and friends to bring their meals from home. Perhaps one of the
most blatant examples of ethnic insensitivity is the Western practice of forcing milk
into patients with substandard diets. Current data indicate that the majority of
Alaskan Natives (Eskimos), American Indians, Chinese Americans, Japanese
Americans, black Americans, and Mexican Americans are lactose intolerant.[12]
Rather than push milk onto persons who cannot tolerate it, hospitals should find
substitutes, such as fermented milk products (buttermilk, yogurt, ripened cheese
and cottage cheese), or other drinks, such as tea.

The manner in which patients express pain also tends to be related to their
ethnic backgrounds. For example, patients of Irish and West Indian backgrounds
are likely to deny or ignore pain, whereas Italians and Puerto Ricans may complain
loudly about their pain.[13] Nurses tend to feel more comfortable with patients
whose expression of pain is similar to their own. Patients who deviate from an
insensitive nurse's cultural pattern of expressing pain frequently are labeled as
"childish," "lacking self-control," or "too demanding."

Making Nursing Care Work

Since all health care facilities exist because of the patient, each institutional activity
impacts on the patient in some way. The nursing service is for all patients—not a
select few. The complexity of the challenge is easily seen in the daily efforts of
nursing service personnel who attempt to plan, carry out, and evaluate patient-

centered nursing care. Grace Peterson lists six similarities in working with others.[14] We have modified the list to fit poor and ethnically different patients.

Courtesy. Courtesy is using socially acceptable manners (for example, being polite or considerate) in a specific situation. In short, it is showing respect for another person. It is extremely difficult to be consistently courteous to individuals whom we define as being in a "lower" or "disadvantaged" subgroup. An example of discourteous behavior includes calling some patients "Mr.," "Mrs." or "Ms." and calling others (usually a person of a lower social class if we do not know them) by their first name. In traditional Spanish cultures, people have two last names. The first last name is from the father's side of the family, and the second is from the mother's. It is in bad taste to drop the first last name when addressing individuals. By extending social courtesies, we acknowledge the other person's dignity. It is important to note that we cannot bestow dignity on other persons. They have dignity by virtue of being born.

Cooperation. Cooperation is working harmoniously with others. To cooperate with poor and ethnically different patients, the nurse must be willing to assist someone whose life style differs from her or his own. It is not easy to push our cultural conditioning into the background to work with culturally different persons. Obviously, the nurse is in a much less humiliating situation, because she or he is likely to be giving to or doing something for a patient. Contrary to popular notion, most poor people would prefer to give help than to receive it. This is especially true in terms of physical or mental health. Social embarrassment or humiliation cuts across all income, social class, and ethnic backgrounds. Sometimes culturally different patients do not cooperate because they have not been told what is expected of them.

Consistency. Consistency is acting the same way in similar situations. A consistent person's behavior is in line with his or her beliefs. Capricious behavior will leave the patient unsure of what to expect. For example, the nurse who jokes about her ethnic identity one day and becomes angry when patients mention it another day is not only inconsistent but also a terror. Of course, not all consistent behavior is functional for an effective nurse-patient relationship. To consistently call minority adults "girls" and "boys" but call white patients "women" and "men" is an example of consistent behavior that requires change. A final example is the nurse who will touch some patients but not others, even though both groups have similar health conditions.

Honesty. Honesty is being truthful. This does not mean that the nurse must know everything, but it does mean that she or he will keep promises to get answers to patients' questions. Dishonesty is the best and quickest way to destroy a patient's trust. Honesty does not mean that nurses have to be destructive when responding to patients' queries. Honesty without tact can be cruel.

Tact. Tact is doing or saying what is appropriate and nonoffensive in a given situation. Unfortunately, many nurses confuse sarcasm and tact; they are polar behaviors. Even hidden in humor, sarcasm can be psychologically damaging. Caustic comments about drunken Indians, wetbacks, and promiscuous Puerto Ricans may get a laugh from patients representing these groups, but the price of the laughter is ethnic embarrassment. Effective patient care cannot be divorced from emotional comfort.

Loyalty. Loyalty is being faithful to one's colleagues, supervisors, and organization. Sometimes nurses join patients in character assassinations aimed at other health personnel. This practice may allow a nurse to feel that she or he is gaining patient acceptance, but this behavior does little to change oppressive situations. Besides, if a nurse confirms the worst fears patients have about other health professionals (such as, "she's a racist," "he's incompetent"), this does little to help the overall organization morale. When co-workers are engaging in dysfunctional behavior, they should be confronted as professionals, not destroyed through innuendo and gossip.

A book focusing on patient care would be incomplete if we did not point out the caregiver's limitations. M. Esther Harding was correct: "We cannot change anyone else; we can change only ourselves, and then usually only when the elements that are in need of reform have become conscious through their reflection in someone else."[15] This places the responsibility for health care where it belongs—with the patient.

Whether we are involved in a helping relationship as professionals or as friends and confidantes, it is inevitable that at some point in the relationship the problem of making choices will arise. Kurt Goldstein believes the right kind of choosing is essential to bringing about a change in a patient:

> Certainly we always try to eliminate suffering and especially pain. But it is not the task of therapy merely to reduce mental and physical suffering. One may be inclined to do this because one assumes that the elimination of suffering is an essential or even *the* essential drive of man, as psychoanalysis proclaims in the form of the pleasure principle. But placing this in the foreground would often *not* help the patient. The idea of the pleasure principle, particularly when applied to normal life, overlooks the enormous significance of tension for self-realization in its highest forms. Pleasure, in the sense of relief from tension, may be a necessary state of respite. But it is a phenomenon of "standstill." . . . One can achieve the right attitude toward the problem of the elimination of suffering in patients and in normal individuals only if one considers its significance for self-realization and its relationship to the value of health. If the patient is able to make the choice we have mentioned, he may still suffer but *no longer feel sick,* i.e., though somewhat disordered and stricken by certain anxiety, he is able to realize his essential capacities at least to a considerable degree. . . . The central aim of "therapy"—in cases in which full restitution is not possible—appears to achieve transformation of the patient's personality in such a manner as to

enable him to make the right choice; this choice must be capable of bringing about a new orientation which is adequate enough to his nature to make life appear to be worth living again.[16]

A general summary for more effective communication with culturally different patients would include the following recommendations:

1. Carefully select the words you use and the signs and signals you transmit.

2. Speak clearly and briefly at a pace that is not so fast that the patient cannot follow you and not so slow that he or she starts daydreaming.

3. Use words that the patient understands.

4. If the patient's words or nonverbal behavior are not clear, ask for clarification.

5. Try to hear what the patient is saying and try to empathize with him or her.

6. Understand the meaning of the patient's gestures.

7. Be alert to congruence and incongruence between what the patient says and what he or she does.

8. Keep an open mind.

9. Increase your knowledge of other cultures.

References

1. Ichheiser, G. 1949. Misunderstandings in human relations. *Am. J. Soc.* 55:40.

2. Branch, M. F.; and Paxton, P. 1976. *Producing safe nursing care for ethnic people of color.* New York: Appleton-Century-Crofts, p. 76.

3. Maslow, A. H. 1968. *Toward a psychology of being.* New York: D. Van Nostrand Co.

4. Rose, H. M. 1971. *The black ghetto: A spatial behavioral perspective.* New York: McGraw-Hill Book Co., pp. 50-60.

5. Martin, P. E.; and Martin, J. M. 1978. *The black extended family.* Chicago: University of Chicago Press, p. 51.

6. Gibson, W. 1980. *Family life and morality: Studies in black and white.* Washington, D.C.: University Press of America, Inc., p. 81.

7. Ingram, G. I. 1974. Families in Crisis. In Hardy, R. E.; and Cull, J. G., editors. *Therapeutic needs of the family.* Springfield, Ill.: Charles C Thomas, Publisher, pp. 20-46.

8. Allport, G. W. 1979. *The nature of prejudice.* Reading, Mass.: Addison-Wesley Publishing Co., pp. 297-324.

9. Vaillot, Sister M. C. 1966. Existentialism: A philosophy of commitment. *Am. J. Nurs.* 66:500-505. Copyright © 1966 by American Journal of Nursing Company.

10. Robinson, L. 1968. *Psychological aspects of the care of hospitalized patients.* Philadelphia: F. A. Davis Co., p. viii.

11. Burton, G. 1970. *Personal, impersonal and interpersonal relations.* New York: Springer Publishing Co., Inc., p. 18.

12. Hongladaron, G. C.; and Russell, M. 1976. An ethnic difference—lactose intolerance. *Nurs. Outlook* 24:764-765.

13. Weisenbert, M.; Kreindler, M. L. K.; Schachat, R., et al. 1975. Pain: Anxiety and attitudes in black, white and Puerto Rican patients. *Psychosom. Med.* 37:123-135.

14. Peterson, G. G. 1968. *Working with others for patient care,* 2nd ed. Dubuque, Iowa: William C. Brown Co., Publishers, pp. 82-85.

15. Harding, M. E. 1965. *The "I" and the "Not-I."* Princeton: Princeton University Press, p. 75.

16. Goldstein, K. 1959. Health as value. In Maslow, A. H., editor. *New knowledge in human values.* Chicago: Henry Regnery Co., p. 182. Used by permission of Regnery Gateway, Inc., 116 S. Michigan Ave., Chicago, IL 60603.

14

Black American
Patient Care

Donna Neal Thomas, B.S.N., M.S.

*Donna Neal Thomas is Assistant Professor at the University of Oklahoma
College of Nursing. She has been a nursing home consultant, a part-time
hospital staff nurse, a nursing administrator, and a secondary school nurse
with the Oklahoma City Public Schools. Ms. Neal is a past President of the
Oklahoma City Black Nurses Association and has been active in numerous
other professional and health-related organizations. Widely spoken on
minority problems in nursing, preventive health care, sickle cell anemia,
societal issues affecting nursing, and dying, her research and special teaching
projects reflect her continuing commitment to the issue of health care in the
minority community. She is currently participating on a Nurse Practice Task
Force for the American Nurses' Association.*

In recent years nursing education and nursing service have begun to recognize the
need to take a holistic, humanistic approach in the planning of nursing care for all
recipients of these services. Even though the focus has been directed toward holism,
there has been a definite lack of information related to the care of Third World
people in nursing journals and textbooks. This deficit in the knowledge base of
nursing graduates has left them lacking in skills to meet the nursing needs of all
clients in a culturally diverse society.

The focus of this chapter is directed toward meeting some of the nursing care
needs of black Americans. Understanding black patients/clients means knowing

their family and community norms. What are the individual and community attitudes toward illness? How does the family respond when a member becomes ill? If the patient is religious, what is his or her denomination? What medicines were used before the patient sought professional help? What does the patient need to know about your job? Do you expect stereotyped behavior from black patients?

SOCIOECONOMIC ASPECTS

Statistics compiled by the U.S. Census Bureau throughout the years have identified the black male as having the shortest life span of any American, and until recently, the black female had the second shortest life span. The white female has the longest life expectancy. Projections for persons born in 1976 forecast a life expectancy of 77.5 years for white women, 72.7 years for black women, 69.8 years for white men, and 61.3 years for black men.[1] Although medical technology is advancing at a rapid pace, a gap still remains between the longevity of whites and black Americans. Much of the disparity between the two groups is directly related to socioeconomic factors.

According to *Black Enterprise,* "whether families are counted or households— defined as any person or groups of unrelated persons occupying one housing unit (house, apartment, etc.) blacks are clustered much more densely toward the bottom of the income range."[2] U.S. Census Bureau statistics for 1977 show the majority of black family/household incomes are $10,000 or less. Another significant statistic is that black Americans have an annual unemployment rate of 11% to 12%.

Many black Americans with extremely low incomes or almost no incomes seek out free clinical health services when the pain, bleeding, fever, or other symptoms become unbearable. The client frequently may have sought assistance from faith healers, practitioners of folk medicine, and home remedies or drugs that may be purchased without prescription. In discussing how his family dealt with illness during childhood, J. Saunders Redding recalls, "When it seemed safe, he [his father] avoided doctors' bills by purging us with castor oil, plastering us with goose grease, and sweating us in flannel."[3]

In many black homes we could find a continued use of the folk health practices that Redding points out. With incomes of $10,000 or less, a family of four or more can ill afford to seek out scientific health care services on a regular basis. These families bear the brunt of runaway inflation in all basic needs—energy, housing, transportation, food, clothing, and utilities. It is highly unlikely that they have enough to meet their health care needs; therefore, it is imperative that illness prevention and health education be promoted as the most effective means of reducing health care costs.

Nursing services must undertake better planning to ensure more effective self-care and long-term health maintenance. Low-income clients in the hospital environment tend to progress well with their prescribed medical regimen. Once they leave this artificial environment and move back into their real world, however, they often return to behaviors that led to the original hospitalization. Nurses and other health providers need to understand each client's life style and how it is likely to affect his or her ability to adhere to a prescribed regimen.

Although medical technology has brought under control catastrophic diseases common decades ago, a gap continues to exist in the knowledge about and health care management of black Americans. Recent studies show an increase in the leading causes of death—diabetes, cancer, and coronary heart disease—among black Americans. These conditions can be reduced considerably with increased awareness by the black population of the risk factors associated with these diseases.

P. Bussey Williams, in discussing coronary heart disease, recommends "an organized, intensive and comprehensive approach that will support adequate training of ethnic allied health manpower and preventive health services ... [who are] able to interpret available health services and needs to the black community."[4] Nurses and other health professionals who are willing to go into black communities and implement health education programs are needed. However, it is essential that these individuals be sensitive, accepting, and aware of physiological, socioeconomic, sociocultural, and psychosocial factors as well as spiritual influences that affect the health care of black clientele.

Earlie L. Jones suggested that care providers evaluate their perceptions:

> The community health nurse who works with black families needs to examine her attitudes toward blacks. For instance, a nurse may comment about the "luxuries" her clients possess which reveals her resentment toward them for using free or low cost clinic services. "A member of their family drove them to the clinic in a new Cadillac!" She may institute punitive measures. For instance, she might notify the social worker of a welfare mother if she misses a routine well-baby clinic appointment without first determining the reason why the appointment was missed. Or she may make negative comments when children go to school the day after Easter or Christmas vacation wearing new clothes. The nurse needs to know and/or attempt to understand what these holidays and possessions mean to black people.[5]

SOCIOCULTURAL ASPECTS

Houston Baker described three major aspects in which black American culture is distinct from white American culture:

1. We are an oral and a musical people.
2. We do not succumb to the "individualistic" ethos "but are committed to a collective ethos with emphasis on common good and sharing."
3. We have developed the capacity and the necessity to repudiate much of what is the American way of life.[6]

Probably the most profound aspects of cultural variation among black Americans pertain to the family and religion. Both are considered by many theorists in cultural diversity as the center of black culture.

Family

Andrew Billingsley, a leading black sociologist, stated that "the family is by far the strongest institution we have. It continues to be the primary component of our effort toward survival and liberation, and it is the key element in our struggle for positive human development."[7] He states further that "the extended family and a multiple variety of nuclear, extended and augmented family forms are an intricate part of what we mean by family."

Strong kinship bonds in the black family are based on cultural remnants of an African heritage modified through experiences of slavery and cross-fertilized with other ethnic groups. Close-knit groups of kin and kith—uncles, aunts, grandparents, boyfriends, brothers and sisters, deacons, preachers, friends of the family, and so forth—may participate in child rearing. This kinship network provides a buttress and support against racism and discrimination during the developmental years.

Usually these strong kin networks are viewed as prevalent among poor and low-income black Americans; however, a recent study demonstrates that this network persists even in prosperous black families.[8] McAdoo's study of middle-income black families in the Washington, D.C. and Maryland area found that these families continue to assist one another with child care, financial help, personal problems, and home reapirs or chores as well as with gifts of clothes and furniture.

Since the family views itself as a buffer against the stress of living, it is not uncommon to find that this network of people are ever present with the family member who seeks health care services. Kin and friends feel a strong urge to "sit up" with the individual to ensure that his or her needs are met. Although black family members are independent, there is usually one individual who must be consulted before the final decision is made regarding any major health care intervention. This person may be the father, mother, aunt, son, or grandparent. Sensitive nurses and other health care providers are cognizant that a decision will not be forthcoming until the key family member has been consulted.

Frequently the nurse making a home visitation may find a multigenerational family living under the same roof. This situation may create problems for the nurse who is not astute in working with extended families. The nurse may find that planned nursing interventions are thwarted if key family members are not included in the planning of nursing care.

Mrs. S and her 3-week-old infant were referred to the county health department for health maintenance care. Upon home visitation, Mr. N, the community health nurse, learned that Mrs. S was adding corn syrup to the commercial formula prescribed for the infant. Mrs. S stated that her mother told her to add the syrup to the formula to make it taste better and to make it stronger. If Mr. N is wise, he will include the grandmother in his plans for health teaching regarding the formula. This strategy will increase the likelihood that the plan will be implemented by the family.

When nursing care is planned, it is necessary to begin assessment by defining the black client's experiential background. The way the client relates to the home, family, and immediate neighborhoods must be determined, and agencies that might directly affect the individual's life must be identified. It is important for the nurse to recognize that the black client or patient, whether child or adult, does not exist in isolation but is part of an elaborate family and community network.

LANGUAGE

Dating back to the period of slavery, black language and speech patterns have been ridiculed by nonblacks. This attitude was graphically apparent in the old vaudeville minstrel acts and later on radio and television through the Amos and Andy show. But there is nothing funny about the way people talk. This type of degradation has contributed to the negative self-images of many black Americans in this country. Only when the care provider realizes that all languages are "standard," will she or he refrain from trying to enforce English-only norms in health facilities.

A non-Anglo, or nonstandard English, language is neither better nor worse than Anglo language; it just is. Clyde Taylor provides a lucid summary of black American language:

> There is increasing evidence that the differences of Afro speech from Anglo speech are mainly due to the survival of characteristics of African languages among black people in America. For instance, the *th* sound is absent in many West African languages, so many Afros substitute *d* as in *de* book or *dis* or *dat.* . . . Another example of some of the differences between Afro dialect and standard English dialect is the tendency to drop final consonants, like *ed, s,* or *t.* So you might hear *tes* for *test* or *col* for *cold.* In some cases the final *th* becomes *f* or *t* as in *oaf* for *oath,* *bof* for *both.* The *r* in *store* or *door* might be left out so you hear *sto* or *do.*
>
> Afro dialect finds uses for double and multiple negatives, usually for emphasis: "You ain't gone find me at no touchie-feelie sensitivity sessions at no time soon!" Still another interesting characteristic of Afro dialect has no counterpart in "standard" English: the use of the verb *to be* in a continuous present tense. Thus, "she be scheming" means she schemed in the past, is probably scheming now, and will most likely be scheming in the future.[9]

Taylor also points out that black Americans are masters of the silent language, nonverbal communication, formerly called *kinesthesia.* Observant care providers notice that black verbal communication is frequently punctuated with gestures.

Whether verbal or nonverbal, communication is the key to a helping relationship. Therefore, it seems obvious that instead of making fun of or bemoaning the unintelligibility of a client's language, the care provider must find a way to communicate with him or her. Until this happens, the effectiveness of a specific health plan is academic.

PSYCHOSOCIAL ASPECTS

Biological and behavioral theorists have demonstrated that when an individual is faced with stress, regardless of its source, he or she attempts to adapt it. Although initially adaptation referred simply to adjustment, today the concept is thought of as: "The whole range of protective adjustments from the simplest motor action to the most complex interaction between individuals or entire nations. . . . With body, intellect and emotion, man attempts to meet the challenge of life actively and agressively."[10]

When black Americans enter the health care system, they may exhibit a range of negative behaviors from very submissive to outwardly aggressive. But this behavior is not unique to black Americans. Other clients enter treatment this way, too. Nevertheless, it seems as though black clients exhibit more paranoid responses, and the resultant hostility creates stress for most nurses, thereby leading to an ineffective nurse-client relationship. It would behoove the nurse to keep in mind that these behaviors usually have their roots in nonhospital interactions. Defensive behaviors are adaptive behaviors that these individuals employ to meet the challenges inherent in their everyday environment. Since these are adaptive mechanisms, it may be the care provider who must learn to cope with them.

Paranoid Responses

Paranoid responses are usually interpreted in Anglo societies as indicative of psychosis. Nevertheless, some behavioral theorists have identified this phenomenon as a coping mechanism black Americans use to adapt to the "realistic discriminatory experiences which they deal with daily."[11] When black individuals who have developed defense mechanisms as a means of coping enter the health care system, they may be hesitant to fully disclose their feelings of paranoia:

> For a black man survival in America depends in large measure on the development of a "healthy" cultural paranoia. He must maintain a high degree of suspicion toward the motives of every white man and at the same time never allow this suspicion to impair his grasp of reality. It is a demanding requirement and not everyone can manage it with grace.[12]

The nurse then needs to develop an awareness that paranoid responses among black Americans may be a means of adaptation to the environment. This knowledge base then enables the nurse to recognize that these behaviors may not be aimed solely at the provider of health care.

Hostility

Hostility, like suspiciousness, has served as a means for adaptation by black Americans to a not so friendly environment. Hostile behaviors may range along a continuum from anger hidden by sweet smiles to overtly acting out aggression and violence. In a crowded environment where high unemployment is the norm, where the primary cause of death among black men between the ages of 21 and 25 is homicide, and where at each critical point the black man's normal masculine development is thwarted, hostility is bound to prevail. Certainly hostility is a means of survival for individuals living in this type of environment. Of course, nurses may find it difficult to establish a therapeutic interaction with clients exhibiting suspicious or hostile behaviors.

RELIGION

The perceptive nurse respects the right of her or his clients to practice their religion in any manner that they see fit. Besides, religion is a vital aspect of health care for many people. In expressing the purpose of religion, Vinton R. Anderson writes that the aim of religion is to help black Americans deal with themselves, examine their motives, and develop wholesome attitudes.[13]

James Comer described the black church in his childhood not only as a place for spiritual and moral development but also as a place where his belongingness need was met.[14] He also saw the church as a place for releasing pent up emotions: the black church provides a catharsis for its members. The intense responses expressed by the people reflected a sense of frustration and helplessness. It was in the church that people could discharge frustration and hostility so that they might face injustice and hardship the following week.

According to Major James black theology is above all else the theology of hope.[15] The mission of Christ was that of liberation—political, social, economic, and religious. Today the black church continues to provide hope, a place for belonging, a place for one to feel esteemed, and a place for releasing pent-up emotions. It is the one place in the community that the individual can feel free of societal pressures and in turn experience a sense of true liberation.

An aware health care practitioner accepts the rituals related to home treatment. Too often, for instance, the "prayer cloth" under the pillow is seen as having nothing to do with health care and is removed. Likewise, tiny bags of pepper pinned to the bottom of the patient's bed or a small piece of garlic found pinned to the patient's clothes are also seen as unrelated—in some instances, unsanitary—and removed. These items which may seem insignificant, if not pagan, to the health care workers, are extremely important to the patient and his psychological well being.[16]

Even though many black adults experience economic deprivation and hold menial jobs, and although many black adolescents are frequently omitted from school activities, they undergo a complete metamorphosis in the church. As deacons, trustees, stewards, ushers, and choir members, they take on a new posture in their positions of leadership and responsibility. In the church they experience a sense of "somebodyness" and a sense of control, pride, and ownership.

The nurse who practices holistic nursing care recognizes the significance of religion to many black Americans for whom they provide nursing services. Areas of religious assessment should include:

1. Religious preference.
2. Sources available for spiritual comfort.
3. Religious writings that may provide comfort.
4. Significant others who may need to be called to meet spiritual needs (a minister, sister, or brother from the individual's place of worship).
5. Possible conflicts of health care regimen with religious beliefs.
6. The individual's perceptions of health and illness relative to his or her religious beliefs.

When members of some congregations are confined to a health care facility, it is not uncommon for other members of the congregation to visit in small groups (missionary circles, brotherhood members, Sunday school classes, choir members, and so forth). These visits reinforce a sense of individual importance and personhood. The sessions may include prayer, singing, and religious readings. The hospital chapel is recommended for religious activities if the client is in a semiprivate room and ambulatory. However, if the client is nonambulatory, curtains may be drawn to prevent infringement on the privacy of other patients.

A minister is a most significant other person for many black Americans. A responsive nurse recognizes the role that the black minister plays in the well-being and restoration to health of his or her parishioners. J. Alfred Smith defines the minister's role in this manner:

> The rich faith of black religion enables black people to call upon the clergy, not to administer the last rites, but to face sickness, suffering, and existential meaningless with calm assurance that they will survive their contemporary existential hell of rats, roaches, and racism. In other words, black religion gives meaning to life.[17]

Just as the nurse collaborates with other members of the health care delivery team to plan care for the client, collaboration with the minister is also vital to meet the client's spiritual needs. The black minister may also be most resourceful in assisting with discharge planning as well as helping the client cope with the stresses in his or her life. In summary, religion provides many black clients with a sense of liberation, hope, and the capacity to endure the stresses of living in a sometimes nonsupporting environment.

PERSONAL HYGIENE AND GROOMING

Ms. M is a 19-year-old black woman who has been admitted to St. Simon's Hospital for abdominal exploratory surgery. On the first day after the operation, Ms. M is confined to the bed with intravenous fluid infusing in her right hand. Ms. T, a new graduate nurse, comes to give Ms. M a bath and to meet her other hygiene needs. She is most attentive and gives Ms. M a complete bed bath, assists her with her oral hygiene, and makes her bed. The nurse then asks Ms. M if there is anything else that she might need. She reassured Ms. M that if she needs anything, she should feel free to press her call signal.

A very important component of Ms. M's nursing care was omitted: hair care was not included in the nurse's plan for meeting her client's personal grooming and hygiene needs. Paul Schilder declares that the touch of others and the interest others take in the different parts of our body are of enormous importance in the development of our self-concept.[18] Although problems with body image are not likely to develop with this 19-year-old young woman because her hair was neglected, what would have been the impact if the client were a black toddler or adolescent confined to a rehabilitative or convalescent institution?

Hair Care

Hair care is essential to good grooming and is ordinarily included in nursing care. As with any other people who are confined to a health care facility, black Americans have a right to expect that their hair will receive proper attention. Caregivers need to be aware of the special quality and requirements for care of black clients' hair.

Black Americans' hair varies widely in texture. It is very fragile and ranges from long, straight hair to short, spiralled, thick, kinky hair. The latter texture is more prevalent among the Negroid race. The hair and scalp have a natural tendency to be dry and require daily combing, gentle brushing, and application of a light oil to the scalp. If the client is female, the hair then may be rolled on curlers, braided, or left loose according to the client's preference. Bobby pins or combs may be used to keep the hair in place. *Essence* recommends the following regime for shampooing the hair:

1. Use a mild shampoo and rinse. (A shampoo containing zinc pyrithione may be used to control dandruff.)

2. Apply protein conditioner if available.

3. Rinse with warm water.

4. Squeeze out excess water and towel dry.

5. Use a widely spaced round toothed comb to comb the hair out before hair dries completely. Part the hair into small sections.

6. Using the fingertips, apply a small amount of light oil to the scalp. If the client does not have his own hair dressing, Vaseline or mineral oil may be used.[19]

If an individual has corn-rowed braids, the scalp may be massaged, oiled, and shampooed, leaving the braids in tact. Several chemical relaxers available are prepared for black hair; however, these chemicals should be used only by a licensed beautician. Hair that has been straightened with a pressing comb will return to its naturally kinky state when exposed to moisture or humidity. Additional information regarding the care of black patients' hair may be obtained from beauticians and from magazines such as *Essence, Blac-Tress,* and *Ebony.*

Facial Hair

Variations of texture are also found in the facial hair of black men. The straighter the hair, the fewer the problems in terms of shaving the client. When an individual who has tightly curled facial hair is shaved, the hair curls back on itself and penetrates the skin. This results in a foreign body reaction in the area, leading to papules, pustules, and multiple small keloid formation. This is the reason that many black men refrain from shaving and instead grow beards.

Before shaving a client, the nurse should determine the client's usual method of facial grooming. Some men use depilatories one to two times a week to remove facial hair. If depilatories are used, the nurse must avoid the chemical's contact with the client's nose, mouth, eyes, and ears. If the skin shows signs of irritation, the depilatory should be discontinued. Straight or safety razors should not be used with depilatories.[20]

Skin Care

The skin color of black Americans ranges from white to black. Distribution of pigment may be uneven, giving a splotchy appearance to the skin. This splotchiness is most evident at birth among a significant proportion of black infants. Mongolian spots range in color from blue to black and may be found on buttocks, the lumbodorsal area, arms, and thighs. These areas of hyperpigmentation vary in size from 0.5 to 12 cm. in diameter.

Parents of infants with such spots should be reassured that they are benign and that they frequently disappear during childhood but may persist into adulthood. Mothers of these infants will often refer to these spots as birthmarks and relate them to some cravings that they experienced during pregnancy. The nurse will need to reassure the mother that there are no adverse effects from the Mongolian spots. They should also be informed that these spots occur in 90% of nonwhite infants but in less than 6% of white infants.

The client's bath is essential to meeting personal hygiene needs. This is a time for the nurse to make a thorough assessment of the client's body to augment or revise the nursing care plan. In preparing the bath water, the nurse may elect to add bath oil or some other moisturizing substance if the client's skin is dry. When bathing any nonwhite client, the nurse may note that the washcloth becomes brown or black. This is not due to dirt but is due to the natural shedding of the pigmented epidermis. This shedding is more evident with nonwhites than whites.

After the black client's skin dries, it is likely to appear ashy. Dryness is much more evident on black skin due to the pigmented background. This white to gray ashiness of the skin may leave the individual with a sense of loss of body integrity. It is therefore necessary for the nurse to apply lotions or creams to restore feelings of body integrity. If the individual does not have lotions or creams among his or her personal belongings, lotions with lanolin base, baby oil, or vaseline may be used to eliminate the ashen look. Alcohol-based lotions are to be avoided.

Doubts as to how the personal hygiene and grooming needs may best be met are best resolved by consulting with the client or his or her family.

DIETARY PATTERNS

Due to cross-cultural interactions and cultural adaptations, few Americans today adhere on a daily basis to the exact dietary patterns of their ancestors. Nevertheless, specific food patterns are followed on a regular basis by individuals according to their ethnic backgrounds. Since the conceptual framework of quality nursing care embraces that of holism and high-level wellness, dietary cultural patterns must be considered a variable for assessment.

It is estimated that more than 70,000 black Americans die each year from diabetes or its complications. The management of diabetes whether it involves insulin or not is directed toward dietary modification.[21] Alterations in diet are difficult for low-income black Americans, because many of the foods included on the diet exchange lists are beyond their economic abilities. Also, most of the foods that they find palatable are not included on standard exchange lists. Some foods included in black dietary patterns are referred to as "soul foods." These foods have deep emotional significance and provide a sense of satisfaction.

When planning or teaching diet modification for any client, the nurse must first take a diet history. In taking a diet history, the nurse should seek the following information:

1. Foods usually eaten
3. Foods that the client finds truly satisfying
3. Methods of food preparation

4. Others who share meals with client and their dietary preferences
5. Frequency and times per meals
6. Utensils used to prepare the food

Inclusion of ethnic foods some of the time in diet planning will promote individualization of the diet and maximize adherence to the dietary plan. If ethnic food preferences are not included on standard exchange lists, they should be added in consultation with a registered dietitian. Barbara Kraus' *Calories and Carbohydrates* can be consulted for assistance with calculating caloric restrictive diets.[22] She includes a listing for foods included in culturally diverse diets.

Mr. T, a 25-year-old black construction worker, has been advised by the medical staff at a local health center that he needs to lose some weight. He is 5 feet, 11 inches tall and weighs 233 pounds. He has hypertension and is a likely candidate for cardiac problems. Mr. T had been instructed on a standard 1500 calorie diet but found it impossible to stay on the diet. He stated that the foods were too bland for his appetite, and furthermore he could not afford them.

The community health nurse assigned to work with Mr. T on his diet conferred with him and his wife on food preferences. Since their food preferences varied somewhat from standard menus, a consultation was arranged with a dietitian for menu planning. The following is a sample of one day's 1500 calorie diet for this family:

Breakfast	*Lunch*	*Supper*
½ c. orange juice or grapefruit juice	Baked chicken (2 pieces)	Boiled neck bones (about 3 pieces)
2 sausage patties (drained on paper towels)	½ c. blackeyed peas	1 c. mixed greens
	½ c. rice (steamed)	1 small slice cornbread
	Sliced tomatoes	1 tsp. margarine
2 slices toast	2 tsp. margarine	¼ c. pudding
1 tsp. margarine	1 slice bread	
1 c. milk	½ c. regular vanilla pudding	
Coffee		
Iced tea or coffee as desired		

By including some of the foods preferred by Mr. T and Mrs. T, greater adherence to the diet was achieved with resultant weight loss. Professional articles focusing on diets frequently ignore the fact that culture greatly influences food preferences and dietary patterns. To ensure a high level of compliance, it is imperative that a thorough diet history be taken. It is also important that modifications of a diet take into consideration cultural variations.

SKILLS FOR INTERVENING

Basic to a therapeutic relationship is the establishment of trust. Individuals whose trusting capacities have been thwarted may find it difficult to establish a trusting relationship with the nurse or any other health care provider. But a trusting relationship must be achieved if the client is to be restored to a state of wellness.

Arthur W. Combs and his coauthors state that the responsibility for establishing trust rests with the individual who is in the helping role (such as nurse, counselor, teacher, or physician).[23] Since the nurse is expected to have the ability to help, it is up to her or him to know how to build client trust. Communication of trust lies with the communicator and not with the person receiving the message. This is known as the client-centered approach to helping.

Rogers and Wood described the client-centered approach as an attitude—a way of being, not a technique—that is nondirective, reflective, or otherwise helpful.[24] They feel that a way of "being" rather than a "theory" is what is facilitative in interacting with clients.

The nurse should use verbal and nonverbal communications that convey acceptance of and respect for the black client. Hostility-producing words, such as "boy," "gal," "you people," and "colored," should be avoided. Initial assessment should be made as to how the client prefers to be addressed. Some younger black Americans prefer to be addressed by their first names, whereas most older black Americans prefer to be addressed by "Miss," "Mrs.," or "Mr." and their last name. Robert LeMaile-Williams chided physicians for similar insensitive behavior:

> Even the initial greeting, the very first encounter, is to treat black patients as children, or as very familiar friends or neighbors. Respect and dignity are promptly forgotten, and you're greeted with, "Hello Sadie," or "How's it going, Sam?" instead of "Good morning Ms. Brown" or "How are you doing, Mr. Johnson?"[25]

Nonverbal interactions that may be construed to mean nonacceptance include refusal to sit down when making a home visit, reluctance to touch the client, physically moving away from the client, or making facial expressions that infer disgust.

When a client exhibits paranoid responses and hostile behavior, a culturally sensitive nurse recognizes these as possible adaptive mechanisms that the client uses to survive in his or her everyday world. The nurse then accepts the client where he or she is and implements an effective means of communication.

In summary, although health care for black Americans is similar in many aspects to the care of the dominant society, there are unique aspects of care that require consideration on the part of the nurse if a high level of holistic individualized nursing care is to be achieved.

References

1. Norment, L. Oct. 1977. How long will you live? *Ebony,* pp. 44-50.

2. Blacks and the economy: an annual review. June 1979. *Black enterprise,* pp. 205-211.

3. Redding, J. 1971. From no day of triumph. In David, J., editor. *Growing up black.* New York: Pocket Books, p. 228.

4. Williams, P. B. 1979. Assessing awareness of coronary disease risk factors in the black community. *Urban health* 8:37.

5. Jones, E. L. 1976. Nursing care of the black patient. In Luckraft, D., editor. *Black awareness: Implications for black patient care.* New York: American Journal of Nursing, pp. 36-37.

6. Billingsley, A. 1974. *Black families and the struggle for survival.* New York: Friendship Press, p. 16.

7. Billingsley, A. 1974. *Black families and the struggle for survival.* New York: Friendship Press, p. 72.

8. McAdoo, H. P. 1979. Black kinships. *Psychol. Today* 12:67-79.

9. Taylor, C. 1976. Soul talk: A key to black cultural attitudes. In Luckraft, D., editor. *Black awareness: Implications for black patient care.* New York: American Journal of Nursing, pp. 1-2.

10. Luckmann, J.; and Sorenson, K. 1974. *Medical surgical nursing.* Philadelphia: W. B. Saunders Co., p. 11.

11. Spurlock, J. 1975. Psychiatric states. In Williams, R. A., editor. *Textbook of black related diseases.* New York: McGraw-Hill Book Co.

12. Spurlock, J. 1975. Psychiatric states. In Williams, R. A., editor. *Textbook of black related diseases.* New York: McGraw-Hill Book Co., p. 161.

13. Anderson, V. Aug. 1979. Religious moral standards can be a cure for crime. *Ebony,* pp. 137-142.

14. Comer, J. P. 1972. *Beyond black and white.* New York: Quadrangle/The New York Times Book Co., Inc.

15. James, E. L. 1971. *Black awareness: A theology of hope.* Nashville: Abingdon Press.

16. Nobles, W. W.; and Nobles, G. M. 1976. African roots in black families: The social-psychological dynamics of black family life and the implications for nursing care. In Luckraft, D., editor. *Black awareness: Implications for black patient care.* New York: American Journal of Nursing, p. 19.

17. Smith, J. A. 1976. The role of the black clergy as allied health care professionals in working with black patients. In Luckraft, D., editor. *Black awareness: Implications for black patient care.* New York: American Journal of Nursing, pp. 13-14.

18. Schilder, P. 1950. *The image and appearance of the human body.* New York: International Universities Press.

19. To oil or not to oil. Oct. 1979. *Essence,* p. 86.

20. McDonald, C. J.; and Kelly, A. P. 1975. Dermatology and venereology. In Williams, R. A., editors. *Textbook of black related diseases.* New York: McGraw-Hill Book Co.

21. Howell, R. O. March 1979. Diabetes: The silent killer of blacks. *Ebony,* pp. 64-71.

22. Kraus, B. 1975. *Calories and carbohydrates.* New York: Signet.

23. Combs, A. W.; Avila, D. L.; and Purkey, W. W. 1971. *Helping relationships: Basic concepts for the helping professions.* Boston: Allyn & Bacon, Inc.

24. Rogers, R.; and Wood, J. K. 1974. Client-centered theory: Carl R. Rogers. In Burton, A., editor. *Operational theories of personality.* New York: Brunner/Mazel, Inc.

25. LeMaile-Williams, R. L. 1976. The clinical and physiological assessment of black patients. In Luckraft, D., editor. *Black awareness: Implications for black patient care.* New York: American Journal of Nursing, p. 17.

Additional Readings

Grier, W. H.; and Cobbs, P. M. 1968. *Black rage.* New York: Bantam Books, Inc.

Liberate your hair. Jan. 1979. *Black-Tress,* p. 30.

15

Hispanic American Patient Care

Ildaura Murillo-Rohde, Ph.D., F.A.A.N.

Ildaura Murillo-Rohde, Professor and Associate Dean at the University of Washington, is Chairperson of the National Coalition of Hispanic Mental Health and Human Services in Washington, D.C. She is also President of the National Association of Hispanic Nurses and has been a family therapist and counselor for Puerto Rican parents and children in East Harlem and the South Bronx. Her many publications focus on drug addiction, family life, family therapy, cultural diversity, marriage and marital therapy, transcultural nursing, child rearing in Puerto Rican families, and health care of Hispanic patients. Dr. Murillo-Rohde has directed psychiatric nursing programs at New York Medical College Graduate School of Nursing, New York University, City University of New York, and Wayne County General Hospital, Eloise, Michigan, and she was Psychiatric Consultant for the Guatemalan government in the World Health Organization.

The United States, unlike many other countries, has a very heterogenous population. President Kennedy put it very well when he said that the "United States is a nation of immigrants."

Source: From Murillo-Rohde, I. 1979. Cultural sensitivity in the care of the Hispanic patient. *Washington State J. Nurs.—Special Suppl. 1979,* pp. 25-32.

There are millions of Spanish-speaking people in the United States who immigrated to this country. However, we have millions of Spanish-speaking and Spanish-surnamed citizens in the West and Southwest of the United States who never immigrated to this country. These are the Spanish-speaking people of Mexican descent whose land was taken over from them by the United States and who suddenly found themselves to be a minority in their own land. Today this group of Mexican-Americans has given itself the name of "Chicanos."

The Island of Puerto Rico became part of the United States in October, 1898, after it had been occupied by United States troops led by General Miles during the Spanish-American War.

Nevertheless, whether they immigrated, migrated, or were taken over, the Spanish-speaking people in this country have retained much of their cultural heritage. The extent to which this cultural heritage is retained is usually in direct relationship to the number of years the family has spent in the United States and to the extent that they have learned the English language and have been acculturated into the Anglo-American culture and its values.

It is commendable and priaseworthy to have the various cultural and ethnic groups retain some of their values and ethnic identity. At this time in our history this is encouraged, and children and adults are being helped to develop pride in their cultural heritage, as evidenced by the bilingual programs in the schools and universities. We can also point to the success of Alex Haley's *Roots*. It is difficult to find any college or university of any stature and prestige that does not have a Black, American Indian, African, Chicano, Puerto Rican or Hispanic Studies Department. It is true that this came about only after the students who came from such ethnic backgrounds forced the universities to make it possible for them and others to know something about their own cultural heritage and past.

It has been estimated that there are close to twenty million Spanish-speaking people in this country. The Hispanic group is the fastest growing ethnic group, as there are 100,000 Latin American immigrants every year to the United States (Cong. Royball, 1976). In addition it has been estimated we have about 10 to 12 million undocumented workers (illegal aliens) who do not report themselves to the authorities but who also need health services.

Spanish-speaking people, like any other group, get sick and become patients in hospitals and clinics throughout the nation. The larger the Hispanic population, the greater the number of Spanish-speaking patients who require health services assistance. The experience of being ill is usually a frightening one under any circumstances. But to be ill and not be able to communicate your problems, your pain, your fears and your needs, or to understand instructions is a traumatic and devastating experience. In a pluralistic society, health professionals in general and nurses in particular must be prepared to respond in a sensitive and effective manner to the needs of all consumers, including Spanish-speaking people.

Life in the United States demands that all nurses have a knowledge base about our cultural pluralism in order to become aware of the human condition of the diverse groups to which they must minister. This knowledge and awareness must be translated into the necessary understanding and acceptance of cultural differences and value systems of the diverse groups in our society. The nursing profession can no longer afford to continue to provide differential care to consumers of nursing care merely because some of the patients differ culturally and physically from the dominant group. Nursing as a profession must include in its scientific knowledge base other cultural and belief-value systems which differ from the majority group.

Research has always been the means through which any profession builds its scientific pool of knowledge. Therefore, nursing and nurses must initiate research projects that will give us the necessary data on which to build safe and effective nursing care that meets the need of our multi-cultural and multi-racial society. We do have some research data as well as empirical data at this time that can help us design educational programs to institutionalize cultural diversity content in nursing curricula.

Although we need to work at many levels to help nurses acquire the necessary knowledge, understanding, and skills to work with and care for the various ethnic groups of color, the most effective and far-reaching program is to start with the School of Nursing curriculum. No nurse should be graduated or nursing school accredited unless it has cultural diversity content in its curriculum.

Trying to speak about the Spanish-speaking people or Hispanics is a very difficult task because this is a very diverse group composed of people from all the countries of South and Central America, Mexico, some of the Caribbean countries, and Spain. The diversity within the group is as great as those within the Anglo-Saxon group. Variations and regionalisms of the Spanish language alone are almost as numerous as there are countries. However, the largest and better known groups in the United States are the Mexican-Americans or Chicanos, the Puerto Ricans, and more recently, the Cubans. The Mexican-Americans are indigenous to the Southwestern United States and are found in large numbers in the Northwest as well. The Puerto Ricans are concentrated mostly in New York and the east coast area and the Cubans in Miami. Of necessity my remarks will be mostly general but there will be some specific ones referring to particular groups which I will identify as such.

To provide effective and safe care to Spanish-speaking consumers we must take into account culture, language, values, and belief systems differences, as these affect health and illness perception of Hispanics. Spanish-speaking people also perceive health care providers in specific ways. In spite of the similarities and commonalities among people there are definitely differences which, if we do not take into consideration, will cause our care to be ineffective and in some instances unsafe. The socioeconomic and educational level of people within the same ethnic group provide the individual with different perceptions of the same values and cultural beliefs. Nurses and health workers need to be aware of and validate this to individualize their care for Hispanic patients. Knowledgeable and sensitive nurses will identify these differences and will plan effective and safe nursing intervention, without offending the sensitivities of her clients or violating their cultural beliefs.

NUTRITIONAL PREFERENCES

Nutritional preferences and habits play an important role, and at times a crucial role, in the lives of people as well as in the outcome of health and nursing care. The nurse with cultural knowledge of Hispanics' food preferences is able to plan nursing care which includes diets that the patient will eat to accelerate the healing process. Hispanic people eat different food and prepare the same food in a different way from the Anglo-American and other groups. They have different likes and dislikes. For instance, Hispanics are rice eaters while Anglo-Americans are potato eaters. Nurses should take this into consideration when planning diets for Hispanic patients if they want them to eat and adhere to the needed diet.

It is almost always possible to substitute foods which Spanish-speaking people like and contain the nutrients prescribed by the physician, and prepare them the way the patient likes them to ensure the desired results. It may take a little more planning and imagination and perhaps a little more time; however, this is what individualized and comprehensive care is all about. Hispanic diabetic patients are a very good example of nutritional preferences being neglected by professionals working with them. The diabetic diet planned for them is the same one planned for members of the majority group; consequently the patients do not eat it and they do a very poor job of substitution, which gets them into problems either because of insufficient amounts of calories or too many calories, to say nothing of wrong foods. All this is avoided when the patient's food habits and preferences are taken into account during the planning stage. This, of course, holds true for all kinds of diets.

HOT-COLD THEORY OF DISEASE AND TREATMENT

Many Spanish-speaking people classify food, illnesses, and medicines according to an etiological and therapeutic system which goes back to ancient times and was also used by Hippocrates in his humoral theory of disease. In the Hippocrates theory, health is the balance among the four humors of the body (blood, phlegm, black bile and yellow bile). Each one of these varies in temperature and moisture from the others. Blood was hot (caliente) and wet; yellow bile was hot and dry; phlegm was cold (frio or fresco) and wet; black bile was cold and dry. When there is a balance among them the body is warm and somewhat wet. In cases of imbalance between the humors, disease manifests itself and the body could be very hot, cold, dry, wet or any combination of these states (Harwood, 1971). Therefore, foods and medications, including herbs that are "hot" or "cold" (caliente-frio), are used therapeutically to restore the body to its normal balance. When "hot" diseases such as rashes, ulcers, or fever occur, the treatment should be "cold" medications and foods. The patient must behave according to expected behaviors inherent in the Hot-Cold theory of disease.

Harwood (1971), in his study of Hot-Cold theory of disease with Puerto-Rican families in New York, found that many Puerto-Rican patients in New York adhere to this classification of illness, medicines, and foods, and this belief system influences whether or not they comply with a medically prescribed therapeutic regime. When a disease is classified as "cold" they are treated with "hot" medicines and foods, while "hot" classified illnesses are treated with "cold" or cool medicines and foods. In New York City there are many *botanicas* in the *barrios* (neighborhoods), wherever Latin Americans live, where herbs are classified according to the "cold-hot" system. This has not only come from the native medicine but also from the medical schools established by the Spanish and Portugese in the 16th and 17th centuries in Mexico and Peru, where the Hippocratic humoral theory was the basis for medical diagnosis and treatment and on which pathology was rooted (Harwood, 1971). According to the humoral theory, body functions were regulated by four humors or bodily fluids which were characterized by heat or cold with wetness or dryness.

The health of the individual depended on the balance of the bodily humors. Any imbalance in these body fluids would result in disease. To restore health and cure the illness it was necessary to correct the imbalances by adding or subtracting heat, cold, dryness or wetness (Taylor, 1963; Currier, 1966; Harwood, 1971). In the Spanish-speaking countries most of the foods, herbs, and medicines are classified as "hot" (caliente) or "cold" (fresco or frio). *Fresco* refers to something being cool.

Currier makes the observation that while the hot-cold syndrome has persisted for centuries as the basis for folk medicine in Latin America, the wet-dry syndrome, which is equally important in the classical theory, has long disappeared. His hypothesis is that the nature of Mexican peasant society is such "that the individual's continuous preoccupation with achieving a balance between "heat" and "cold" is a way of reenacting, in symbolic terms, a fundamental activity in social relations" (Currier, 1978, p. 139).

Diseases caused by cold imbalance in the body are ailments which disable the individual by disrupting or stopping the sensory and motor functions of the body, and this comes about by the intrusion of coldness into a given part of the body (Currier, 1966). For example, earache is due to a cold draft of air which enters the ear canal; rheumatism is the result of cold from outside the body lodging in the affected bones; tuberculosis is caused by cold air or beverages entering the overheated body. On the other hand, there are other diseases which are believed to be brought about by the excess of heat in the body. Kidney diseases are caused by an abundance of heat in the body, and a kidney pain is a "hot pain." On many occasions it is accompanied by itching of the feet and ankles, redness of the palms, and fever.

These few examples suffice to give an idea of what can happen in the treatment of these diseases, if a physician who is not aware of these cultural medicine beliefs prescribes medications and diets which the patient and the family believe will have adverse effects on the body. The nurses, who are the ones who usually administer the medications and oversee the consumption of diets in the hospital, will be confronted with the patient's refusal to eat or to take the medications prescribed by the physician. When the patients are in their homes they will simply not take the medication or not give it to the children, as it was found in the South Bronx study done by the Martin Luther King, Jr. Neighboorhood Health Center. In the case of the common cold, which is believed to be caused by a cold draft entering the body and must be treated by restoring the body balance by using "hot" (caliente) remedies, the physician's recommendation for "plenty of fruit juices" will not be followed because these are "cool" or (fresco) liquids and therefore harmful to the body by adding more coldness to the body. If physicians and nurses are aware of this cultural medicine system they can get fluids into the system by recommending hot teas, soups, broth, etc., which are acceptable and will be followed by the patient and the family.

There is need to understand and respect the cultural beliefs of patients. We must appreciate that a cultural belief that has survived and served the Latin American people for so many centuries must have some "functional significance" in their lives and cannot be lightly dismissed. Currier makes the point that if this were not the case the hot-cold concept would have disappeared the way the wet-dry concept has almost vanished.

The hot-cold (caliente-frio) theory plays a very important role in the etiology of diseases in the Latin American countries. The hot-cold syndrome, Currier states, has been reported for Mexico (Beals, 1946; Foster, 1948; Lewis, 1960; Redfield, 1934), for Mexican-American communities (Saunders, 1954; Clark, 1959; McFeely, 1949; Rubel, 1960), for the Guatemalan Highlands (Gillin, 1951; Adams, 1952), for coastal Colombia (Reichel-Dolmatoff, 1958; Velasquez, 1957), for the Colombian Highlands (Reichel-Dolmatoff, 1961), and for coastal Peru and coastal Chile (Simmons, 1955). Currier also states (1978) that D'Harcoutr in 1939 in Paris stated that the hot-cold concept appears in a discussion of Inca medical practices at the time of the Spanish Conquest. By personal observation the writer has been able to experience the same hot-cold (caliente-frio) theory of etiology of disease in Panama and in Costa Rica.

Temperature and changes in temperature play a very important role in the causation of diseases according to the Latin American belief, as in the case of the common cold outlined above. For instance there is a condition very common among Hispanic people called *Pasmo*. The term *pasmo*, according to Currier (1978), describes two different conditions, both related to the hot-cold theory. In one it refers to *pasmo* as a tonic spasm of any voluntary muscle, after exposure to cold air and becoming chilled when the body is in an overheated condition. In the other use, *pasmo* refers to a cough, stomach pain, or any other cold-classified manifestation which has become chronic. There is a third use of *pasmo* which could or could not be related to the hot-cold theory. The physical growth and development of a child could be arrested for long periods of time as a result of *pasmo,* which can be brought about by *desarreglos* (negligency) of the mother in exposing the child to extreme temperature, especially cold, when the child is overheated. Then it is said that the child *está pasmado* (its growth is stunted).

If the etiology of diseases is connected to the hot-cold theory, it then follows that the correction or cure of illnesses is also interconnected with medicines and nutrition which follows the same classification. Therefore, illnesses brought about by exposure to cold and chilling are cured by "hot" medicines and the patient should only ingest "hot" foods and "hot" beverages. The reverse is true of diseases and conditions that are brought about by exposure to hot temperatures. This presents a great deal of difficulties for physicians and nurses when treating Hispanic patients.

Hispanics use of the principle of "neutralization" or neutralizing the nature of the medicine or the food; this could be very useful to the health professionals. Currier (1978) gives us a good example of "neutralization" in the use of penicillin as a prophylactic in the case of former rheumatic fever patients. Because rheumatic fever involves joint pains, it is classified as a "cold" illness, and "hot" penicillin is therefore an accepted treatment. However, if the patient is having diarrhea or constipation at the time that he is participating in a maintenance program, this treatment will be contraindicated by the patient's standards because diarrhea is considered a "hot" disease. The way to neutralize the "hot" effect of penicillin is to advise the patient to take the penicillin with fruit juice or any other cold substance. This will insure that the patient will indeed take the penicillin he needs to avoid reappearance of rheumatic fever symptoms.

It is possible to use the hot-cold theory beliefs to reinforce regular treatments used by physicians and nurses. One example given by Harwood (1971) is the recommended bland diet in the case of an ulcer, which prohibits most of the foods which are considered "hot" and would therefore be avoided by the patients because of their belief system. The same is true of the prescription of aspirin for colds or arthritis; both are considered "cold" diseases. Aspirin, being a hot medication, is good to restore the balance in the body, and therefore in agreement with both therapeutic systems.

It is very important to take into account the hot-cold classification of foods in pediatric care, especially in the feeding of infants. Harwood makes the point of evaporated milk being classified as a "hot" food, while whole milk is considered "cool" or fresca. Hospitals usually recommend for mothers a formula with an evaporated milk base. Because infants tend to develop rashes, and these are believed to come from "hot" foods, mothers prefer to give whole milk formulas to their babies. Harwood describes a study with a sample of 27 Puerto Rican mothers in New York in which 41 percent of the mothers, almost immediately upon return home from the hospital, changed the babies' "hot" formula. The strategies used to accomplish this were of two types: five mothers, or 19 percent, merely discontinued the evaporated milk formula after a few weeks and gave the babies whole milk only. Because it is believed that it is dangerous to switch too fast from "hot" to "cool" food, mothers usually fed their babies weak tea and mannitol (cool substances) for 24 hours before starting whole milk. However, six mothers (22 percent), rather than switching milk, decided to use the "neutralizing" principle to resolve the conflict. They added a cool substance to the evaporated milk formula or fed something cool to the baby as a supplement. The substances used were barley water, magnesium carbonate, and mannitol. The latter two substances are cathartic and diuretic, respectively, and were given to the babies in sufficient amounts to cause diarrhea. The study suggested a source of diarrhea in Puerto Rican babies in New York that Harwood felt should be rigorously investigated. At the same time, if the nurse and the physician working with these mothers knows about the "hot-cold" theory system, they will encourage the mothers to use barley water as a neutralizing agent instead of the other two, which are harmful to the babies.

If the nurse and the physician are knowledgeable about the "hot-cold" theory of disease and treatment, they can design their treatment regime and management to be within this principle to ensure that the patients will carry out the prescribed treatment procedures and therefore have success in recovery [Table 15-1]. In pediatrics it is good to keep in mind that the usual childhood diseases which include skin eruptions or rashes are classified as "hot" in the nosology of this system. Therefore, in cases of measles, chickenpox, etc., cool medications are used in the home to "cool" the internal organs and bring the rash to the surface. Raisins soaked in warm milk or water are given to the children. In order to get fluids into the system, the nurses can recommend "cool" drinks, such as fruit juices, be given to the babies, and they can be sure the mothers will follow instructions which will benefit the children.

Harwood (1971) states that pregnant women avoid hot foods and medications during this time to avoid the baby being born with an "irritation" (red skin or a rash). They also "refresh" themselves repeatedly by taking Milk of Magnesia (1 to 3 tablespoons a day) or use commercial antacids and take two to four doses a day during the first two trimesters of gestation. This is done even more if they have used abortifacients unsuccessfully to prevent irritation. It is essential that they take "cool" preparations.

La cuarentena, or the period of 40 days after the delivery, is traditionally observed by women. They avoid "cold" or "cool" foods because it is believed these impede the flow of blood and will prevent the emptying of the uterus and the birth canal. Care must be taken that the lochia does not flow toward the head as it is believed that this will cause nervousness or even insanity (purga del parto), which literally means the "purge of parturition" (Harwood 1971). To help prevent all these possible dangers, hot foods and tonics are made of "hot" foods such as chocolate, garlic, cinnamon, rue (ruda), mint and pieces of cheese. It is believed that "cool" or "cold" foods must be avoided while menstruating because it is

Table 15-1. The hot-cold classification among Puerto Ricans*

	Frio (cold)	Fresco (cool)	Caliente (hot)
Illnesses or bodily conditions	Arthritis Colds Frialdad del Esomago Menstrual period Pain in the joints Pasmo		Constipation Diarrhea Rashes Tenesmus (pujo) Ulcers
Medicines and herbs		Bicarbonate of soda Linden flowers (flor de tilo) Mannitol (mana de manito) Mastic bark (almacigo) $MgCO_3$ (magnesia boba) Milk of magnesia Nightshade (yerba mora) Orange flower water (agua de azahar) Sage	Anise Aspirin Castor oil Cinnamon Cod liver oil Fe tablets Penicillin Rue (ruda) Vitamins
Foods	Avocado Bananas Coconut Lima beans Sugar cane White beans	Barley water Bottled milk Chicken Fruits Honey Raisins Salt-cod (bacalao) Watercress	Alcoholic beverages Chili peppers Chocolate Coffee Corn meal Evaporated milk Garlic Kidney beans Onions Peas Tobacco

*From Harwood, A. 1971. The hot-cold theory of disease: Implications for treatment of Puerto Rican patients. *J.A.M.A.* 216:1153-1158.

important for the flow of blood from the womb to be complete. The author remembers that as a young girl when her own menses started she would not take baths which would chill the body (there was no hot water plumbing) or walk in the rain or even wash clothes because soap was considered "cool" and so was the cold water in which the clothes were washed.

La matriz debil or "weak" womb is believed to "jump" around in the abdomen looking for something hot to fortify it. Thus it is customary to give "hot" foods and beverages to strengthen the womb. *Ruda* or rue, an herb, is one used very often for this condition, mixed with cocoa, black coffee, or rum.

The cultural belief of "hot-cold" theory of etiology of disease is one that should not and cannot be ignored by nurses or other health professionals if they want to be effective when caring for Hispanics. They should familiarize themselves with the theory and cultural beliefs, as well as the "hot-cold" classification of diseases, foods and medications.

Currier (1966) gives a list of some diseases considered "cold," because they are caused by cold entering the body, such as chest cramps, earache, headache, paralysis, pain due to sprains, stomach cramps, teething and tuberculosis. He also gives a list of some of the illnesses considered to be caused by an overabundance of heat in the body: *algodoncillo,* erysipelas, dysentery, sore eyes, *fogazo,* kidney ailments, *postemilla,* sore throat, warts and rashes. He also gives a group of diseases which can be caused by either heat or cold, which means that each one has its "hot" and "cold" form and remedies must be applied accordingly. He gives three examples of these: diarrhea, which is usually caused by cold but may also be "hot." You can differentiate them by observation. If feces are merely loose it is caused by cold; if feces are green and steam when fresh, then it is caused by heat. With enteritis or *torzon,* a more serious form of diarrhea, again it is the appearance of the feces that tells you its etiology. If they are streaked with blood, it is a "hot" illness, if they are white and covered with mucous, they are caused by "cold." Toothache, when in the molar teeth are "hot," caused by improper diet, but those in other teeth are usually caused by a draft of cold air.

There are long lists of classifications of foods and medicines into "cold" and "hot" and a couple are included here, but they would be too long to be part of this paper. It will suffice to say that "cold" foods include most fresh vegetables, most tropical fruits, dairy products and low prestige meats, such as goat, fish and chicken (Currier, 1966). "Hot" foods include most of the chili peppers, most temperate zone fruits, goat milk, cereal grains, high prestige meats, such as beef, water fowl, and mutton, most oils, hard liquor and aromatic beverages (Currier, 1966).

It is believed that warm or hot foods are more easily digested than cold foods. Because the inside of the body and the stomach are warm, all foods have to be warmed before they can be digested. If food is hot or warm, it is ready to be digested upon entering the stomach, while the cold food requires more work of the stomach to warm it before being able to digest it. According to some Hispanics, it is easy to identify food as to whether it is easily digestible or not.

Currier goes on to outline the aspects of life other than those of disease and nutrition which relate to the qualities of hot and cold. In this other context the symbolic meanings of hot and cold are more patently revealed. Cold is associated with threatening aspects of life while warmth is associated with reassurance. This is a practice that has been observed and reported in several of the Latin American countries, such as Mexico, Guatemala, Peru and Chile (Simmons, 1956; Rubel, 1960; Adams, 1952). Men or women in those countries, if they are to go out at night, pull a portion of their *ponchos, sarapes,* or blankets over their noses and mouths to prevent the cold night air from getting into their bodies and causing illness. Cold is more likely to be introduced into the body when it has been particularly warm, such as coming out of a warm house into the cold air of night. Nursing mothers must be very careful of extreme temperatures, cold or hot. Cold decreases the flow of milk, but extreme heat makes milk curdle in the child's stomach and it cannot be digested. When this happens it is said that the child is *enlechado*.

Nurses and health workers need to familiarize themselves with the "hot-cold" theory of disease of the Hispanic population to give effective care to the largest minority group (unofficially) in the United States, if we count the millions of undocumented workers. Sooner or later we all will care for some Hispanic clients. It is not necessary for the health professionals to accept this etiology of illness but it is necessary to understand it and respect it as part of the belief system of a group of people for whom this is a cultural institution that has persisted and served them well throughout the centuries. There must be something to it. Like parapsychology, we need to research it. In the meantime health professionals need to take this into account when caring for Hispanic patients, if they want their patients to follow their treatment and advice. I certainly utilize it and modify it by using the neutralizing concept. I am convinced there is utility for the group in the "hot-cold" theory and we could use it judiciously to help our Hispanic clients.

LANGUAGE BARRIER

With the influx of newly arrived Latin Americans to the various parts of the United States, the number of Hispanic people who have difficulty speaking and understanding English has increased. Even those who have been longer in the country are not too proficient in the English language. Grebler, Moore and Guzman (1970) referred to this problem and its extent. In Los Angeles and San Antonio, in a comprehensive study of Mexican-Americans, it was found that over half of the subjects chosen at random had difficulty with English. The subjects were representatives of the lower socioeconomic class.

This has tremendous implications for health care and treatment of all diseases but it becomes even more acute when we deal with meantl illness and its treatment because of the traditional psychotherapy, or "talking therapy." There is no way that an Hispanic with no English or very limited English could establish a therapeutic relationship with a therapist who can speak no Spanish. Health education schools, including nursing, must recruit and graduate bilingual, bicultural Hispanics to help alleviate this very common situation in areas where Hispanics are found. The other alternative is that more Anglo-American nurses and health professionals learn the Spanish language. They are certainly as intelligent as the Hispanics who learn English. Then the question of how effective they would be with Hispanic clients needs to be validated by research.

However, we must deal with this problem as it now exists and make sure that health service agencies that have Spanish-speaking clients who have problems with English have bilingual, bicultural interpreters who can not only interpret the words but also the cultural meanings and symbolism in order to serve the Hispanic patients effectively. Acosta Johnson (1964) makes the point that interpreters who work with Spanish-speaking patients must be hand-picked. Spanish-American interpreters who have recently risen from the lower ranks into a white collar job "may be disdainful of the plight of their uneducated countryman." This is quickly picked up by the patient "who wears his supersensitive pride on his sleeve, and a further strain may be added to the treatment process."

PSYCHOLOGICAL ASPECTS

Hispanics are very emotive people and it is very interesting to observe the group in interaction between and among themselves. Their gestures are very expressive, and while to us they are second nature, they are disturbing to the more sedate and less expressive Anglo-American counterpart. Personal observation has revealed that at times the emotivity of the Hispanics is distracting to the Anglo-American who may be involved in an interaction with a Spanish-American. Therefore, some of us have had to learn two styles of interacting with people—one with the majority group, and our natural one with our own group.

Among the cultural values of the Latin American or Hispanic is the firm belief that you do not reveal personal or family information to strangers, or even friends, if this has no relevance for them. Personal and family affairs are a private matter and must be kept within the family group. At times even individual matters are not told to the family if they cannot help and will only bring them worry and anxiety. This is in contrast to the Anglo-American group who are much more open and willing to discuss private and family matters freely. It used to be a matter of amazement to me that upon casually meeting an Anglo-American person, within minutes I would be told the family history and at times the most intimate problems of this individual. This, of course, has a great deal of value in relation to psychotherapy, as the individual can easily disclose self and family problems to a therapist. On the other hand, the Hispanic's reluctance to self and family disclosures makes him a poor candidate for psychotherapy or "talking therapy." Jourard and his associates (Jourard, 1971) studied the self-disclosure styles and evaluation of comparative cross-cultural levels of self-disclosure and his findings indicated that Black and Puerto Rican college students are less inclined to reveal personal information to others, including friends and parents, than are Anglo-Americans. This may be partly responsible for the reason that Hispanics are less involved in psychotherapy even when there are free clinics located in the areas where they live (Kline, 1968; Yamamoto et al., 1968). This is partly because there are other studies (Rendon, 1974) that have indicated that discrimination permeates even the psychiatric agencies. Psychiatrists assign Puerto Rican adolescents in New York State to psychiatric hospitals more than twice as often as adolescents from the majority group. Another factor is the insensitivity of agencies and health professionals to the problems of Hispanics and therefore the mistrust of Hispanics for institutions and professionals who practice racism, overtly or covertly. . . .

The expressions of pain and anxiety may take different forms than from those of the majority group. Patients in pain may groan and moan to let those around them know they are uncomfortable and suffering. This brings contempt, and at times reprisals, from the Anglo-American nurses because they "cannot stand babies." This is a cultural way of expressing pain and suffering. If understood in this context, it would be easier for nurses to accept it without ridicule or retaliation.

CULTURAL BARRIERS

Stenger-Castro, in his research to study how the effect of cultural barriers affects the treatment of Mexican-Americans, investigated cultural barriers between Mexican-Americans and Anglo-Americans. He found that there is a definite cultural barrier between the Mexican-Americans and Anglo-Americans (I think this can be generalized to include Hispanics in general). He found that all the Mexican-American patients interviewed for the study were alienated from their therapists because of the cultural differences. Consequently, they did not trust them and did not reveal all the facts even after several years of treatment, no matter how important this was for their treatment.

Perhaps this may remain forever thus; however, this can be minimized by the Anglo-American professional being aware of and sensitive to cultural values of Hispanic patients and by being genuinely concerned about their well-being in general and by having respect for the cultural differences and utilizing them for the benefit of the client.

SUMMARY

The Hispanic group is unofficially the largest ethnic minority group in the United States, if we include all the undocumented workers in the nation. They are found in all states of the Union with large concentrations in the east, west and certain parts of the southeast and southwest. This means that all these consumers at one time or another are in need of health and nursing services. What kind of service they will receive and how effective nurses and other health professionals will be in their treatment of Hispanics will depend upon their knowledge base of Hispanic cultural values, their genuine concern and caring for Spanish-speaking patients, and their willingness to respect their cultural values and utilize them whenever these values are not dysfunctional to the individual.

Many Hispanics adhere to the "hot-cold" theory of disease and treatment. Congruent with this belief, their health and illness conception is dominated and permeated by the "hot-cold" theory, and their behavior to promote health and eradicate disease is in conformity with it. If health professionals understand this cultural concept and respect it they can utilize it to ensure the patients will follow the treatment regime, and they will be more effective in working with Hispanics.

Language and cultural barriers can be minimized by employing bilingual, bicultural interpreters who can not only interpret the language but also the culture.

The Anglo-American professionals can do much to modify the image Hispanic patients hold of them by being more knowledgeable about Hispanic cultural values and beliefs, and utilizing them to become more effective in their treatment of the Spanish-speaking patient.

References

1. Royball, E. Sept. 1976. COSSMO First National Hispanic Conference on Health and Human Services, Los Angeles, California.

2. Harwood, A. 1971. The hot-cold theory of disease: Implications for treatment of Puerto Rican patients. *J.A.M.A.* 216:1153-1158.

3. Taylor, H. O. 1963. *Greek biology and medicine.* New York: Cooper Square.

4. Currier, R. L. 1978. The hot-cold syndrome and symbolic balance in Mexican and Spanish American folk medicine. In Martinez, R. A., editor. *Hispanic culture and health care: Fact, fiction, folklore,* St. Louis: The C. V. Mosby Co.

5. Rubel, A. J. 1960. Concepts of disease in Mexican-American culture. *Am. Anthro.* 62:795-814.

6. Simmons, O. 1956. Popular and modern medicine in mestizo communities of coastal Peru and Chile. *J. Am. Folklore* 68:57-71.

7. Grebler, L.; Moore, J. W.; and Guzman, R. C. 1970. *The Mexican people.* New York: The Free Press.

8. Johnson, C. A. 1964. Nursing and Mexican-American folk medicine. *Nurs. Forum* 3:104-113.

9. Jourard, S. M. 1971. *Self-disclosure: An experimental analysis of the transparent self.* New York: John Wiley & Sons, Inc.

10. Kline, L. Y. 1969. Some factors in the psychiatric treatment of Spanish-Americans. *Am. J. Psychiatry* 125:1674-1681.

11. Yamamoto, J.; James, Q. C.; and Polley, N. 1968. Cultural problems in psychiatric therapy. *Arch. Gen. Psychiatry* 19:45-49.

12. Rendon, M. 1974. Transcultural aspects of Puerto Rican mental illness in New York. *Int. J. Soc. Psychiatry* 20½:18-19.

Bibliography

Beals, R. L. 1946. *Cheran: A Sierra Tarascan village.* Publications of the Institute of Social Anthropology, Smithsonian Institutions 2:1-225.

Clark, M. 1959. *Health in the Mexican-American culture.* Berkeley, Calif.: University of California Press.

Foster, G. M. 1948. *Empire's children: The people of Tzintzuntzan.* Publications of the Institute of Social Anthropology, Smithsonian Institutions 6:1-279.

Lewis, O. 1960. *Tepoztlan: Village in Mexico.* New York: Holt Rinehart & Winston, Inc.

McFeeley, F. 1949. *Some aspects of folk curing in the American Southwest.* Berkeley: University of California at Berkeley (M.A. Thesis).

Redfield, R. 1934. *Chan Kom: Amaya village.* Washington, D.C.: Carnegie Institute, Publication 448.

Reichel-Dolmatoff, G.; and Reichel-Dolmatoff, A. 1962. *The people of Aritama: The cultural personality of a Columbian Meztizo village.* Chicago: University of Chicago Press.

Reichel-Dolmatoff, G.; and Reichel-Dolmatoff, A. 1958. Nivel de salva y medicina popular en una aldea mestiza Colombiana. *Revista Colombiana de Antropologia* 7:199-249.

Saunders, L. 1954. *Cultural differences and medical care.* New York: Russell Sage Foundation.

Velasquez, R. 1957. La medicina popular en la costa Colombiana del Pacifico. *Revista Colombiana de Antropologia* 6:193-241.

16

American Indian
Patient Care

Martha Primeaux, R.N., M.S.N.
George Henderson, Ph.D.

For many years Americans espoused the "melting pot" philosophy in an attempt to minimize the differences among the wide variety of cultural groups in our society. Many culturally distinct groups have now proclaimed a different philosophy. American society can be compared with a tossed salad: each element is mixed with others, yet each maintains its own unique characteristics, customs, values, and belief systems. Each group makes a unique contribution to the total quality of the American experience, and no one element is seen as better or worse than any other. In such a culturally diverse society the health care delivery system should demand that its practitioners be prepared to carry out their professional tasks with full understanding of the significance of multiculturalism in promoting meaningful health care for every citizen.

In the evolution of the health care professions, the emphasis historically has been on the care of the majority population. As noted in Chapter 2, it was not until the late 1960s that Madeleine Leininger and other nursing professionals saw the critical importance of understanding cultural values and beliefs and developing a body of theory and skills to facilitate the delivery of care to people of different cultures.[1] These theories and practices were to have special emphasis on values, beliefs, and practices of a group regarding the issues of health and illness.

It was not until the early 1970s, however, that groups of Third World nurses began to emerge, emphasizing the right to health care for Third World people of the four federally defined groups (black American, American Indian, Mexican

American, and Asian American). This trend was a part of an affirmative action movement across the United States. The aim of the nursing profession now is that all people receive better health care, regardless of age, sex, color, or religion. Inherent in this goal is a system of values that includes respect for cultural differences, respect for economic, political and social rights of others, and affirmation of the right to seek and maintain an ethnic identity.

Marie Branch and Phyllis Paxton point out that knowledge of cultural differences requires a set of responses that are directed toward cultures as distinguished from social needs of clients.[2] We contend that health care services cannot provide adequate, effective, comprehensive, safe care unless cultural aspects of health and illness are given full consideration. An individual's reaction to illness, health maintenance, daily activities, and various curing and caring treatment practices are closely linked with cultural beliefs, values, and past experiences. Thus, attitudes and reactions to health and illness require cultural understanding on the part of the caretaker to provide effective and safe health care.

This chapter addresses the unique characteristics and health care needs of American Indians, with special emphasis on the interrelatedness of religion and medicine. Further, this chapter shares with health care providers practical knowledge and nursing interventions. It is our aim to help the reader understand how certain rituals, values, and customs of American Indian cultures shape members' attitudes, behaviors, and beliefs regarding health care. In addition, social forces that largely determine the quality of life of American Indians are examined.

SOCIAL FORCES

Each decade ends with a larger number of Native Americans living in metropolitan areas such as Chicago, Denver, Los Angeles, New York, and San Francisco. The major reason for this relocation from reservations and often rural areas is the search for jobs. Few well-paying jobs can be found on reservations and in rural areas.

Rural or urban, Native Americans face a special set of health care problems and concerns. The types and multitudes of disease processes in any given population have direct correlation to the population's environment, economic status, education level, and traditional values. These variables in turn influence individual Native Americans' health and nutritional status as well as the availability and demand for health services.[3] The social conditions of Native American communities such as impoverished socioeconomic conditions, limited educational levels, substandard housing, poor sanitation, malnutrition, and inadequate health services all contribute to the high incidence of deaths by accident, suicide, and disease. Diseases that are nonexistent in other populations are still leading causes of death in the Native American population.[4] As noted in the final report on Indian health to the American Indian Policy Review Commission, "While there has been striking improvement in mortality from diseases of acute and chronic infections as well as cardiovascular disease, these results are overshadowed by the increased deaths associated with accidents, alcoholism, cirrhosis of the liver and suicides."[5]

These social forces on health must be considered within the framework of health care delivery. No one can dispute the fact that environment plays a very important role in maintaining and improving the health of any group. Poor housing conditions have had a negative impact on the health of American Indians and have significantly contributed to the high incidence of preventable diseases. Poor housing is only one cell of a cluster of adverse conditions affecting American Indians:

> Nutritional deprivation due to inadequate or nonexistent sanitary facilities, lack of conventional utilitarian services, geographic isolation, lack of transportation, low income and unemployment all contribute to malnutrition and create a situation in which it is difficult for many American Indians to have good nutritional habits.[6]

As a result, in general the diet of Native Americans is high in carbohydrates and fats and low in proteins, essential vitamins, and minerals.

If health care providers understand the impact of these social forces, they can be in a better position to assist Native American families and direct them to health resources as well as assist them when they encounter barriers to services. Specifically, nurses and other health care workers employed in the public health sector can utilize the Indian Health Service, local Housing and Urban Development offices, agencies in the Bureau of Indian Affairs, and state health departments.

IMPORTANCE OF FAMILY

Health workers must respect the value system of the group that they work with to have open, reciprocal communication. According to Edward T. Hall and W. F. White, major conflicts in transcultural situations center on communication.[7] Any breakdown in communication leads to a breakdown in the level of health care given. Transferring one's own cultural expectations of how individuals should behave in certain situations is bound to lead to miscommunications. Consider the following example:

> An elderly woman had a small bag attached to a necklace. The nurses thought the bag had an offensive odor, and, after much protest from the patient, they removed the necklace and placed it with other personal items away from the bedside. When family members visited, the elderly patient told of the incident. The family became extremely upset over the breaking of a taboo and the certainty that their elderly family member would now die. The family members were chided by the nurse for thinking such a "silly" thing. The patient became critically ill within a few hours and did indeed die within a few days.[8]

Clarissa S. Scott states that social distance is created when Third World consumers and health care providers subscribe to different sets of values.[9] For example, understanding the kinship system of American Indians will assist the health care worker to offer better services, avoid needless confrontation, narrow the "social distance," and avoid a breakdown in communication. The value of the family is exceedingly important to American Indians. *To be poor in the Indian world is to be without relatives.* The community health worker will likely find many people living in small quarters in the Native American community. To the American Indian, family is an extended part in the truest sense. All blood relatives are considered part of the family and will extend over several generations. Grandparents, uncles, aunts, and cousins may live together under one roof at various times. It is more unusual to find a Native American nuclear family living alone, even in urban areas where Native Americans have migrated for employment purposes. Sometimes it may not even be a blood relative but a tribal person (someone from the same tribe) who is considered part of the family.

> I remember an incident in a municipal hospital in which a young American Indian was a patient in the intensive care unit. His visiting privileges were limited to immediate relatives only. Three different Indian women came at different times, all professing to be the young man's mother. The Anglo nurse did not understand that all three women were instrumental in his developmental process and were all indeed called "mother" in his Indian language. He distinguished among them by certain descriptive words.[10]

Family structure becomes exceedingly important during periods of crisis; family members are a source of security, strength and emotional support. This kinship system has implications if the American Indian client is hospitalized. A variety of relatives will come to the hospital expecting to visit with the hospitalized relative only to find that visiting privileges are limited to certain close relatives. The American Indian does not distinguish between close and distant relatives. To have many people visit you in the hospital is an expectation of the ill person as well as the family members. If relatives are limited to parents, brothers, and sisters, it will soon become apparent that the Native American has several sets of parents and grandparents and a host of brothers and sisters.

One may wonder how Native Americans could have such a large family. First cousins are treated as brothers and sisters; uncles and aunts become grandparents and are accorded the privileges thereof. This kinship system exists in all American Indian tribes we have come in contact with, even for the urban American Indian who may have assimilated many values of the Anglo culture. Creative approaches to including family members in actively caring for the patient would be beneficial to all concerned—the patient, the family, and the nurse. It is not uncommon for patients to be discharged earlier than their conditions merit because family members were incorporated into their care. If given the opportunity and a little assistance from professional workers, the Indian family is and can be extremely resourceful.

INDIAN MEDICINE AND RELIGION

Through the study of linguistics and anthropology one learns that different groups of people not only think in different ways but also see things differently. Cultural differences then lead individuals to view all things around them in specific ways. Attitudes toward disease and cure vary considerably with all groups of people. Ari Kiev states that culture greatly influences both the form of illness and the treatment.[11] Furthermore, methods of treatment are culturally defined and culturally specific. Lyle Saunders further contends that illness and disease are social as well as biological phenomena, and the relationship that the ill person has to other group members is also culturally prescribed.[12] These concepts are especially applicable to American Indians, who like other Third World people, have repertoires of culturally defined patterns of behavior that assist them in maintaining a specific level of survival.

In the Western world religion is generally perceived as a discrete body of knowledge practiced in a specific place. The religious experience to the American Indian is something that surrounds the being at all times.[13] In fact, most American Indians believe that nothing could be classified as nonreligious. We believe that it was these beliefs that maintained American Indians against all odds of survival and that consequently religion has had a profound influence of their entire being.

The intimacy of religion and medicine is seen in the Native American theory of disease and illness causation, treatment, and prevention. Native American medicine is based on ages of tradition and trust. Disease causation is not related to the germ theory. In fact, a recent survey of American Indian registered nurses from 23 different tribes found no tribal word for "germ." Health embraces a broad category of forces beyond the treatment of diseases and the healing of wounds. These forces are intertwined in all aspects of the physical, social, psychological, and spiritual being. It employs a reciprocal relationship of individuals or groups and the process of what is happening in the environment. Religion is integrated with a distinct way of living and interpreting life. This view can best be classified as holistic health care.

Holistic health care is the total of those factors that affect the life of the individual in the prevention of disease. Consequently this concept rejects the idea of treatment based on the germ theory of causation. Utilizing the holistic concept, healing ceremonies differ from tribe to tribe with varying degrees of complexity. Despite tribal variations, most healing ceremonies take place in the home with participation of family members, other tribal members, or both. If the patient should be hospitalized, nurses should be cognizant of the wishes of the Indian patient or family to seek traditional healers and make them feel that their services are legitimate. Providing space and privacy for ceremony is in order. The nurse can ask family members what their needs might be and how the system may assist.

The family may want to leave objects in the room that were used in the healing ceremony because these objects are associated with the elements identified with the cause of illness. It is the agent responsible for the illness that determines the cure. The ritual is just as important as the medicine used. The specific treatment will depend on the social, physical, emotional, or spiritual component. For example, if cornmeal is used, it may need to be left in place for a specified time, or an object may be requested by the family to be placed on the bed of the ill person.

> The encouragement and acceptance of curing practices as legitimate rather than witchcraft will help to reduce anxiety and alienation that many Indian patients experience with hospitalization. In some instances, the meal may be removed immediately after the ceremony and placed in a container provided by the family. At no time should the meal be removed and tossed into a waste can without family permission. If the family does not provide a container for the meal, it may be removed and taken outside of the room for disposal after the family has given permission for the removal.[14]

Although most American Indians recognize the value of Western medicine, many continue to use traditional medicine and cures. These treatment regimes are both symbolic and concrete for the ill person and are therefore trusted. In many instances American Indian patients will turn to native healers when they are dissatisfied with results of other treatment regimes. It is not infrequent that the Native American patient perceives the medical treatment to be improper. Scott believes that understanding the underlying reasons for the selection of certain therapies and therapists will enable the majority health care system to develop an appropriate delivery system.[15] Certainly the nurse is in a strategic position to obtain information regarding choice of systems.

Belief in how to maintain health and how one became ill is deeply ingrained from cultural beliefs and will influence whether a patient decides to follow or not follow a particular medical regime. This concept has implications for nurses in health teaching. *Indian medicine and religion cannot be separated.* In fact, Native American medicine makes no distinction between physical and mental illness. It is important to remember that we are talking about curing systems that predate scientific medicine. Furthermore, as pointed out in earlier chapters, we are talking about religious practices proven to be effective long before hospital procedures were established. We have also noted in earlier chapters that the separation of mind and body is not characteristic of Indian and other Third World cultures. The issue is not the legitimacy of this approach; instead, it is respect.

Failure to respect a people's religious beliefs and practices will ultimately lead us to treat them as nonpersons. Tribal healing ceremonies are not pagan orgies. On the contrary, they are highly ritualistic religious ways to deal with sickness and death. Extending the rituals to include family members is the way Indians share in all aspects of life—even suffering. This concept of group healing has been briefly discussed in Chapter 12. Interestingly, most health practitioners have little difficulty accepting the religious healing ceremonies of their own sects. Native Americans will utilize their own healing ceremonies with or without orthodox institutional permission.

The amount of time devoted to curative ceremonies may vary from tribe to tribe and according to symptoms expressed, but causation is central to the process. It is the agent responsible for the illness that determines the cure. Some rituals may be carried out by the family or one healing person, or the family may seek the assistance of more than one specialist from the traditional culture.

> Privacy for the ceremony is in order. Such a ceremony may be frightening to other patients and families who do not understand it. Nothing elaborate is needed. Space requirements depend upon the number of family members present. There is nothing wrong in asking an Indian family member whether the patient's room is big enough. In most instances, it will be. . . . Rituals or ceremonies held in hospitals are relatively short—from 30 minutes to two hours. While the elaborate sing or healing ceremony that is prevalent in some Indian tribes could last one to nine days, these are usually held in the community. Rituals carried out in hospitals are done in such a manner that they may go unnoticed by many.[16]

Nurses can do much to allay the fears of non-Indian patients who are within close proximity of the ceremony. It is hardly comforting to be told, "I don't know what's going on." Nurses should know and be able to interpret to non-Indian patients and hospital personnel the importance of Indian curative ceremonies.[17] Ignorance, not the ceremonies, is to be feared.

The most prevalent pattern for the American Indian is the alternate use of traditional medicine and modern Western medicine, either independently of each other or simultaneously. In most instances the two systems of care are complementary, and choosing between the two does not produce ambivalence. However, Native Americans will not totally give up a health care system that has worked for generations for a system that practices fragmented care. When there is "cultural fit," there is no reason to give up either system. Lack of cultural fit occurs when two or more health cultures are dissimilar in crucial ways that make it impossible for a member of one tradition to accept certain beliefs and behavior of another. The result is dissatisfaction by both the provider and the receiver. Nurses and health care practitioners can help to implement a cultural fit between Native American and modern Western medicine.

CULTURAL FOODS AND DIET

The use of food items in the Native American population goes beyond a consideration of nutritional value. Each tribe has foods that have symbolic meaning. Two of the most common food items are corn and squash. As noted earlier, cornmeal is used in a variety of curative rituals and commands utmost respect. Cornmeal is used to sprinkle on the shoulders before entering a home to ward off bringing in illness. This practice has significance for health care workers who may be administering care in the home. During winter months when colds and influenza epidemics may be more frequent, or when a highly susceptible person is being cared for in the home, cornmeal may be used as a preventive measure.

Cornmeal is also used in hospitals—sprinkled around the bed of the Native American patient or sprinkled directly on the patient. Respect for these beliefs must be evident even though the health care worker may not view them as scientific. Any other attitude will certainly alienate the patient and the family, leading to noncooperation with the Western medical therapy regime.

Diet is a function of the culture and plays a vital role in most ethnic groups. If nurses and other health care providers have a knowledge of cultural food patterns, they can adapt diets to include ethnic foods and still maintain daily dietary requirements even for specialty diets. Dietary regimes should be constructed in light of the available food resources. If hospitals cannot provide such foods or do not have knowledge in preparation, family members are usually more than happy to be able to do this for their ill family members.

Utilization of community members as a resource for knowledge and expertise in food preparation or cultural customs pays large dividends. The University of Oklahoma's College of Nursing collaborates with four ethnic community groups to produce a cultural food festival. The ethnic groups prepare and serve the food to 150 nursing students and 20 faculty members. Everyone has a good time eating, and the ethnic groups enjoy sharing part of their culture on which they are the experts. Creative nurses can utilize other approaches in providing ethnic food for their clients.

For American Indians, eating is a social function; they eat with social equals. If the environment has been one of sharing, respect, and mutual exchange, a Native American will want to serve food to a nurse visiting in the home. Initially only fruit or coffee may be offered. Sharing is a concept within American Indian cultures that crosses tribal lines. Food, money, or other material possessions are of value only when shared with family and friends.

URBAN INDIANS

Few studies have been made of the life styles of urban American Indians. Steve Unger compiled a book of readings that details the culture shock, alienation, and destruction of American Indian families.[18] John G. Red Horse and his coauthors take issue with the assumption that the urban American Indian family is disintegrating.[19] Instead, they argue that diverse family network interlockings and life styles represent different ways of coping with environmental stress.

Red Horse and his coauthors distinguish three urban Chippewa family life style patterns: traditional, bicultural, and pantraditional. Traditional families are characterized by parents and grandparents who speak Ojibway as the conversational language, whereas the children are bilingual. Midēwiwin is the religion, and Native American cultural activities (feasts and powwows) are still part of family life. English is the conversational language of bicultural Chippewas, but some Ojibway is retained. Anglo religions, mainly Catholicism, prevail, and bicultural Chippewas engage in all of the Anglo society's activities. Pan traditional Chippewas speak either English or Ojibway as their conversational language. Religion is a mixture between Midēwiwin and Anglo systems, such as the Native American Church. Pantraditional Chippewas openly and aggressively pursue both Indian and Anglo culture activities.

Traditional Native Americans have a difficult, if not impossible, time relating to Anglo-oriented health system. They tend to politely listen to care providers but seldom accept their advice. Bicultural Native Americans relate quite well to care providers. They accept and expect scientific medical treatment. Pantraditional Native Americans are likely to denounce health care providers. This latter group is largely comprised of Native Americans seeking to redefine themselves and recapture their identity within urban realities.

OTHER IMPORTANT TRAITS

The Anglo custom of looking someone in the eye to show that you are paying attention is considered disrespectful in many Native American tribes. Folk culture prescribes that looking into an individual's eyes is to look into his or her soul. In some folk cultures, looking into the eyes may result in a loss of the soul for the person being looked at. Consequently, Native Americans who do not look directly at care providers should not be labeled "inattentive" or "disinterested."

Shaking hands is very much a part of Native American tradition. However, there is an art to giving a proper hand shake; it should not be a vigorous handshake, which is interpreted by American Indians as a sign of aggressiveness. Both the manner of paying attention as well as shaking hands reflect the cultural traditions of respecting the other person's space and personal existence.

The Navajo, for example, place special emphasis on individual rights. Each person has the right to speak only for himself or herself, and each person's action should be self-initiated. "This has implications for Anglo health care," Mary Kniep-Hardy and Margaret A. Burkhart write. "Trying to obtain a patient's history from others is difficult, because even close family members may believe they have no right to give personal information concerning another."[20] Modesty is another characteristic Navajos share with other Native Americans.

> The morning after Ms. Z's admission, the nurse wishes to give her a bath and comb her hair. Because modesty is important to a Navajo, she asked permission. Asking permission of any adult patient prior to beginning a bath is good common sense, but it is especially important to Navajos because

disrobing in front of strangers discomforts them. After the bath the nurse helped Ms. Z comb her hair. Then she removed all hair from the brush and saved it in the bedside stand. The Navajo dispose of it appropriately later.[21]

Traditional American Indian cultures not only view life differently from most Anglo cultures but also view death differently. Native Americans define death as a part of the life cycle: the old *must* die and the young may die. Grief counseling for Native Americans who cling to their traditional culture should not focus on rewards in death for good deeds during one's life. To the traditional American Indian, death consists of joining one's ancestors. Good deeds or bad deeds have nothing to do with this reunion.

The American Indian's concept of time also differs from most Anglo cultures. It is viewed as a continuum with no beginning or end. Thus to prescribe medical treatment according to rigid time sequences would conflict with the Native American preference to do something spontaneously instead of doing something within a specific period of time. The major focus is on the interaction, not when the interaction occurs. Frequently, insensitive care providers complain about Indian patients being late for appointments. This proclivity for not being punctual according to Anglo standards has resulted in some Native Americans jokingly referring to being on "Indian time" (late). Most, however, keep appointments and are punctual.

It should be clear by now that care providers who understand the verbal and nonverbal languages of Native American patients will be the most effective in bridging cultural gaps. Of course, there are Native Americans who believe that only pure-blooded American Indians can effectively help them.

It is also important for care providers to understand the educational history of Native Americans. This aspect of American history is seldom found in professional curriculum. In the early years of the reservation system, children were made to enroll in schools located on reservations. They were herded into the schools, stripped of their native clothing, and had their hair cut. Having their hair cut was a painful operation, because the children had always worn their hair long. Native American children were punished for speaking their native languages. Books that contained Native American subjects were either absent or removed from the schools. It was very difficult to become adjusted to the clothing of the Anglos. The schools tried to teach the children an entirely new set of values and morals.

The Indian Education Act of 1972 was created to help American Indians on or off the reservation participate in the planning, development, and implementation of special programs designed to help American Indian students. The act is divided into four parts. Part A provides for a parent committee made up of 50% American Indians in the local public schools. This is to help provide communication between parents of Native American children and the school. Part B provides for Indian tribes and organizations. Part C is for adult education, and Part D provides for an office of Indian Education within the U.S. Office of Education.

Too few teachers or health care providers understand child-rearing practices and learning styles of Native Americans. Children are taught by example rather than by precept. This educational process is person centered. The object of learning is not, to Native Americans, the competitive struggle characterizing Anglos; therefore, children are taught to share in activities and rewards. Competition is acceptable if it is not to hurt someone. Native American children are seldom, if ever, struck by an adult. Furthermore, talking in a loud voice to correct a child is not a cultural norm.

The following case history vividly illustrates some of the ways care providers fail to understand Indian culture.

A CASE HISTORY*

A two-month old Indian male, C.P., was referred from the Indian clinic to a specialized pediatric hospital in a large medical center because of "abnormal white blood count, anemia and fever of unknown origin." The possibility of a battered child was diagnosed upon his arrival at the hospital.

When he arrived at the hospital the infant was accompanied by his grandmother. The abnormal white blood count and anemia were verified by laboratory findings. The diagnosis of possible battered child was never confirmed. It had been suggested by a funny red lesion on the left side of the infant's face near the eye. "It looked like an old cigarette burn and trauma to the eye." The eye was reddened with large hemorrhagic areas. Above the infant's buttocks, midway on his back, were reported bruises. These were later identified as Mongolian spots, prevalent on most dark-pigmented infants. C.P. just happened to have a deeper pigment and larger spots than are usually seen.

Although the infant was being admitted to the hospital by the grandmother, it was learned that he had two live parents, not present at the time. The admission was delayed at length by officials conferring with the grandmother as to why she had possession of the infant and the whereabouts of the parents.

The Anglo health care workers (physicians, social workers, and admitting clerks) were unaware that quite frequently a grandmother will care for children of young parents. In this instance, they were in another town where they had sought employment. In some Indian tribes it is the grandmother who will give permission in such circumstances as a child's being admitted to the hospital. The Indian grandmother, who could not read English but could speak English, could not understand why the health care workers were so upset that she should have possession of her own grandchild. On the progress report was written, "Suspect that the infant has been abandoned."

The infant was admitted to the hospital. While the grandmother stayed in the admitting office signing official admitting forms, the infant was taken to the ward.

*From Primeaux, M. 1977. American Indian health care practices. Nurs. Clin. North Am. 12:61-63.

All children are given baths as a standard procedure. For this purpose a small leather band with a small bag attached was removed from the child's wrist. Since the infant had diarrhea, an abnormal white count, and high temperature, intravenous therapy was started. The infant's thick, black hair was shaved from temple to temple since the scalp is the "site of choice" for I.V.'s in infants. These acts of shaving the infant's head and removal of the leather wristband were the beginning of many cultural conflicts between the grandmother and the hospital personnel.

The nursing and medical staff were unaware of the cultural taboo of cutting an infant's hair. In many tribes, a baby born with long, thick hair (as most Indian children are) is a sign of a healthy child. To cut the hair is in violation of a taboo, and something surely will happen to the infant. This act of cutting the hair upset the grandmother more than did the removal of the leather band with a preventive herb. The grandmother confided to the nurse's aide, "My grandbaby will die now because his brain will become sick."

After three days of hospitalization of her grandchild, the grandmother was labeled as "schizophrenic and uncooperative." She was asked to leave the bedside of the infant as she was "in the way" while nurses attempted to care for the infant. When she was obviously absent from the ward window for one full day, there were remarks about "the poor Indian infant—no one to care about him."

It was noted the next day that many family relatives came "to see" the infant, but none were permitted to be with him. They held a special curative ritual outside the hospital for the infant. When attempts were made to leave a significant item used in the ritual to be attached to the bed, this was not permitted. What looked like "a charcoal-burned item (stick) and a small bundle" were considered unsanitary for the nursery. The Anglo personnel were unaware of the intimacy of religion and health in this culture. To place this item on the bed of the ill infant would have had positive effects for both the family and the personnel. First, the family saw this as curative in nature and reaffirmation of their faith that the infant would recover. Acceptance by the hospital personnel would have shown the family that their practice was legitimate and not "mockery, magic or witchcraft."

As the treatment regime continued, the family members kept a vigil in the hallway outside the nursery. After extensive diagnostic procedures, cancer of the eye was confirmed. According to reports, hospital personnel made attempts to locate the parents to communicate the new diagnosis and obtain permission to begin therapy. Most hospital personnel chose to ignore the grandmother because her behavior was not within the normal expectations of the Anglo culture.

After five days of hospitalization, there was a notation that the grandmother wanted the infant discharged so that she "could consult a Medicine Man." This request was apparently refused. The last notation was "The grandmother takes child AMA" (against medical advice). After the grandmother had kept the child "in hiding" for almost three months, they were found and the child was rehospitalized. The parents were present for this hospitalization. Unfortunately the infant was listed in critical conditions and prognosis was poor.

As the American Indian attempts to use the Anglo health care system, the system providers must make this service relevant and recognize that many American Indians use their traditional system for health care. The two systems need not be in competition. If trust and rapport are established with mutual respect, the systems will complement each other, and both the provider and the client will benefit.

SUMMARY

Culture and language variations among the Native American preclude a single approach to health care for Native Americans. American Indian beliefs and attitudes about health and illness are often in direct conflict with the Anglo society, and frequently these differences cause a great deal of hardship and frustration. Differences in perception and orientation are culturally determined. What is considered unacceptable behavior in one group may be an accepted practice in another group. An opportunity to learn components of a particular culture should be viewed by health providers as an opportunity for professional and personal growth and enrichment.

It has been shown that culture influences forms of illness and the subsequent culturally specific treatment. Illness has both social and biological meanings to group members. It is of paramount importance for nurses and other health care providers to be open minded and have nonjudgmental attitudes, which are more likely to develop the trusting relationship needed to enhance the delivery of optimal health care. Hence, major challenges for health care providers are to seek out, experience, and understand cultural diversities and apply these findings in culturally specific and relevant manners.

The following letter written by a traditional American Indian parent to her child's non-Indian teacher provides vital tips for nonteachers, especially health care professionals. The acceptance and respect she wished for her child is nothing less than what is needed by all Native Americans, young and old.

Dear _____:

Before you take charge of the classroom that contains my child, please ask yourself why you are going to teach Indian children. What are your expectations? What rewards do you anticipate? What ego needs will our children have to meet?

Write down and examine all the information and opinions you possess about Indians. What values, class prejudices, and moral principles do you take for granted as universal? Please remember that different from is not the same as "worse than" or "better than," and the yardstick you use to measure your own life satisfactorily may not be appropriate for their lives. The term culturally deprived was invented by well-meaning middle-class whites to describe something they could not understand.

Too many teachers, unfortunately, seem to see their role as rescuer. My child does not need to be rescued; he does not consider being Indian a misfortune. He has a culture, probably older than yours; he has meaningful values and rich and varied experimental background. However strange or incomprehensible it may seem to you, you have no right to do or say anything that implies to him that it is less than satisfactory.

Our children's experiences have been different from those of the "typical" white middle-class child for whom most school curricula seem to have been designed. I suspect that this typical child does not exist except in the minds of curriculum writers.

Nonetheless, my child's experiences have been as intense and meaningful to him as any child's. Like most Indian children of his age, he is competent. He can dress himself, prepare a meal for himself and clean up afterward, and care for a younger child. He knows his reservation like the back of his hand.

He is not accustomed to having to ask permission to do ordinary things that are part of normal living. He is seldom forbidden to do anything; more usually the consequences of an action are explained to him and he is allowed to decide for himself whether or not to act.

His entire existence since he has been old enough to see and hear has been an experimental learning situation, arranged to provide him with the opportunity to develop his skills and confidence in his own capacities. Didatic teaching will be an alien experience for him.

He is not self-conscious in the way many white children are. Nobody has ever told him his efforts toward independence are cute. He is a young human being energetically doing his job, which is to get on with the process of learning to function as an adult human being. He will respect you and expect you to do likewise to him. He has been taught, by precept, that courtesy is an essential part of human conduct and that rudeness is an action that makes another person feel stupid or foolish. Do not mistake his patient courtesy for indifference or passivity.

He doesn't speak standard English, but he is in no way linguistically handicapped. If you will take the time and courtesy to listen and observe carefully, you will see that he and other Indian children communicate very well. They speak functional English, very effectively augmented by their fluency in the silent language, the subtle, unspoken, communication of facial expressions, gestures, body movement, and the use of personal space. You will be well advised to remember that our children are skillful interpreters of the silent language. They will know your feelings and attitudes with unerring precision no matter how carefully you arrange your smile or modulate your voice. They will learn in your classroom because children learn involuntarily. What they learn will depend on you.

Will you help my child learn to read, or will you teach him that he has a reading problem? Will you help him to develop problem-solving skills, or will you teach him that school is where you try to guess what answer the teacher wants? Will he learn that his sense of dignity is valid, or will he learn that he must forever be apologetic and trying harder because he isn't white? Can you help him acquire the intellectual skill he needs without at the same time imposing your values on top of those he already has?

Respect my child. He is a person. He has the right to be himself.

References

1. Leininger, M. 1976. First Regional Conference on Transcultural Nursing. Salt Lake City: University of Utah, College of Nursing (unpublished).

2. Branch, M.; and Paxton, P. 1976. *Providing safe nursing care for ethnic people of color.* New York: Appleton-Century-Crofts.

3. See Primeaux, M. 1978. Health care and the aging American Indian. In Rhinehardt, E. M.; and Quinn, M., editors. *Current practices in gerontological nursing.* St. Louis: The C. V. Mosby Co., p. 133.

4. Primeaux, M. 1977. American Indian health care practices—a cross-cultural perspective. *Nurs. Clin. North Am.* 12:59.

5. American Indian Policy Review Commission. 1976. *Task force six: Indian health.* 1976. Washington, D.C.: U.S. Government Printing Office, p. 40.

6. American Indian Policy Review Commission. 1976. *Task force six: Indian health.* 1976. Washington, D.C.: U.S. Government Printing Office, p. 63.

7. Hall, E. T.; and Whyte, W. F. 1976. Intercultural communication: A guide to men in action. In Brink, P. J., editor. *Transcultural nursing: A book of readings.* Englewood Cliffs, N.J.: Prentice-Hall, Inc.

8. Primeaux, M. 1977. Caring for the American Indian patient. *Am. J. Nurs.* 77:92. Copyright © 1977 American Journal of Nursing Company.

9. Scott, C. S. 1974. Health and healing practices among five ethnic groups in Miami, Florida. *Public Health Rep.* 89:256.

10. Primeaux, M. 1977. Caring for the American Indian patient. *Am. J. Nurs.* 77:92.

11. Kiev, A. 1968. *Curanderismo: Mexican-American folk psychiatry.* New York: The Free Press, p. 176.

12. Saunders, L. 1954. *Cultural differences and medical care: The care of the Spanish-speaking people of the Southwest.* New York: Russell Sage Foundation, p. 144.

13. Capps, W. H. 1976. *Seeing with a native eye: Essays on Native American religion.* New York: Harper & Row, Publishers, Inc.

14. Primeaux, M. 1977. Caring for the American Indian patient. *Am. J. Nurs.* 77:92.

15. Scott, C. S. 1974. Health and healing practices among five ethnic groups in Miami, Florida. *Public Health Rep.* 89:526.

16. Primeaux, M. 1977. Caring for the American Indian patient. *Am. J. Nurs.* 77:91-92.

17. Primeaux, M. 1977. Caring for the American Indian patient. *Am. J. Nurs.* 77:92.

18. Unger, S., editor. 1977. *The destruction of American Indian families.* New York: Association of American Indian Affairs.

19. Red Horse, J. G.; Lewis, R.; Feit, M.; et al. 1978. Family behavior of urban American Indians. *Soc. Casework* 59:67-72.

20. Kniep-Hardy, M.; and Burkhardt, M. A. 1977. Nursing the Navajo. *Am. J. Nurs.* 77:95.

21. Kniep-Hardy, M.; and Burkhardt, M. A. 1977. Nursing and the Navajo. *Am. J. Nurs.* 77:96.

17

Asian-American Patient Care

Betty Chang, R.N., D.N.S.

Nurses in the United States today are more likely to have contact with Asian patients than ever before. The latest available figures from the 1970 census represent a gross underestimate, because those figures are 9 years old and of course did not take into consideration the influx of new immigrants in recent years. Also, Asians are wary of census takers; many fear deportation and hide from the census takers, which results in an inaccurate census count. According to the 1970 estimates, the largest Asian groups in the United States were Japanese (589,000), Chinese (435,000), Filipino (340,000), and Korean (215,430). As of October 29, 1979 (*Los Angeles Herald Examiner*), Vietnamese (200,000) ranked fifth, making a total of 1,779,430 Asians in the United States. When Pacific Asians other than those already cited are included, the total may be closer to 2 million.*

If we accept the premise that human beings have universal feelings but that the expression of those feelings may be modified by cultural and social conditioning, we open the way for the discovery of different behaviors for the expression of such universal feelings as anger and pain. When nurses assess patients for care, then, they must take into consideration cultural aspects as well as biological, social,

---

*In addition to the 1970 census, this figure is based on estimates from the Union of Pan Pacific Community Publication, including 10,000 Cambodians, 10,000 Guamians, 100,000 Hawaiians, 20,000 Laotians, and 48,000 Samoans in the United States.[2] Thais were estimated only for Los Angeles at 10,000, with relatively large populations in Chicago, New York, San Francisco, Houston, and Denver.

psychological, and environmental aspects. Kluckhohn and Mowrer in a discussion of personality and culture suggest that for each of the biological, physical, social, and cultural determinants of personality, individuals may manifest behavior that is universal, communal, role, or idiosyncratic.[1] *Universal traits* or *components* are those properties of social stimulus, value, or traits that all humans have in common. *Communal traits* refer to those that the members of any given society share with each other to a greater extent than with members of other societies. *Role components* consist of the social behavior of persons within certain categories of people that remain constant. *Idiosyncratic determinants* refer to that behavior in which members playing similar roles differ among themselves.

Because of the wide diversity of groups of Asian Americans, the two largest Asian populations in the United States—Japanese and Chinese—are used as specific examples in this chapter.

The chapter reviews some of the common themes in the history of Chinese Americans and Japanese Americans in the United States as a background for understanding their behavior within a historical content; describes major cultural values and concepts that may underlie communal and role behaviors manifested among Asians, particularly traditional Chinese and Japanese patients; and suggests approaches for nurses in the care of Asian patients that take into consideration the patients' value systems.

ASIAN AMERICANS DEFINED

The term "Asian American" refers to persons of American citizenship whose parents or ancestors came from any one or a combination of Asian countries, including China, Japan, Korea, Southeast Asia, and Vietnam. More recently, the term "Pacific Asian" has come into vogue. This category includes people whose ancestors came from Asian countries as well as such Pacific Islands as the Philippines, Samoa, and Guam.

Americans generally view people of Asian descent as a homogeneous group sharing the same physical characteristics, personality traits, and behaviors. Although there are certain physical, cultural, historical, and social similarities among the groups, differences also exist. Asians for the most part view themselves as belonging to particular ethnic groups and subgroups. For example, Chinese or Koreans may view themselves as American born or from various regions of other countries; Japanese may view themselves as belonging in subgroups according to the number of generations in the United States—Issei (first), Nisei (second), Sansei (third), Yonsei (fourth), or a subgroup of Nisei educated in Japan (Kibei). The Chinese and Japanese in Hawaii feel that they are different from those in the United States (mainlanders). But even subgrouping does not adequately describe the Asian population. Many Asian Americans are difficult to classify because they are of mixed ethnic or generation parentage (for example, parents may be Chinese or

Korean, Nisei and Sansei, or Japanese and Filipino). Individuals of one ethnic group generally dislike being mistaken as a member of another group.

BACKGROUND

To understand Asian Americans within their historical context, a brief summary of the history of Chinese and Japanese immigration to the United States is necessary. There were similarities in the immigration patterns of the two groups as well as differences.

Early Chinese and Japanese settlers in the United States were predominantly men who came here to further their economic situation. Besides being inadequately educated and having little or no capital, many were further handicapped by an inability to speak or understand English.

The original intent of these people had been to come to the United States, make a fortune, and then to return to their native land; however, racial discrimination against Asians in the United States beginning in the 1850s restricted the freedom of Asians and limited their socioeconomic well-being. At various points in history, masses of Chinese and Japanese were deported, relocated, or tragically murdered. Surrounded by hostility, small enclaves of ethnic groups evolved into Chinatowns and Little Tokyos. From 1924 until the passage of the McCarran-Walters Bill in 1952, Asian immigration almost came to a halt, with only a few qualified businessmen, preferred professionals, and scholars allowed to enter the United States. Asians were aliens "ineligible for [U.S.] Citizenship" and ineligible for immigration to the United States.[3,4]

In spite of these hardships, many of the pioneers managed to survive and to make contributions in agriculture, mining, railroading, and other areas of the economy. Some managed to start families, and today there are first, second, third and fourth generation Chinese and Japanese in the United States. The enactment of Public Law 89-232 in 1965 eliminated discrimination against Asians in immigration laws, thus lifting the restrictions that had been enforced for over 80 years.[5] The way was then open for an influx of new immigrants. The immigration section of the Southeast Asian Supportive Service sponsored by the Archdiocese of Los Angeles further estimates that Southeast Asian refugees are coming to the Los Angeles area at the rate of some 50 persons per week.[5]

The newer generations of Asians for the most part have not been faced with the overt discrimination and harassment suffered by pioneers. Many of the communal traits among traditional Asians may have had their origins in their minority status in America.

The Chinese

Chinese immigration began with the Gold Rush in 1849, and since the venture was viewed as a temporary economic enterprise, wives and children of married men were left behind. With the rise of anti-Sinoism dating as early as 1852, laws were enacted to restrict the opportunities of the Chinese. These laws were followed by personal harassment, violence, and mass murder. Subsequent restrictions placed on immigration prevented wives from joining their husbands, resulting in the "mutilated" family: families remained legally intact, but the wives and children were physically separated from the husbands and fathers. The mutilated family had become the dominant form of Chinese family life in America until 1946, when several legislative acts permitted the reunion of some families. Many Chinese went to Hong Kong to seek wives through their elders or contacted marriage brokers who obtained wives for them. Their only acquaintance with the wives was through a picture or a surreptitious look when the prospective bride walked down a street as the go-between pointed her out to her prospective husband.[4] Nevertheless, some men remained single all their lives, and to this day there are many elderly patients in Chinatown—single men who live alone maintaining a mutilated family (if indeed it could be called a family at all) all their lives.

Another group of Chinese were the businessmen, members of professions, and scholars who came to the United States around 1920-1930. They were college educated and came for business graduate school or advanced professional preparation. Their families often came with them, and they were accustomed to varying degrees of traditional thinking and behavior in their daily and family lives. With the beginning of the communist regime in 1947, this group chose not to return to China, and today they are called the "stranded" Chinese.[6]

The most recent influx of Chinese from Hong Kong, Taiwan, Vietnam, and the People's Republic of China came to the United States with backgrounds and purposes different from the earlier pioneers. Their ability and desire to adhere to traditional values and behavior will depend to a great extent on the sociocultural environment or their country of origin.

The Japanese

Japanese immigration to the United States began later than the Chinese. Some of the differences between the early Chinese and Japanese immigrants were summarized by Yip and her coauthors. First, the Japanese were a more welcome group than the Chinese. Since they had been better educated in Japan, the Japanese were felt to be more able to assimilate. Second, the Japanese were expected to teach the United States how to produce teas and silks and to perhaps provide lessons in frugality and politeness. Third, Japan maintained a paternalistic attitude toward its emigrants. Finally, wives and children of Japanese laborers were permitted passage to the United States. Thus they did not suffer the plight of the "mutilated families" of many of the Chinese pioneers.[2]

Beginning in 1885, thousands of Japanese men came to the West Coast from both Japan and Hawaii (during a time when Chinese exclusion had been successful). Immigration from Japan was limited from 1908-1913 because of a Gentleman's

Agreement whereby Japan would voluntarily limit immigration to the United States. After 1913, war brides and wives came to the United States, and Japanese immigration continued until 1924, when the passage of the American immigration bill halted Asian immigration. The first Japanese immigrants were generally young men with about 4-6 years of education who came from what may be considered rural Japan. They were soon joined by Japanese women.[3]

Since most of the early immigrants were from agricultural backgrounds, they gravitated naturally toward farming in this country. Some others also found work as laborers on the railroad or in canneries, mining, meatpacking, and the salt industries. Japanese also did gardening and landscaping and launched small businesses such as stores, banks, and fruit and vegetable markets.

Anti-Japanese legislation in 1913 prohibited the Issei from owning land, and unsuccessful attempts were also made to restrict their American-born children from owning land. The Nisei children were brought up with a strong emphasis on education, obedience to the teacher, and competitiveness among each other. They were not forced to attend segregated schools as were Chinese, Indian, and Mongolian children (partly because the Japanese Americans had the backing of the government of Japan, which was a first-class military power at that time). The Niseis were encouraged to work hard and to achieve academically in schools. However, more recent generations are placing importance on being an "all around person," which includes but is not limited to academic achievement.[3]

As is well known in American history, during World War II Japanese Americans on the West Coast were evacuated from their homes and placed in "relocation" centers. This policy caused the Isseis to lose their homes, businesses, and farms and created a disruption of their families. The relocation camps were declared unconstitutional in 1945, and the Japanese Americans had a new start in life. One of the many consequences of the relocation was that Japanese Americans came in closer contact with whites, and the Isseis lost some of the strong emotional and economic hold they may otherwise have had on the Niseis.

Since that time, Japanese Americans have seen an increase in population due to the immigration of postwar brides and the arrival of new Isseis, which began in the 1950s. There has also been an influx of Japanese tourists, students, and businessmen representing large corporations. These new arrivals, like the new arrivals of Chinese Americans, are vastly different in their education, socioeconomic status, and purpose for being in the United States. They have also experienced a very different social climate than their predecessors in the United States.

TRADITIONAL VALUES AND BEHAVIORAL NORMS

Since values in America as well as in China and Japan today are in a state of transition, it is difficult to attribute specific values and behaviors to all Asian Americans or even to all Chinese Americans or Japanese Americans with any degree of certainty. An attempt is made to describe some general traditional Asian values and norms as a point of reference while acknowledging that a wide range of behavior may exist within as well as between groups. Major topics selected for discussion are concepts related to: (1) the family; (2) the "situational orientation"; (3) filial piety; (4) the control of feelings, such as anger and pain, (5) inconspicuousness; and (6) death and dying.

The Family

The form of extended household associated with rural China and Japan in the early 1900s in which grandparents, parents, siblings, uncles, aunts, and cousins lived under the same roof is rare in the United States today. Social scientists regarded the extended kinship family in China as commonplace.[4,7] Families also varied by locality (urban versus rural) and individual circumstances. The new immigrants interviewed by Wu preferred to live alone rather than with their married sons and daughters.[7] Kitano and Sung have noted that by the 1970s Asian families had become as diverse as any American group in their structure, size, and closeness.[3,4]

Though they may not live under the same roof, members of a traditional family often maintain strong emotional bonds. Frequent visiting and get-togethers are common when geographical distance permits. A sense of family pride remains intact, as does a sense of responsibility for mutual aid in times of need.

To varying degrees, the more traditional Asian family has a male-dominated household consisting of a man, his wife, and their children. Occasionally there may be elderly persons present, in which case they are probably the man's parents or his surviving mother. Exceptions may be made in families in which economic circumstances force large numbers of related and unrelated people to live in crowded conditions, such as the Chinatowns of New York City, San Francisco, or Los Angeles.[4,8]

A traditional Asian wife devoted herslef to care of the home, children, and husband. If her husband were unhappy or if the children misbehaved, she would blame herself. Asian women historically have occupied an inferior position to men. Sons were more welcome in a family than daughters. Women were usually thought of as liabilities, because they were generally raised to marry into someone else's family and transfer their loyalties to their new family. Once married, the woman became integrated into the man's family, rarely visiting her own home except for special occasions. Even in modern families, among American-born Chinese and Sansei Japanese, young women state that in their homes their brothers received preferential treatment.

In the traditional Asian family, family members had well-defined roles and obligations. The head of the family was the father, with the authority passed to the eldest son when the father was absent. In many families, major issues were discussed, and the male member was responsible for decisions affecting the family.[9,10] There were also well-defined roles for the aged, and young people were expected to follow patterns of deference to their elders. In America, in many ways the ethnic community as well as the family has become a reference group acting as a norm that exerts social control over its members. The community also provides recreational and ethnic educational opportunities.[3]

Interactions in the Asian family tend to be less verbal than in the white middle-class family. Family members have well-understood means of communicating the fact that they care about each other. One occasion during which members can show their love for a person is by caring for that person during times of illness, no matter how minor. Caudill describes the use of hypochondriacal illnesses and minor discomforts as excuses to refrain from work among men in Japan.[11] Caudill contends that such illnesses provide an opportunity for the family members (wife or mother) to show their true feelings of love and affection for the men. However, in Hawaii, where the nuclear family is predominant and where many working wives may not be available to care for the men at home, a religious (Tensho) sect has discouraged the use of the sick role as a means of legitimizing one's dependency and affiliation needs. Through conversion to Tenshoism, recovery is expected to follow the ritual efforts of the individual (sick) person, and contact with other persons is avoided.

In spite of recent changes and diversity in family structure and function, it is not unusual for hospitalized Asian patients to have many family members and colleagues visit them. This behavior often causes friction between the nursing staff and the family because the hospitals in the United States, unlike those in parts of Asia (such as Taiwan), generally do not provide for family members who wish to stay in the patient's room for prolonged periods (days or weeks at a time). The following situation illustrates the involvement of the parents and extended family with a hospitalized child.

> An 8-year-old boy, a second generation Asian, was hospitalized on a pediatric unit of a large metropolitan hospital with a diagnosis of multiple fractures following a bicycle accident. The 35-year-old mother, a first generation Asian, spent most of the day in the hospital, and the father came after work each evening to visit the child. A stream of other visitors were in and out of the room all day bringing various foods for the young patient. Members of the staff expressed a variety of concerns, ranging from "the boy is being disturbed too much," "he is old enough to accept the separation from his parents," to being afraid the food would clutter up the room too much.
>
> The staff made a special effort to talk with the parents, because they were at first incommunicative even though they spoke some English. It was discovered that this was the only son and first grandson in the family. The mother had felt she was to blame for "not watching him carefully enough." Rather than further discuss her feelings, she wanted to be able to "live in" at the hospital to ensure that the son was well taken care of, and her husband encouraged her to stay at the hospital to pay full attention to the child's needs.*

---

*Clinical situation, 1974, San Francisco, Calif.

The nurse's assessment of the cultural determinants of behavior in this situation included her knowledge of the universal component of the structure and function of families in the rearing of the young. The communal component included the nurse's knowledge of the traits shared by other members of the group. In this instance, the situation was that of a close-knit family and community of extended kin and friends. The initial reluctance of the parents to discuss their feelings may be another manifestation of the norms shared by traditional Asians, which is described in greater detail later in the chapter. An additional communal norm was that of seeking a situational solution (that of mother staying overnight) rather than a psychodynamic analysis of how they were feeling.

The nurse's knowledge of the prescribed roles in a traditional Asian family can be invaluable as a frame of reference in assessing the role component of behavior. Here the high regard for the male of the family, the reliance on his carrying on the family name and inheritance, may be playing a large part in the indulgent role of the parents in their care of the son.* Because Asian households may often be patriarchal, it is a good idea for the nurse involved to ascertain the opinion of the father on issues requiring decision making.

The nursing plan for this patient and his family included: (1) allowing the mother to sleep on a cot in the child's hospital room, (2) indicating sensitivity to the parents' expressions of feelings even though they may be nonverbal, (3) clarifying "sensed" feelings but refraining from unwelcome probing, (4) allowing the extended family members to visit and bring food to the boy, and (5) making some arrangements for the storage of food brought by the visitors.

Possible Language Barrier

The patient and his parents in the preceding situation spoke some English. Had the patient and his parents been non-English speaking, the situation would have been further complicated by a language barrier. A nurse confronted with a language barrier must do some creative problem solving. Several sources of assistance may be sought. The nurse may (1) request a bilingual staff member or interpreter at the hospital. This may be an ideal solution; however, the number of such personnel available is rarely adequate. She or he may (2) recruit relatives and other visitors to help to interpret, or she or he may (3) contact local ethnic community organizations, social service centers, or senior citizen centers for bilingual persons

---

*Although parents cosleeping with children is a common occurrence in Japan, as reported by Caudill and Plath, Kitano's impression in the United States is that it is not widespread among the Japanese Americans.[3,12] Judging from my personal acquaintances, I would say that parent-child cosleeping is also uncommon among Chinese Americans. The child's behavior may also be explained in terms of the Japanese concept of "Amae," which is difficult to translate but includes the desire for love and attention and to "depend and presume upon another's benevolence."

who may be able to assist. Community residents who are bilingual and who are in good health may be able to form a "pool" of interpreters if, in turn, they can be remunerated for their services. Some bilingual "young-old" (age 60-75) senior citizens who are active and alert may derive a great deal of satisfaction and increase their sense of self-esteem if they can render such services and receive some monetary recognition.

Even if an interpreter can be found, a method of communicating between the patient and the nurse is still required for the period of time that the interpreter is away from the bedside. A method with which nurses are already familiar is the use of bilingual "picture cards" containing such statements as "I need a bedpan" and "I have pain." At the present time, residents of the Chinatown in Los Angeles are preparing a deck of cards for non-English speaking Chinese persons who are either clients at the center or who attend the health fair scheduled for December 1979. As useful as these cards are, they tend to be rudimentary in their content of communication. Two other alternatives that are more efficient consist of an "electronic communication board" and a pocket-size "foreign language processor." The former is composed of an electronic board that uses "content sheets," each of which contains about 100 concepts, or messages, with or without pictures. The messages on the content sheets are determined by the buyer (such as hospital) and produced by the engineering firm.* Different "content sheets" with different messages or languages can be inserted into the board depending on the nature of the patient situations. Patients can select the messages they wish to convey to another person by turning the board on, which activates a scanner and a pointer. As the messages are scanned, patients may point to the message of their choice. Patients may also point to a series of messages and store them in a memory until the nurse has time to come into the room. The memory can then be recalled in the nurse's presence, and the series of messages from the communication board can be read.

The foreign language processor contains over 3000 words in four languages: English, French, German, and Japanese. However, the use of this processor requires that patients know how to spell in one of these languages. Words in any one language can be translated into any of the other three and read in the display case, much as one would read the answers on a pocket calculator.

Of course, these picture cards and mechanical gadgets cannot replace an interpreter, but they do provide means for supplementing the services of an interpreter in the care of non-English speaking patients. Nurses may find further that the generous use of gestures and demonstrations can help convey messages. As a nurse who was taking care of a non-English speaking infant and mother on a pediatric unit related to me, "I use plenty of 'monkey shine' to talk to her [the mother] when the interpreter isn't here."

---

*Zygo Co., Portland, Ore.

SITUATIONAL ORIENTATION

The "Asian situational orientation" has been emphasized by a number of authors.[3,4,14,15] In the United States, the individual is important, but in Asia, the total situation must be considered. Often the behavior and course of action do not benefit the individual, but the realization that the behavior is best for the situation and for others in the group is vital. Asians strongly emphasize harmony and avoidance of conflict in groups.

Traditional Asians established harmony and avoided conflict in part by behaving toward people according to prescribed roles and statuses. Specifically, the norm of the Japanese *enryo* governs much of the behavior in interpersonal relationships. This norm consists of a collection of behavior (*enryo* syndrome) that calls for restraint, reserve, and lack of assertiveness in social interactions.[2] These behaviors were originally conceived as an expression of modesty in front of those in power and authority; however, the meaning has been broadened to encompass a collection of behaviors to be used in ambiguous, embarassing, or anxiety-producing situations. Individuals in such situations may remain quiet or simply nod to indicate they do not want to cause any embarrassment.[3]

To illustrate, if a professor should ask an Asian student the question, "Is this clear?" The student who has high respect for the teacher may answer, "Yes," meaning "I don't want to cause any embarrassment." The student would not wish to be impolite by saying, "No, it is not clear," implying that the teacher is either confused or unable to communicate, or both.

In a clinical situation, an instance occurred where a nurse gave a thorough explanation of the importance of a low-sodium diet to a female Asian patient, which the nurse felt the patient understood. The patient had nodded and said "yes" throughout the interchange. Later the nurse discovered that "yes" meant the patient was listening, and the kinds of foods they had disucssed were not included in the patient's usual diet and were not preferred foods. The patient simply did not want to be so impolite as to interrupt (or disrupt) by saying "no" or by asking questions.

In the preceding situation, the communal behaviors related to restraint and reserve can be identified. The restraint may be more pronounced in women than in men because of the former's inferior status in Asia as well as other societies. A nursing approach could consist of using communication skills learned in other situations to ask the patient to clarify her understanding in her own words. The nurse can also ask the patient to give some examples from her own diet related to the principle being discussed. The nurse can then determine whether "yes" is being used in the Asian or American sense.

In addition, during the course of an interchange, it is a good idea to phrase questions in such a way that they require more than a "yes" or "no" answer. More important, the use of negative questions should be avoided because of the confusion that arises due to differences in the Asian-English grammatical use of "yes" and "no" in answering negative questions.*

Another behavior that Kitano indicates is related to the *enryo* syndrome is the manner in which an Asian may respond to praise or positive reinforcement.[3] If the praise is directed at the person directly or about a member of his family, he may respond by saying, "No, I did not do this very well," or "No, my children are bad," or in Chinese, a formalized "Where?" Meaning "Not true, where did you see this happening?" The praise of self or members of one's own family is considered poor manners, and the accepted behavior of the one offering the praise is to ignore the denial. This Asian behavior may be mistakenly interpreted as a lack of self-esteem or as belittling family members.

Another means of preserving harmony among Asians is the avoidance of direct confrontation. A direct confrontation forces a showdown in which one or the other of the parties must lose face or self-esteem. One of the techniques used by more traditional Asians to avoid confrontation may be one of blaming themselves for the mistake, when in fact the mistake was the other person's. The correct behavior is for the second person to say, "Oh, no, it is not your fault." However, it seems likely that Asians in America quickly learn to avoid using this technique after a few trials in which they find that indeed they have become the scapegoat.

In relation to the expression of feelings, some traditional Asians feel that it is not always helpful to express negative feelings directly. Such expressions can only damage relationships among persons who must continue to interact with each other. Some believe that, given time, there may be "situational solutions," that is the situation may change so that the need for confrontation will no longer exist.

Nurses often use confrontation as a positive means of helping patients to face their own feelings or situations. This technique may result in withdrawal and silence on the part of the Asian-American patient. First, the patients would find it difficult to respond to this technique, and second, they might find it difficult to let a nurse an authority figure, know that they do not wish to participate in any type of confrontation. The natural response will be "impassiveness" or "nonresponsiveness."

Filial Piety in the Family

Filial piety as a duty and obligation is presumed to be emphasized in all Asian families. The term most frequently refers to the duty of a child (usually the son) to respect and care for his or her parents in their old age. It is when they reach that

---

*The use of "yes" and "no" may cause confusion due to differences in the grammatical structure between English and many Asian languages. A "yes" to a negative question in the Asian sense means a "no" in English. For example, the nurse asks, "Haven't you gone for x-ray?" The Asian patient answers "yes," meaning, "Yes, you are right, I have not gone for x-ray." The patient has answered in English but has used an Asian grammatical syntax for doing so.

time of life that the parents reap the harvest of their lifelong hard work in raising their children. In precommunist China, the teachings of Confucius explicitly outlined the duty of a son to his parents. These obligations have been translated into specific laws in Taiwan.[16] This is not to say the ideal was or is a reality in every family. A number of researchers have noted that reverence and respect for the elderly by the young may be on the decline.[3,4,14,17] Thus the expectations of some of the elderly immigrants may not be fulfilled. However, the Niseis, who are primarily well educated and financially successful, have shown a continued sense of caring for the elderly Isseis.[3,17]

A study of how the elderly are perceived by young people of Chinese descent measured the attitudes of 400 nonrandomly selected college-age students (male = 225; female = 175) in Los Angeles in three major subgroups: American born (N = 108); those from Taiwan (N = 149), and those from Hong Kong (N = 121).[18] (Twenty-two were "other," which included Chinese from Cambodia, Singapore, Malaysia, or Vietnam). Two scales were used: the Attitude Toward Old People (OP) Scale, which measures the degree to which young people hold to stereotypes of the elderly, and the Needs of Old People (NOP) Scale, which ascertains the degree to which young people agree with statements related to such everyday needs of old people as housing, nutrition, transportation, and physical care.[19,20] In addition, a voluntary group of 80 students was asked some open-ended questions to explore whether they would choose to live with the elderly if they had a choice and what they (the young people) felt would be an ideal environment for the elderly.[21]

In general the subjects' scores were positive on the Attitude Toward Old People Scale, in which they disagreed with many of the negative stereotypes about old people and agreed with statements attributing more favorable characteristics to the elderly. The scores of the subjects of Chinese descent were not significantly different from the scores of white students at Boston University.[19] On the Needs of Old People Scale, the subjects of Chinese descent indicated they agreed with many of the practical everyday needs of the elderly and felt the elderly were entitled to care.

Some differences, however, were found between subgroups. The American-born groups showed significantly more favorable OP scores (reflecting nonstereo-typical thinking toward the elderly) than the subgroup from Hong Kong. No differences were found between the subgroup from Taiwan and the other two subgroups. On the other hand, the subgroup from Hong Kong had a significantly higher score (reflecting an agreement with the practical everyday needs of the elderly and a feeling that the elderly are entitled to care) than the subgroup of American-born Chinese. Again, the subgroup from Taiwan did not differ from the other two subgroups. Interestingly, the women were more in agreement with the needs of old people (had significantly higher scores) than the men in the study. The level of income, number of years in the United States, occupational and educational level of the father, and educational level of the mother all failed to be significant in explaining the variance in stereotypical thinking about the old people (OP scale) or the agreement regarding the needs of old people (NOP scale).

In response to the open-ended questions, most of the American-born Chinese and those from Hong Kong responded "no" to the question of whether they would live with the elderly if they had a choice. The majority of those from Taiwan, however, indicated they would prefer to live with the elderly. The societal supports and laws in Taiwan may have influenced these answers. Nearly all subjects indicated that they thought a peaceful, quiet environment with easy transportation for visiting children, grandchildren, shopping, entertainment (Chinese operas, *mahjong*), and exercise (*Tai Chi Tuan* or gardening) would be ideal. Many mentioned that if they did share a household, the house must be large enough for privacy and separate cooking facilities. That is, the house must be large enough for "in-law" apartments. This form of housing is reported to be popular among Japanese families who absorb their elderly.[3]

The preceding study on young people of Chinese descent illustrates two points: (1) on standardized scales, the attitudes of Asian subjects in the study were not significantly different from those of the white subjects in Kogan's study, perhaps pointing to a change in the Asian Americans' attitudes related to filial piety; and (2) diversity exists in ethnic groups to the extent that significant differences are found between subgroups of the same ethnic group.[19]

This diversity in Asian groups is reinforced by the following situations from my personal and professional experiences:

Situation 1. Mrs. G, a full-time housewife and second generation Asian in the United States, lives with her husband, three children, and her husband's mother in their ranch-type house. She said that when she was young, her parents' parents were not living in the United States; however, her father had an elderly aunt who lived with them. Mrs. G always considered it a privilege to have an elderly person in the home when she was growing up.

She very much wanted her children to have the privilege of living with grandparents in the household. When her husband's mother was widowed, she moved into Mrs. G and her husband's home and lived there for about 10 years until her death at the age of 79. During those 10 years, the elderly mother-in-law spent 2-4 weeks twice a year at the home of another son "for a change." Although there were some inconveniences and minor disagreements, she felt that they lived more or less harmoniously, and Mrs. G felt she was able to help her mother-in-law in visits to the doctor and medications and treatments for her high blood pressure and arthritis.*

Situation 2. Mr. and Mrs. H and their four children live in an apartment in a metropolitan area. Mr. H's mother passed away, and Mrs. H's father lives with the young couple. Mr. H's father suffered a stroke and has been discharged from the hospital with residual paralysis. Both Mr. and Mrs. H work, but Mrs. H took some time off work to make arrangements with a

---

*Interview, 1974, San Francisco, Calif.

homemaker's service and a home-health service for limited care. When their resources were low, they were hesitant to apply to a social service for assistance. They felt guilty that they even mentioned their difficulties to any "outsider."*

Situation 3. Mr. I, age 68, had been in a rehabilitation unit for 2 weeks following a fracture of the hip. He had recovered sufficiently to be discharged from the rehabilitation unit but needed supportive care in the home. Mr. H was living alone in a second floor walkup apartment and spoke enough English to make himself understood in daily situations.

The social worker had talked to Mr. I's son and daughter-in-law to effect a "placement" for him in their home until he could be completely independent. To the social worker's surprise, the son and daughter-in-law refused. A conference was called to discuss the "problem." It was the staff's impression that the Asians had a strong, cohesive family that stressed filial piety. The staff felt that the son or the family clan should take care of their own.

In talking with the son and daughter-in-law, the social worker learned that they felt remorse for "letting their family down," but they were working their way through graduate school. They had neither "extended family" nor "clan." They did not live near Chinatown where they might have been able to enroll their father in the day-care center for the elderly for physical therapy, social service, one hot meal per day, and recreation. They themselves felt they could not be excused from their own responsibilities at work or school to meet the obligations of taking care of their ill father. They were willing to visit the father after school or work daily.**

All three situations illustrate that there are expectations from the majority society and from Asian Americans themselves to care for the elderly in their homes. However, the extent to which members of the group are willing to do so depends to a large extent on the young people's own socioeconomic status and life style. In all three situations one can see the daughter-in-law is important in the care of the mother-in-law or father-in-law. This is in line with traditional communal values in Asian American families; however, this demand is relaxing, and in some instances today daughters also participate in the care of elderly parents.

Situation 1 most closely follows the communal traits one would expect in Asian families with respect to filial piety. It can be seen that the family had adequate financial resources. There were also additional family members (another son's family) who could give Mr. and Mrs. G's nuclear family a "respite" in caring for the elder Mrs. G.

In situation 2, there is a discrepancy between the expectation of the young couple that they should care for the elderly and their lack of financial and human

---

*Interview, 1978, Los Angeles, Calif.

**Clinical experience, 1976, San Francisco, Calif.

service resources to do so. The nurse can build on the family's strengths and provide positive feedback for what the family has done so far. The nurse can further assist the family to gain a new perspective regarding the sources of help available. This may include an educational program to make it clear to the family that social services are not "charity" but rather a positive effort to help families who are in need.

Situation 3 illustrates that the cultural, communal norms that dictate that the son and daughter-in-law take care of the elderly do not exist for some Asian American families. The young people themselves are part of the work force in the economy, and their situation does not permit them to fulfill the role of both worker and full-time caretaker for their ailing father. They also lack the support of the extended family network. Mr. I's son and daughter-in-law need the supportive services of the majority community of which they have become a part, and they should receive some emotional support for their daily visits.

Mr. I may be observed for signs of disillusionment, because his expectations may be that the son would be more traditional in his expression of filial piety. The nurse may assist Mr. I in his expression of feelings and acknowledgement of his feelings. Mr. I can be gradually assisted in understanding the different means by which the needs of the elderly in our society are met. Specific services and agencies (such as home health care, visiting nurses, and homemakers services) applicable to Mr. I should be mentioned as examples. Ethnic community organizations, neighbors, and senior citizen centers are additional sources of support that are vital to include. They may assist by (1) providing much needed visiting, (2) assisting with the more complex translations, (3) completing bureaucratic forms, and (4) providing recreational opportunities.

Social Control: Use of Guilt and Shame

In traditional Asian families, a high degree of family and community stability existed that was conducive to social control of family members. The family units, with their code or hierarchy that respected age and men and their practice of ancestral worship, exerted a strong influence on family members to conform to appropriate behavior. Emphasis was placed on one's obligations and duties, such as being obedient to parents and giving the family (and therefore the community and the ethnic group) a good name.[9] Guilt was related to failure to meet expectations in a system based on duties and obligations. A result of such failure is shame to the family and the larger community. Undesirable behavior, such as low achievement, psychopathology, divorce, disobedience to parents or other authority, brought shame to the family, community, and ethnic group. Parents made extensive use of guilt-arousing techniques, such as threatening to disown the child or verbally censuring individuals to obtain conformity in behavior.[9]

In interviews with second generation Asian Americans, it was apparent that guilt and shame had been used in their childhoods to make them conform to family expectations. One person stated that although he was not encouraged verbally to excel in school, he was made to feel guilty for having brought shame to the family for not achieving as well as a cousin. Expectation was implied by such comparisons as "Your cousins are doing so well in school."

Certain characteristics, however, may be viewed as signs of weakness. In a hospital situation, a second generation Asian woman had "major surgery." Following the operation, she was given a blood transfusion. She did not inform her mother-in-law that she was receiving the transfusion because she felt it may have been misinterpreted as a sign of weakness.

In situations such as this, the nurse can acknowledge the patient's feelings in relation to the transfusion and clarify the need for it to the patient. The relationship of the mother-in-law to the daughter-in-law is deeply rooted in Asian tradition. The mother-in-law is an authority figure to the younger woman, and the latter must not behave in a way to bring shame to her family by marriage (which plays a more central role than her family of origin).

Control in the Expression of Feelings:
Examples of Anger and Pain

There is evidence in the literature as well as through personal interviews that the family encourages the individual to learn patterns of self-control and bravery in the face of pain, hardship, and other emotional situations.[3,9] From a young age, Japanese boys are taught to be ashamed of emotional outbursts, and Asian girls are taught to be submissive and to suppress their feelings. The Japanese language itself involves the use of tonal control and indirect terms so that individuals may conceal their feelings. The lack of any outward signs of feelings is also practiced by the parents themselves. As one second generation Asian reported, "My parents showed little signs of emotion. Sadness and disappointments or even the happy moments were not accompanied by much expression. I knew, however, that there were times when they experienced these feelings."

Expression of Anger

Anger is seldom expressed, particularly not in a hospital if an Asian should happen to be a patient. Individuals of any race are robbed of much of their dignity and identity when they are admitted to the hospital. To be a "good" patient, they must not complain, much less show anger, and most important must be grateful to the staff for the care they receive. When I was engaged in participant observation and interviews in a hospital setting, white patients indicated to me that they did not want to complain or turn on their call-light too often for fear of subtle retaliation. If white patients who have no "language problem" and no fear of racial discrimination express this feeling, minority Asian patients may try even harder to be the "good" patients. Thus, it is unlikely nurses will ever observe outbursts of anger in Asian patients.

If anger is expressed at all, it will be by way of information expressed to family members. Some sex differences may be seen, for example, men are more likely to express anger than women, because the culture finds such behavior more acceptable in men. The nursing staff may see and hear little expression of anger from the patients themselves, particularly the female Asian patients.

A nurse assessing the patient's feelings should take into consideration the universality of feelings in human beings under certain conditions. The communal behavior in handling anger may be control of self-expression, but an acceptable avenue of release may be through family members. However, the nurse may note differences in role behavior in the expressions of anger. Those in more responsible positions (particularly men in higher echelon occupations with higher socio-economic status) may be more overt in expressing anger than those in a lower status. Nursing intervention in situations involving anger may include: (1) heightened sensitivity to situations that may elicit strong emotions, particularly in reactions to illness; (2) inclusion of the family in discussions of the patient's care and feelings; and (3) acknowledgement of feelings when they are expressed, no matter how mildly stated.

Reactions to Pain

In a class project, nursing students interviewed a nursing supervisor at a general hospital that had a large number of Japanese patients.[22] The supervisor informed them that, "Demanding or critical verbalization will never be encountered with a Japanese-American patient. He will not respond to pain with the usual behaviors, crying for help, thrashing out, etc., but will instead, deny its intensity. He may say, 'It doesn't hurt so much. It's all right'."[23] Because of Asian American patients' stoic reaction to pain, the nursing supervisor indicated to the students that in relation to pain medications, "one-half the dose is sufficient" for an Asian patient.[24] However, the "sufficiency" of reduced doses was not suggested by patients I interviewed, particularly not by an Asian registered nurse who herself had had a cholecystectomy. The following three patient situations illustrate various reactions to pain. All of these patients were Asian Americans (Chinese or Japanese).

> *Situation 1.* Mr. B, a second generation Asian American, was hospitalized for "major surgery." He retold his postoperative pain experiences as follows: "I endured a lot of pain before asking for anything. I knew that pain medications were available, but I asked them (nurses) to bring them to me at their convenience. I was hurting pretty badly, but I didn't make a big fuss or ask them to call my doctor."
>
> He went on to say that in his opinion, an older patient may have an even more difficult time, because he (1) did not want to bother anyone, (2) had difficulty with the English language, and (3) was ashamed to admit he has pain and felt it must be endured.*

---

*Observations as research assistant, 1976, San Francisco, Calif.

Situation 2. Mrs. C, a first generation Asian American had the following comments about pain during labor and delivery: "I think it is shameful and vulgar to yell when you are in pain, even during labor and delivery of a baby. Also, I don't think patients want anything for pain because they associate it with habit-forming opium. As anyone who knows Chinese history is aware, opium is harmful and destructive to people.*

Situation 3. Mrs. D is an Asian American registered nurse who has been in the United States about 20 years and is presently an instructor of nursing. She had a recent experience as a patient when she had a cholecystectomy. Her statements indicate she is an insider to the health care system. In relating her pain experience, she stated: "When I had pain, I turned on the light early to call the nurse. Then I told her I had pain like this." The interviewee then wrinkled her face in a grimace, placed her hands over her epigastric region, and groaned loudly. She said that her husband, who is also a first-generation immigrant Asian was ashamed of her. He thought that she had "too loud a mouth," "lack of self-control," and was "indecent" in her expression of pain. She went on to say that if she did not express herself in that manner, she would either not have received any medication or she would have received too small a dose, much too late."†

In the preceding situations, the nurse should utilize her knowledge about universal components of pain. She must assess the location, intensity, duration, quality, associated manifestations, whether they are aggravating or alleviating dimensions, and the like. In addition, communal behavior in Asians suggests that it is shameful to give any expression to pain, and patients may be reticent about their own needs. Men may have a particularly difficult time expressing pain because of their role-related training in response to a masculine image. The nurse may also note idiosyncratic characteristics, such as the personal use of meditation or other relaxation techniques, as adjuncts to medications in the relief of pain.

In the situations of Mr. B and C, the nurse may have helped the patients further by providing some anticipatory guidance to the patient and family, explaining that pain is to be expected and describing the means available for the relief of pain. If the measure can be repeated every 3-4 hours, the nurse must be sure to inform the patient and the family. An explanation to patients about the short-term use of pain medications may be necessary if the patient has fears about opiates associated with addiction or the opium dens of China. The nurse needs to be sensitive to the patients' anticipated pain and offer relief before the pain reaches its peak. We are reminded that when medications are used, the maximum effectiveness can be obtained if given before the intensity of pain is at its acme.[25] In addition, the nurse might make a special point of asking the family how the patient says he or she is feeling. Complaints often are given to the family rather

---

*Interview, 1979, Los Angeles, Calif.
†Interview, 1979, Los Angeles, Calif.

than to the health care staff. Offering nursing measures such as deep breathing, back rubs, and a soothing environment, the same measures one would institute for a patient of any ethnic group, would be especially helpful to Asian patients. It is unlikely that the traditional Asian American patient will ask for these services. Inquire of the patient and family whether the patient has any personal practices that he or she performs regularly at home for relaxation. If so, he or she can be encouraged to use the techniques in addition to medication.

The assessment of pain in situation 3, Mrs. D, will not be difficult for non-Asian nurses. Mrs. D has obviously learned the same cues that health professionals read in assessing pain. In her expression of pain, she may be leaning more toward the American norm; she is also breaking away from the traditional role of women as inferior to men by persisting in her clear expression of feelings, in spite of her husband's admonitions about her behavior. She may be influenced in part by her feeling of confidence in a hospital setting, where she knows that her behavior is within the accepted norms of the majority population, most important, the staff. Mrs. D's situation indicates that the number of years a person has been in the United States is not necessarily an accurate indicator of the degree of acculturation in relation to the expression of feelings. Other features such as a person's previous experience, education, and sense of confidence in a situation surely must be taken into account.

Inconspicuousness

Inconspicuousness, or the avoidance of attracting special attention to oneself, has been a typical characteristic associated with Asians. There are several reasons for this attitude: (1) a culture that emphasizes situational harmony, consideration of other people's rights and feelings, and an avoidance of behavior that would bring shame and dishonor to the family; (2) respect and obedience to those in authority; and (3) the discrimination and persecution experienced by early Asian settlers in the United States. At one time in U.S. history, Asians accused of misdeeds were unable to obtain a fair trial, thus evolved the expression "a Chinaman's chance," meaning no chance at all. Also, in the pioneer days, Asian Americans reasoned that if the majority population did not notice you, there was less likelihood of being harassed or killed.

A health care situation implies a superordinate-subordinate relationship, with the patient in the subordinate position. With their background of cultural, historical, and role expectations, it is no wonder that traditional Asian Americans are often reluctant to ask for anything when they become patients. If nurses find that they are taking care of quiet, reticent, agreeable Asian patients, they may try some of the following approaches to make the patients aware of nursing care available to them. The nurses may take a greater initiative in providing the patient with anticipatory guidance. They may provide the patients and their family with an orientation to the hospital or clinic services and the treatment and care program for the particular patient. They may also assist the patient and family in using the system, for example, the nurses may inform them of the usual mode of communication to obtain certain services that the patient will probably need. In a hospital situation, the nurses may simply go into the rooms of Asian American patients more often for a personal assessment of the patient's needs. One patient mentioned that he waits until the nurses have time to come; he did not want to bother them by calling with the light. Calling with the light would create too much of a disturbance for the nurses.

Death and Dying

Asian American patients exhibit a wide range of behaviors concerning death and dying. Some persons may have come from families where a discussion of death was taboo, as it is in many American families. Other patients may take a more religious or philosophical view.

Many Asians believe in a form of Buddhism that teaches that death in all living things is inevitable. Human beings are believed to be an aggregate consisting of the body, senses, perceptions, consciousness, and intellect, which taken together form the person. All things, including human lives, will inevitably disintegrate and come to an end. Thus people are instructed by Buddha not to make plans in this world without reckoning with death.[26] One Asian patient stated that according to her Buddhist religion, death is not something to fight against, for it will defeat you; it is rather something to accept with confidence. However, the ideal is not always practiced in reality.

Nurses may encounter situations in which a patient may be dying of cancer, but an aura of "closed awareness" surrounds the patient, family, and staff. That is, the staff and family realize that the patient is dying, and the patient realizes he is dying, but each will be careful to avoid any discussion of death. One graduate nursing student who had completed a course about death and dying noted an instance when she was caring for a patient in which "closed awareness" was operative. She first established a trust relationship with the patient. The nurse then suggested that patients who are seriously ill often have concerns about death. The patient then acknowledged that she had been thinking about "what might happen to some people with cancer" and proceeded to discuss the subject of death, initially offering other people's experiences.

By working with this patient over a period of time, the graduate nursing student was able to identify various stages of dying as described by Kübler-Ross; that is, stages of denial, rage and anger, bargaining, depression, and acceptance.[28] The graduate nursing student felt that these universal feelings were expressed more subtly in an Asian patient than in a non-Asian patient, particularly feelings of anger, bargaining, and depression. She felt that seminar discussions dealing with her own feelings about death and dying and the extensive readings available in the regular curriculum were most helpful in her interventions. The only modifications she suggested were that the nurse develop a hypersensitivity to expressions of the patient and family, develop an ongoing relationship at the patient's pace, and avoid confrontations with the patient, even in the stages of denial. The nurse may acknowledge the patient's feelings and from time to time provide gentle suggestions that serve as a stimulus to the patient's own thinking.

SUMMARY

The foregoing discussion has described some of the major values and norms in traditional Asian behavior. In assessing the Asian American patient, one should remember that varying degrees of acculturation as well as individual idiosyncrasies may be present. Some of the examples in this discussion have illustrated different degrees of acculturation; however, the spectrum of Asians and Asian Americans described in this chapter was by no means complete. In Sue and Sue's discussion of intrapsychic conflicts experienced by Chinese, they describe the traditional Chinese, the Chinese American (whom they saw as militant), and the marginal man (whom they defined as one who has become westernized and has lost his Chinese identity).[9] Even this conceptualization, in my view, does not cover the gamut of Asian Americans.

My conceptualization of Asians in America consists of four major typological characters (see Figure 17-1). Asians in America have been exposed to both Asian and dominant Western values and behavior. They may choose to assimilate certain values and reject others. In this process, they may become (1) *traditional Asians* and adopt Asian values and behavior associated with first generation immigrants;

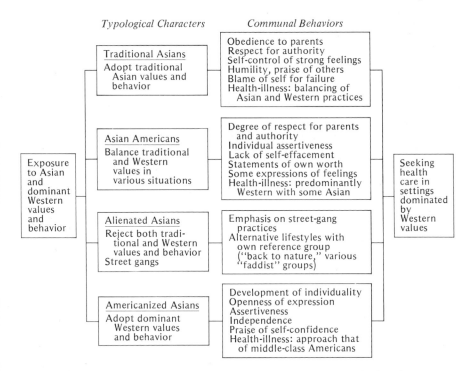

Figure 17-1.   Conceptualization of four typological characters of Asians in America.

(2) *Americanized Asians* who have adopted the dominant Western values and behavior generally associated with white, middle-class America; (3) *Asian Americans* who have integrated selected Asian traditional values and Western values and behavior for various situations; and (4) *alienated Asians* who have rejected both the traditional Asian and dominant Western values and behavior.

The communal behaviors that may be observed for each of the four typological characterizations are also shown in Figure 17-1. For example, traditional Asian behaviors may include obedience to parents, respect for authority, self-control, humility and praise of others, and self-effacement and self-blame for failures. In terms of health-illness behavior, however, they may blend varying degrees of their beliefs in traditional illness causation and treatments and Western scientific beliefs. They have developed a complex coexistant system for dealing with illness.[29,30]

In contrast, dominant Western behaviors in the Americanized Asian include an emphasis on the development of individualty, assertiveness, openness of expression of feelings, and praise of oneself. Their health-illness behavior will approach that of the American middle class. This is not to say that there is not an overlap of values between the traditional Asian and Americanized Asian and Asian American groups. Often the Asian values of hard work, achievement, and so forth coincide with the Protestant work ethic of the Americans.

The Asian Americans can be seen to continue certain traditional Asian behaviors but to modify them to their situations. In their social interactions with the dominant society, for example, they may not be as reserved and passive as the traditionalist. They can speak with pride about their own abilities, thoughts, and feelings. At the same time, they may avoid outward expressions of success and self-acclaim considered normal in the Western culture but ill mannered in the Asian tradition. In terms of health care, persons who balance Asian and Western values may follow a predominantly Western practice but use some traditional or family treatments for selected illnesses.

Alienated Asians who reject both Asian traditions and dominant Western values may be those we think of as deviants from any dominant or minority society. They would include the dropouts in society and those who may join street gangs. Others may choose to live an alternative life style, such as joining certain faddist groups and religious cults. They develop their own values and behaviors compatible with their own reference group.

Asians in any one or any combination of the four typologies may seek health care in a setting dominated by Western values. Nurses and other health professionals will be confronted with the task of assessing Asian patients' needs, formulating care plans, and intervening in a manner that will facilitate recovery. In considering the cultural determinants of behavior (along with the biological, physical, and social determinants) the nurse must be aware that acculturation may result in a blending of values, the acceptance of majority values, the rejection of both Western and Asian values, or the acceptance of a deviant reference group. In addition, the degree of acculturation may vary in different situations in the same individual. In an example previously cited, Mrs. D, and Asian American nurse, may perhaps have been more acculturated in a health care situation than in other situations. The practicing nurse, therefore, needs to be aware of a wide range of differences when caring for Asian Americans, should identify which behaviors are Asian communal role behaviors and which are American, and should differentiate communal and role behaviors from those that are idiosyncratic.

Armed with information about different cultural groups, nurses can develop greater cultural sensitivity in their care of people of varied ethnic backgrounds. Only with increased sensitivity and understanding of other cultures can we truly address the nursing care needs of our multiethnic population.

References

1. Kluckhohn, C.; and Mowrer, O. H. 1976. Culture and personality: A conceptual scheme. In Brink, P. J. *Transcultural nursing, a book of readings.* Englewood Cliffs, N. J.: Prentice-Hall, Inc., pp. 93-125.

2. Yip, B. C.; Lim, H.; Fung, V. H., et al. 1978. *Understanding the Pan Asian client.* San Diego, Calif.: Union of Pan Asian Communities.

3. Kitano, H. H. L. 1976. *Japanese Americans: The evolution of a subculture,* 2nd ed. Englewood Cliffs, N.J.: Prentice-Hall, Inc.

4. Sung, B. L. 1971. *The story of the Chinese in America.* New York: Collier Books.

5. Yamamoto, Y. 1979. Evaluation of Pacific/Asian elderly health services. Los Angeles County.

6. Lee, 1958. The stranded Chinese in the United States. *Phylon* 19:13-194.

7. Wu, Y. T. 1975. Mandarin-speaking aged Chinese in the Los Angeles area. *Gerontology* 15:271-275.

8. U.S. Department of Health, Education, and Welfare, Bureau of Community Health Services. 1973. *Home health service in Chinatown.* Washington, D.C.: U.S. Government Printing Office.

9. Sue, S.; and Sue, D. W. 1973. Chinese-American personality and mental health. In Sue, S.; and Wagner, N. N., editors. *Asian Americans: psychological perspectives.* Palo Alto, Calif.: Science & Behavior Books, pp. 111-124.

10. Okamoto, N. I. 1978. The Japanese American. In Clark, A. L., editor. *Culture, childbearing, health professionals.* Philadelphia: F. A. Davis Co., pp. 64-86.

11. Caudill, W. 1977. The cultural and interpersonal context of everyday health and illness in Japan and America. In Leslie, C., editor. *Asian medical systems: A comparative study.* Berkeley: University of California Press, pp. 159-177.

12. Caudill, W.; and Plath, D. W. 1974. Who sleeps by whom? Parent-child involvement in urban Japanese families. In Lebra, T. S.; and Lebra, W. P., editors. *Japanese culture and behavior selected readings.* Honolulu: The University Press of Hawaii, pp. 277-312.

13. Doi, T. 1974. Amea: A key concept of Understanding Japanese personality structure. In Lebra, T. S., and Lebra, W. P., editors. *Japanese culture and*

behavior. Honolulu: The University Press of Hawaii, pp. 145-173.

14. Hsu, F. L. 1971. *The challenge of the American dream: The Chinese in the United States.* Belmont, Calif.: Wadsworth Publishing Co., Inc.

15. Lyman, S. 1971. *An Asian American reader.* Los Angeles: Continental Graphics.

16. Chang, W. 1979. Filial piety and the criminal law of the Republic of China (typewritten translation).

17. Kiefer, C. W. 1974. *Changing culture, changing lives.* San Francisco: Jossey-Bass, Inc., Publishers.

18. Chang, B. L. Nov. 25-29, 1979a. Perceptions of elderly grandparents held by Chinese Americans in Los Angeles. Washington, D.C.: paper accepted for presentation at the Thirty-second Annual Scientific Meeting of the Gerontological Society.

19. Kogan, N. 1961. Attitudes toward old people. *J. Abnorm. Soc.* 62:44-54.

20. Kilty, K.; and Feld, A. 1976. Attitudes toward aging and toward the needs of older people. *J. Gerontology* 31:586-594.

21. Chang, B. L. Dec. 5-7, 1979b. The relationship of ethnicity and attitudes toward aging and needs of old people. San Antonio, Tex.: paper accepted for presentation at the American Council of Nurse Researchers Annual meeting.

22. Brunton, E.; Estradas, L.; Fellner, P., et al. 1972. A study of Japanese-Americans with regard to health and illness. San Francisco: Department of Nursing, San Francisco State College (class presentation).

23. Brunton, E.; Estradas, L.; Fellner, P., et al. 1972. A study of Japanese-Americans with regard to health and illness. San Francisco: Department of Nursing, San Francisco State College (class presentation), pp. 15-16.

24. Brunton, E.; Estradas, L.; Fellner, P., et al. 1972. A study of Japanese-Americans with regard to health and illness. San Francisco: Department of Nursing, San Francisco State College (class presentation), p. 16.

25. McCaffery, M. 1979. Nursing intervention on the relief of pain. Los Angeles: class presentation to the graduate medical-surgical student, School of Nursing, University of California.

26. Long, J. B. 1975. The death that ends death in Hinduism and Buddhism. In Kübler-Ross, E., editor: *Death: The final state of growth.* Englewood Cliffs, N.J.: Prentice-Hall, Inc.

27. Glaser, B.; and Strauss, A. L. 1965. *Awareness of dying: A study of social interaction.* Chicago: Aldine Publishing Co.

28. Kübler-Ross, E. 1972. On death and dying. *J.A.M.A.* 221:174-179.

29. Campbell, T., and Chang, B. 1973. Health care of the Chinese in America. *Nurs. Outlook* 21:245-249.

30. Louis, T. T. T. 1976. Explanatory thinking in Chinese Americans. In Brink, P. J. *Transcultural nursing, a book of readings.* Englewood Cliffs, N.J.: Prentice-Hall, Inc., pp. 240-246.

18

Biological Variation: Concepts from Physical Anthropology

Teresa Overfield, R.N., Ph.D.

Theresa Overfield, Associate Professor and Director of Research at the College of Nursing, Brigham Young University, teaches "Biological Variation in Health and Illness" in the Medical Anthropology Program at the University of Utah. Her publications, papers, and talks have dealt with disease among Eskimos and American Indians, nursing research, and nursing education. Her ongoing research concentrates on Eskimos in the areas of racial variation, population genetics, and demography, with a recent excursion into botany.

People differ biologically as well as culturally. We are all aware of differences in skin color and facial features, but biological variation encompasses more than the obvious surface characteristics of individuals. Nurses need to be aware and knowledgeable about such differences in order to give effective care.

The majority of nurses and physicians in the United States have been members of the dominant white culture and have, unconsciously or not, incorporated their own ideas of normal into their management of patients. Studies of biological baselines in growth and development, nutrition and other areas have been done on whites, thus setting standardized norms that do not apply to other racial groups.

Source: From Overfield, T. 1977. Biological variation: Concepts from physical anthropology. *Nurs. Clin. North Am.* 12:19-26.

This paper will attempt three things: to indicate the necessity for inclusion of concepts of biological variation into nursing practice; to give an indication of what needs to be learned, and finally to give a few suggestions on how these concepts might be integrated into a curriculum.

THE IMPORTANCE OF CONCEPTS OF
BIOLOGICAL VARIATION FOR NURSING

Nurses are increasingly becoming aware that cultural differences must be considered while providing care.[7] Initiating health intervention that opposes a cultural practice may not be successful even if it is a "good" health measure. More efficient use of time and energy results if the health measures advocated are culturally relevant.

This same awareness must be developed in the realm of biological variation. A "good" health practice that produces biological problems may result in nurses promoting ill health. A prime example of this is encouraging pregnant women to drink milk without taking into consideration that most racial groups other than whites cannot tolerate milk in adulthood.[1]

An adult complaining of diarrhea, a bloated feeling and a great deal of discomfort from flatus might actually be ill as a result of nursing intervention. These symptoms may be due to ingestion of milk or milk products by a person deficient in lactose enzyme. When the lactose enzyme is missing, milk lactose ferments in the intestinal tract, causing gas production.[1] Nurses are involved in nutrition counseling and might easily recommend the very thing that produces these symptoms. "Drink milk, eat cheese for calcium and protein needs of the body"—good advice for a small portion of adults in the world, but 90 percent of blacks, Orientals and American Indians, plus 10 percent of whites, are lactose-enzyme deficient. To improve nutrition, a nurse can suggest using cheese aged over 60 days—the sharper cheeses—since the lactose sugar has been changed to lactic acid during the aging process.

Again in the realm of foods, fava beans (also called the broad or horse bean) can cause severe hemolytic anemia in persons with G-6-PD deficiency. Over 100 million people have this hematologic deficiency, which evolved as a protection against malaria, as in the case of sickle cell trait. It should also be known that G-6-PD deficient people develop anemia after taking various drugs, particularly oxidant drugs. These include aspirin preparations, sulfa drugs, and certain vitamin K preparations, to name a few.[14] Persons with G-6-PD deficiency appear normal, except when exposed to malaria, when they are protected from some of its severe consequences, or when exposed to fava beans or certain drugs, when they become ill.

Overcoming Culture Shock and Discomfort

Ethnocentrism and cultural shock can be alleviated to some extent in a person who has an understanding of how groups vary biologically. Part of ethnocentrism relates to a feeling of biological superiority. Understanding how different races evolved, in relation to their environment, makes it clear that our features, skin color, body size and shape, even our enzymes are the result of the biological adjustments our ancestors were able to make to the environment in which they lived. It is postulated that the original skin color of man was black, and that white skin was the result of mutations and environmental pressures incurred by those living in cold, cloudy northern Europe.[11] Light skin was better able to synthesize vitamin D on the few sunny days and, conversely, black skin became a neutral trait where protection from the sun and heat of the tropics was not a factor.

Familiarity with external and internal biological variation helps one to make an easy transition from discomfort to comfort in the presence of people who differ in their appearance. Knowledge of why people differ in their external characteristics helps one to get beyond the "all Chinese look alike" phenomenon and to intellectually satisfy one's desire to stare. Part of the discomfort dissipates with time and familiarity, but the process can be speeded up considerably by being informed concerning biological variation. It is better to have a nurse's energies concentrated on the individual and his health problem, rather than on her own problems of culture shock and discomfort. With biological differences put in perspective, a nurse becomes comfortable and thus may give better care to her clients.

To illustrate the above point: the first two babies I delivered in Alaska looked as though they might have Down's syndrome. Fortunately, I said nothing. After seeing a few more Eskimo babies, the next white babies I saw looked strange. Even today, for me, a normal baby is an American Indian or Eskimo baby because most of my experience as a nurse has been with Indians and Eskimos.

Understanding Variations as the Basis for Health Care

Perhaps the strongest argument for including biological variation concepts in nursing practice is the provision of scientific facts to aid in giving knowledgeable health care. A nurse who cares for people of another culture needs to know certain basic biological concepts, in order to give not only adequate care, but also nonharmful care. Human beings vary tremendously in how they appear externally, and in what genetic variations have occurred internally. White values for many factors related to growth and development, nutrition and response to disease are not normal for blacks, Orientals or American Indians. Some of what is labeled non-normal might better be called nonwhite.

Assessing Physical Differences. Physical assessment skills have become a part of basic nursing. Independent gathering of knowledge about patients is necessary in order to give thorough and logical care. Physical assessment skills require that a nurse must be aware of normal variation in all ages and types of persons.

When a nurse is assessing a *newborn*, she may find mongolian spots, body proportions different from white norms, or unusual fingerprint patterns. She must know the ranges of expectation, or at least be aware of the possibility for variations. Mongolian spots, bluish discolorations on the lower back, are a normal hyperpigmented area in many Oriental, American Indian, and black groups. They are most prominent in babies, but gradually fade with age. Newborn body proportions differ by race, and appear to be genetically programmed to conform to the differences in pelvic shape of the mothers. A study of this phenomenon, relating it to maternal pelvic measurements, is being done at the University of Utah. This information will be valuable to nurse midwives and physicians in assessing cephalopelvic proportions in various racial groups. Fingerprint patterns vary by group and also by syndromes. Another study is being conducted at the University of Utah on fingerprint patterns in prematures, to see if these patterns are different from those of normal newborns. If there are differing fingering patterns, this may indicate that there are genetic causes of prematurity.

In assessing a pre-school child, *ear wax type* might play a role in determining whether there is ear disease. Ear wax comes in two genetically determined varieties, wet ear wax and dry ear wax. Dry ear wax is recessive; American Indians and Orientals have this type. Most blacks and whites have wet ear wax. These two types of ear wax differ in their composition. Studies have shown that wet wax is approximately 50 percent lipid, while dry wax is around 18 percent lipid. Wet wax contains 16 percent cholesterol, dry wax, 3 percent.[9] Wet wax is brown and sticky, while dry is gray and brittle.

Use of underarm deodorants is generally unnecessary for people with dry ear wax. Body odor comes from deterioration of apocrine sweat, especially in the underarm area. Dry ear wax individuals have only a few apocrine glands when compared with wet ear wax individuals, hence, do not smell as much as those with wet ear wax. Body odor is considered a pathological condition in Japan.[9] A nurse should not use body odor as an indicator of personal hygiene. It really is related to ear wax type and/or the desire to cover up a natural process.

Growth and development scores in very high or low categories must be assessed. Blacks are generally advanced, Orientals generally retarded in growth rates when compared with white norms.[2] High scores are expected to occur in black children, while low scores are common in Oriental children. The reasons for differential growth rates are not known, but they do occur and are part of normal human variation.

Physical assessment at any age should include awareness of the fact that certain *muscles* are absent in some groups of people. The peroneus tertius muscle in the foot and the palmaris longus muscle in the wrist are absent in some individuals. Muscle absence does not seem to be more prevalent in any particular racial group, nor does absence of one of these correspond with absence of the other. Studies have shown an absence of the peroneus tertius muscle in up to 24 percent of the people studied.[15] The absence of either muscle in a child might be of concern to a mother; a nurse, knowing that this phenomenon was a fairly common variant, could alleviate her worry.

Similarly, a mandibular or palatine torus might be of concern to a nurse inspecting a mouth. A torus is a bony protuberance. The palatine torus occurs on the midline of the palate, while the mandibular torus occurs as a lump on the inner side of the mandible near the second premolar. Tori are fairly common; palatine *tori* occur in up to 25 percent of many racial groups studied. Mandibular *tori* occur in approximately 7 percent of whites, 2 percent of blacks, and up to 40 percent of Orientals.[5]

Teeth are also subject to variation. For example, peg teeth, congenitally missing teeth, additional teeth, and natal teeth all occur at varying frequencies in different racial groups.[5] Tongues also vary; a few of the more common variants are "scrotal" tongues (5 percent of some groups), geographic tongues (3 percent of some groups), fissured tongues (5-40 percent of groups).[16]

Nurses helping pregnant women might have noticed the different patterns of superficial veins on the anterior chest. There are two patterns of venous drainage in the mammary region, called the transverse and longitudinal types. These two patterns occur in both sexes and appear to be caused by a single dominant gene. The only known alterations in the vein patterns are due to breast tumor.[15]

Variations in Susceptibility to Disease. Susceptibility to disease varies among groups. Urban Jews are the most resistant to tuberculosis. Blacks and American Indians are most susceptible. Persons with type O blood have more duodenal ulcers. Those with blood type A have more cancer of the stomach. There is information that women with type O blood have less chance of venous thromboembolic disease than women with other ABO blood types, especially when taking birth control pills.[6] The present author has been working on a study that indicates that the amount of tooth decay is related to blood type and to a specific blood enzyme.

Sickle cell anemia is most commonly found in blacks. It is also present in other groups of people whose ancestors lived in malaria-plagued areas; Mediterranean peoples may also have the disease or the trait.

Blacks have a tendency toward overgrowth of connective tissue components concerned with protection against infection and repair after injury. Keloid formation is one manifestation of this tendency. Other lesser known results of this overgrowth have been suggested, namely: greater incidence of Burkitt's lymphoma, multiple myeloma, and systemic lupus erythematosus; increased susceptibility to tuberculosis (a granulomatous infection); increased tendency toward endomyocardial fibrosis after myocardial infarction.[13]

Certain eye problems are more common in specific groups. Europeans and East Indians have more color blindness than other racial groups. Approximately 19 percent of Chinese are myopic; fewer whites and even fewer blacks and American Indians have this problem.[2]

Variations in Body Structure. Here we are concerned with normal human variation in the area of body size and shape. There are no specific health implications but such information should be of interest to anyone working with people and intellectually curious about individual and social differences. As mentioned previously, understanding biological differences helps one to achieve comfort in working with other racial groups.

Faces have many fascinating parts that go on to produce a whole, which people are prone to categorize racially. For instance, eyelids come in a few varieties: those with skin droops over the cartilage plate above the eye and those whose skin does not droop. Another variation is the epicanthic fold, which is predominantly an Oriental characteristic but occasionally is present in other groups.

Ears are fascinating. Ear lobes can be free and floppy (handy for earrings), or attached, which means the lobe does not hang free, or soldered, in which it looks as though someone wanted to make sure the lobe stayed there. This type has the least defined ear lobe.

Noses—no need to mention their variety, but it might be of interest to know that nose size and shape correlates strongly with the homeland of an individual's ancestors. Small noses were produced in cold regions—the classic Oriental nose. Dry areas produced high bridges and roots—the classic Iranian and American Indian noses. Moist warm areas gave us the broad flat noses characteristic of some blacks.

Tooth size helps to shape the lower face. Groups differ in tooth size. Australian aborigines have the largest teeth in the world, plus four extra molars. Orientals and blacks generally have large teeth, whites smaller teeth. Larger teeth cause some groups to have prognathic lower faces; this is a normal variation, not an orthodontic problem. There is also a growing tendency among all racial groups for tooth number to decrease; gradually people are not producing third molars or maxillary lateral incisors. Peg teeth are sometimes a step in the evolution from presence to absence of a particular tooth type.

Blood Group Variations. Blood groups help to differentiate people. American Indians are predominantly blood type O, some blood type A, and virtually no type B. Japanese and Chinese people have almost equal amounts of A, B, and O type blood, and around 10 percent AB type. American blacks and whites have similar percentages of ABO blood types, mostly A and O, with fewer AB and B type.

RH negative blood is most common in whites, much rarer in other groups, and absent in Eskimos.

It is interesting to know that the incidence of dizygote twinning is highest in blacks (up to 4 percent of births); it is around 2 percent in whites and ½ percent in Asians.[3]

WHAT NEEDS TO BE LEARNED

Once the necessity of knowing about human biological variation has been explained, the next step is to suggest ways to gain the knowledge. Since the very existence of race is debated, the controversy should be discussed with arguments from both sides of the question. Once one knows where the notion of race stands in present-day scientific thinking, and some time is given to understanding the controversy over race and intelligence, racial biases should disappear.[4,12]

Specific biological differences occurring in different social groups and in different regions should be studied. There is no need to cover all differences in exhaustive detail. The important concepts to emphasize are that biological variations exist, and these variations are responses to past environmental influences; that present-day differences represent a map of our evolutionary past, not some sort of innate biological difference. Concepts of human variation, especially those related to health and illness, are not collected together in any one book or article, but many papers are available on the subject. As a nurse becomes aware of biological differences and has searched out a few specific variations in the literature, perhaps related to patients she has seen, the notion of biological variation will color her future observations.

An acquaintance with genetics as related to populations would help make some of the above-mentioned concepts clear. Although mentioned last, population genetics need to be studied before the race concept. An understanding of natural selection, mutation, random mating, genetic drift and breeding population is necessary to an understanding of the whole notion of race and general biological variation.[10] These concepts have been taught in anthropology departments by physical anthropologists. An obvious suggestion is to take an introductory physical anthropology course, but the realities of full schedules would suggest picking up the concepts through selected readings.

INCORPORATING THIS KNOWLEDGE INTO
THE NURSING CURRICULUM

At the present time, these concepts are not incorporated into the nursing curriculum in any organized way. Some of the dramatic variations such as sickle cell anemia and sickle cell trait are probably included, but the more mundane ones are ignored. If this is so, and there is not a built-up tradition of incorporating such concepts, a suggested beginning for nursing faculty would be to teach a course to students on these concepts related specifically to nursing and health. Faculty should be encouraged to take human variation courses in anthropology departments to sensitize themselves to these concepts. Hopefully, once normal variation becomes more widely appreciated among faculty and nurses in general, specific courses could be dropped and the concepts taught where they fit in the curriculum.

At the College of Nursing, University of Utah, baccalaureate curriculum is built on an adaptation model. Students learn throughout their schooling how man adapts socioculturally, biologically, and psychologically to various stimuli. Several faculty are interested and excited about incorporating both biological and cultural variation concepts into the day-to-day teaching of students. Even with this group of interested faculty and the encouragement and support of the administrators, biological variation concepts have not been fully incorporated. To help with the immediate problem and to add to the transcultural nursing program, the author is offering a graduate level course entitled "Biological Variation and Health Care Delivery." It will give graduate students and interested faculty an opportunity to formally incorporate the information into their nursing repertory.

References

1. Bayless, T., et al. 1975. Lactose and milk intolerance: Clinical implications. *N. Eng. J. Med.* 292:1156-1159.

2. Brues, A. In press. *People and races.* New York: Macmillan, Inc.

3. Bulmer, M. 1970. The biology of twinning in man. New York: Oxford University Press.

4. Goldsby, R. 1971. *Race and races.* New York: Macmillan, Inc.

5. Jarvis, A., et al. Minor orofacial abnormalities in an Eskimo population. *Oral Surg.* 33:417-427.

6. Jick, H., et al. 1969. Venous thromboembolic disease and ABO blood type. *Lancet* 1:539-542.

7. Leininger, M. 1970. *Nursing and anthropology: Two worlds to blend.* New York: John Wiley & Sons, Inc.

8. Matheny, A. 1975. Sex and genetic differences in hair color changes during early childhood. *Am. J. Physical Anthro.* 42:53-56.

9. Matsunaga, E. 1962. The dimorphism in human normal cerumen. *Ann. Hum. Genet.* 25:273-286.

10. McKusick, V. 1969. *Human genetics.* Englewood Cliffs, N.J.: Prentice-Hall, Inc.

11. Neer, R. 1975. The evolutionary significance of vitamin D, skin pigment and ultraviolet lights. *Am. J. Physical Anthro.* 43:409-416.

12. Osborne, R. 1971. *The biological and social meanings of race.* San Francisco: W. H. Freeman & Co. Publishers.

13. Polednak, A. 1974. Connective tissue responses in Negroes in relation to disease. *Am. J. Physical Anthro.* 41:49-57.

14. Sapeika, N. 1974. *Food pharmacology.* Springfield, Ill.: Charles C Thomas, Publisher.

15. Spuhler, J. 1950. Genetics of three normal morphological variations: Patterns of superficial veins of anterior thorax, peroneus tertius muscle and number of vallate papillae. *Cold Spring Harbor Symposium on Quantitative Biology* 15:175-189.

16. Witcop, C., et al. 1963. Oral and genetic studies of Chileans 1960: I. Oral anomalies. *Am. J. Physical Anthro.* 21:15-24.

19

Color Changes in
Dark Skin

Lora B. Roach, R.N., M.S.N.

Lora B. Roach, Associate Professor of Nursing at the University of Texas at Arlington, has had fourteen years of clinical experience in psychiatric, tuberculosis, medical-surgical, and pediatric nursing. While practicing and teaching in Dallas, Texas, she developed particular interest and skill in observing and interpreting color change in persons with dark skins. In 1972 she began to fill the gap in the literature on assessment of color change in dark skin and has since published numerous articles on this topic.

Have you ever wondered how you would recognize the pallor of anemia in a dark-skinned American Indian boy? Or the jaundice of hepatic obstruction in a dark-skinned Mexican-American? Or cyanosis in a Negro?

Such dermatoligic signs are usually difficult, and sometimes impossible to see when the patient's skin is heavily pigmented. Since a generous portion of our population is dark-skinned, either by genetic factors or suntanning, many young nurses express concern about failing to recognize important signs of pathology. There are very few signs, however, that cannot be recognized despite dark skin provided the nurse has good color sensitivity and observes her patient's usual color and behavior.

Source: Reprinted with permission from the January issue of *Nursing 77.* Copyright © 1977, Intermed. Communications, Inc.

PROBLEMS OF OBSERVATION

Poor color sensitivity, or even color blindness, accounts for the difficulty that many nurses have in recognizing color changes. In addition, descriptions of skin colors are at best highly subjective. Each of us has a very personal interpretation of the various colors and tones—yellowish, livid, ashen, dusky, etc.—and find it quite impossible to convey that interpretation accurately to another person for the purpose of subsequent comparison. Attempts to develop standardized skin color comparators have not been successful because of the myriad variations of skin tones among persons of each skin color. Assessment of skin color is, therefore, still based on individual skill. If you are an alert observer with good color sensitivity and if you spend a few minutes with each patient observing the basic color tones and behavioral characteristics, you will have the basis necessary for recognizing even subtle changes. But conditions for observation must be right.

Inadequate lighting often prevents accurate observation of even light-skinned individuals, so color changes that are ordinarily observable despite heavy pigmentation will be missed if poorly illuminated. The best illumination is nonglare daylight, but when this is not available, a stand light with at least a 60-watt bulb may be satisfactory. One of the newer lights that simulate sunlight would be better, however. Flashlights and the soft illumination of many overbed lights are totally inadequate for identifying subtle color changes.

The position of the individual, and especially of his extremities, also strongly influences the accuracy of evaluation of color change. Not only must you position the part being inspected for correct light reflection, but you must consider the effects of gravity as well. Particularly in conditions involving vasomotor changes, the force of gravity on an elevated or lowered limb may induce a false color change or enhance the subtle color change of early pathology. Accurate evaluation of color change necessitates careful consideration of the relationship between color and position as well as a good understanding of the contributing pathophysiology. A good method of assessing the relationship is to examine the part while it is at heart level, then (assuming there are no contraindications) to elevate the part about 15 degrees for at least five minutes, and finally to lower it 30 to 90 degrees for at least five minutes.

The temperature of the environment and the patient's emotional state may mask color changes or create temporary but misleading changes. Air-conditioned rooms frequently cause "cold cyanosis," in which the lips and nail beds of sensitive individuals become cyanotic. The condition is not harmful, but it effectively masks any pallor that may exist. Lying on a cold examining table may cause blanching of the skin of the back, which is noticeable even in moderately pigmented areas; anger and fright may cause a similar but a more generalized pallor. In contrast, an excessively warm room or embarrassment may cause an increased redness of the skin resulting from superficial vasodilation. Obviously, temperature and emotional factors should be controlled when possible, and their influence duly noted when not controlled. When assessing very subtle color changes in the nail beds, you should determine when the patient last smoked a cigarette (if he smokes); the vasoconstrictive effect of smoking can be quite marked.

Collections of sweat and sebum may hinder accurate assessment of skin color, particularly when one is attempting to locate petechiae and other localized changes. A thorough cleansing of the skin before inspection may be indicated, taking care not to create additional distortions through the use of vigorous friction, harsh soaps and so forth.

Edema of the skin reduces the intensity of skin color by increasing the distance between the surface and the pigmented and vascular layers. As a result the darkly pigmented skin becomes lighter, but pathologic color changes such as pallor of anemia, jaundice and erythema are also obscured so that the lightened pigmentation sometimes gives a false pallor. When edema precedes the development of jaundice, the jaundice cannot be seen even in the light-skinned individual. Thus, awareness of the presence or absence of edema is essential to accurate assessment of color changes.

The normal distribution patterns of pigment in dark-skinned persons may obscure certain color changes, and lead to misinterpretations by inexperienced observers. For example, some dark-skinned people, particularly of Mediterranean origin, have very blue lips, giving a false impression of cyanosis. Full-blooded blacks often have normal bluish pigmentation of the gums, distributed evenly or in splotches; the portion of the sclera exposed in the lid slit may contain deposits of brown melanin that could be misinterpreted as petechiae. Also, blacks commonly have brown freckle-like pigmentation of the gums, buccal cavity, borders of the tongue and even of the nail beds. Babies of genetically dark-skinned persons are lightly pigmented at birth, but grow progressively darker with age until pigmentation peaks after six to eight weeks. Color changes in both the adult and child are best observed where pigmentation from melanin, melanoid and carotene is least: the sclera, conjuctiva, nail beds, lips, buccal mucosa, tongue, palms and soles. However, heavily calloused palms and soles usually have an opaque yellowish cast (carotene), which decreases their value to the observer.

SPECIFIC TECHNIQUES

Petchiae, although only pinpoints of reddish-purple color, are sufficiently dark to be seen readily in moderately dark-skinned persons, particularly if inspected over the areas of lighter melanization: the abdomen, buttocks, and volar surface of forearm. When the skin is black or very dark brown, petechiae cannot be seen in the skin. However, petechiae usually occur in the mucous membranes as well as the skin in most of the diseases that cause bleeding tendency and microembolism (e.g., thrombocytopenia, subacute bacterial endocarditis and other septicemias). Therefore, inspect for petechiae in the mouth, particularly the buccal mucosa, and the conjunctiva (both the bulbar conjunctiva covering exposed surface of the eyeball and the palpebral conjunctiva lining the eyelids) for petechiae. Do not be misled by the presence of the blue or brown pigmentation previously described: in most cases, it is patchy enough to allow for visualization of petechiae.

Ecchymotic lesions caused by systemic disorders can be observed in the same areas as petechiae, although their larger size makes it possible to see them on rather dark-skinned individuals. Detecting localized ecchymosis from trauma is rarely a problem because the history and the accompanying discomfort suggest its presence; unless a complication such as hematoma is developing, the question of its presence or absence tends to be academic anyway.

When differentiating petechiae and ecchymosis from erythema in the mucous membrane (and in moderately pigmented skin), pressure on the tissue will momentarily blanch erythema but not petechiae or ecchymosis.

Pallor in the dark-skinned individual is observable by the absence of the underlying red tones that normally give the brown and black skin its "glow" or "living color." The brown-skinned person will therefore appear more yellowish-brown, and the black-skinned person will appear ashen-gray. Admittedly, it takes an experienced eye to identify the change, but any nurse (without visual perception defects) who practices can quickly become experienced.

Generalized pallor can also be observed in the mucous membranes, lips and nail beds. The palpebral conjunctiva and nail beds have long been the sites of choice for observing the pallor of anemia. When inspecting the conjunctiva, you will get a more accurate idea of the amount of color if you pull down the lower lid sufficiently to see the conjunctiva near the other canthus as well as the inner canthus; the coloration is often lighter near the inner canthus.

If the nail beds are not pigmented, a slight pressure on the free edge of the second or third fingernail blanches the nail bed, giving you a color comparison for assessing the presence of, or degree of, pallor or cyanosis. The speed with which the color returns following slow release of the pressure indicates the quality of vasomotor function; slow return, as compared with a test of your own nails, indicates diminished quality. The lips and earlobes, if not too darkly pigmented, can be observed in much the same way, using digital pressure to create color comparison.

The pallor of impending shock is accompanied by other subtle manifestations such as increasing pulse rate, oliguria, apprehension, and restless movements. Anemias also often announce their presence in ways other than pallor: "Spoon" (concave) nails often accompany chronic iron-deficiency (microcytic) anemia. Lemon yellow tint of skin (especially of the face) and slight yellowish sclera accompany pernicious anemia; so do sensory neurologic deficits and red, painful tongue. Easy fatigability, dyspnea on exertion, rapid pulse, dizziness, and impaired mental function accompany most severe anemias.

Since most of the conditions causing pallor also cause diminished oxygenation of the brain, you need not rely totally on color change. Relatively acute behavioral change—for example, a person normally alert becomes drowsy and forgetful—

provides reliable evidence of hypoglycemia, internal bleeding, shock, and so forth.

Erythema is generally associated with increased skin temperature (as in a localized inflammatory process), but you cannot rely on warmth of the skin to denote erythema any more than you can assume that coolness indicates pallor. The degree of redness is determined by the quantity of blood present in the subpapillary plexus, whereas the warmth depends primarily on the rate of blood flow through all the vessels of the skin (arteries, arterioles and venules as well as the subpapillary plexus).

When you suspect inflammation in persons with very dark brown or black skin, you will usually need to rely on your skills of palpation: feeling for increased warmth of skin; for "slick," tight skin suggesting edema; and for hardening of deep tissues or blood vessels. The dorsal surface of your fingers will be more sensitive to subtle temperature differences than will the palmar surface. Curve your fingers into a relaxed flexion and gently rest the middle phalanges on the skin to be tested; then move them to another skin surface for comparison.

The erythema of rash is not always accompanied by a noticeable increase in skin temperature. With a little practice in palpating different skin textures, you can usually identify papular rash by palpating gently with the fingertips. In the case of macular rash, you may have to rely on the patient's complaints of itching or on evidence of scratching. Keep in mind, though, that itching may result from a number of other conditions such as jaundice, dry skin, irritating clothing or chemicals, etc. When the skin is only moderately pigmented, a macular rash may become recognizable if the skin is gently stretched between the thumb and finger (as for administering an injection). This maneuver decreases the normal red tone, thus brightening the macules. Some generalized rashes can be seen in the mouth, so inspect the palate especially.

The increased redness (flushing) that accompanies carbon monoxide poisoning and the polycythemias can usually be seen in the lips when the skin is too dark to show it. Of course, the masking effect of lipstick must be considered. Lipstick can be removed gently with a cream or lotion, but allow 20 to 30 minutes for the lips to resume their "at rest" color before making a final assessment of color.

Cyanosis remains the most difficult clinical sign to observe in the darkly pigmented individual. The usual sites of observation (lips, nail beds, skin around the mouth, over the cheekbones, and the earlobes) may have just enough pigmentation to obscure beginning cyanosis. Nevertheless, close inspection of the lips, nail beds, palpebral conjunctiva, palms and soles at regular intervals will usually enable recognition of cyanosis when it develops. The palpebral conjunctiva demonstrates generalized cyanosis as readily as it does pallor, but you will need to become thoroughly familiar with the precyanotic color or you may not recognize early changes.

When cyanosis is questionable, apply light pressure to create pallor. In cyanosis, the tissue color returns slowly by spreading from the periphery to the center. Normally, the color returns in less than one second, and it appears to return from below the pallid spot as well as from the periphery.

Cyanosis of an extremity may become more recognizable if the position of the extremity can be changed (from elevated to dependent or vice versa). Remember to control influencing factors such as smoking and excessive air-conditioning throughout the observation period. Peripheral vasoconstriction can prevent cyanosis even though serious anoxia is present. Also, for cyanosis to be evident, the blood must contain 5 grams of reduced hemoglobin or 1.5 grams of methemoglobin per 100 ml of blood.

Jaundice in the dark-skinned person is more readily observed in the sclera, just as it is in the light-skinned person. However, be wary of misinterpreting other forms of pigmentation as jaundice. Many darkly pigmented individuals have heavy deposits of subconjunctival fat containing enough carotene to mimic jaundice. The fatty deposits become heavier as the distance from the cornea increases, so inspecting the portion of the sclera revealed naturally by the lid slit may provide the most accurate assessment of color. When the sclera are yellow even to the edges of the cornea, inspect the posterior portion of the hard palate in bright daylight. If the palate does not have a heavy malanin pigmentation, jaundice can be detected there quite early, i.e., when serum bilirubin is 2 to 4 mg per 100 ml. The absence of a yellowish tint of the palate when the sclera are yellow would indicate carotene pigmentation of the sclera rather than jaundice. Light or clay-colored stools and dark golden urine often accompany jaundice and may help in interpreting the significance of yellow tones.

Observation and evaluation of color change in the dark-skinned person is not the insurmountable problem that some nurses believe. The rules are: accurately observe color and behavior for comparison with later changes, anticipate and look for changes using the techniques described, and know and recognize behavior changes that accompany disorders causing color change.

20

In Retrospect

George Henderson, Ph.D.
Martha Primeaux, R.N., M.S.N.

Most of the good intentions of nurses go to waste because of their lack of understanding as to what is helpful to Third World patients and what constitutes a helping relationship. To the affected patients, this waste of effort may be so negative that it causes them to have a revulsion against all forms of helping. When this happens, helping is seen as a process that benefits nurses more than patients, and nurses are seen as neurotic "do-gooders." Although this book has focused on ethnic minority groups, the analyses and suggestions are relevant to all ethnic groups.

PRELUDE TO HELPING

Most definitions of help are based on subjective values—something tangible or intangible discovered in a relationship between a helper and the person receiving that help in which the helper aids the recipient in achieving a measure of self-fulfillment. In actuality, help is something that a person discovers for himself or herself. Each person must accept and act on helpful information with the knowledge that the ultimate responsibility belongs to him or her. In final analysis, help cannot be given to patients; it can only be offered.

The helping relationship has qualities that are the same whether it is between therapist and client, counselor and client, or nurse and patient. The psychological equilibrium underneath the heatlh care roles resides at a much deeper, more fundamental level. This is true for both the nurse and the patient. Numerous studies suggest that effective help is initiated not so much by technique or special knowledge of the nursing profession but rather by positive attitudes of the nurse. Furthermore, research findings suggest that experienced nurses have a better conception of what constitutes a helping relationship than their colleagues who have mastered theoretical concepts but have little work experience.

Some health professionals see the helping process as one in which they make intricate diagnosis of patients and then use a wide variety of helping methods on them. Still other professionals define patients as being sick and themselves as being well. These are not really helping relationships. On the contrary, they are controlling relationships. When the patient becomes an object rather than the subject, he or she is no longer the person who acts but instead becomes the person acted on. Conceptually, a thin line separates wanting to help another person from wanting to change him or her to conform with our cultural norms.

There is an underlying assumption in the health professions that trained persons can make a significant contribution to the lives of others if their training has instilled a commitment to effectively using oneself in the helping process. The primary technique or instrument in the helping relationship is the ability of the nurse to become an instrument to be used by the patient to achieve health needs that must be met (at least from the patient's perception) and to achieve some measure of self-fulfillment in doing so. From the nurse's point of view, this goal of self-fulfillment means that the patient will become more realistic and self-directing.

One of the most important aspects of helping in health care settings is that some patients do not seem to want to be helped. At least they do not appear to want to be helped by health professionals. Many patients who ask for help are afraid that it will not be given. There are many ways of asking for help. For example, missing appointments may be a plea for help. Consequently, nurses must be aware of these subtle pleas and be prepared to enter into a growth-producing rather than punitive relationship with patients.

> Patients learn to mask their feelings. They do not openly or directly express their anger toward people on whom they depend; instead, they often agree to any request: "Yes, I will keep the appointment." This is what the professional wants to hear. The patient does not deliberately lie: It may be a response a mother has learned to protect herself and her family. It could also be interpreted as passive aggression toward those in authority and an attempt to exercise some control over her life.[1]

Carl R. Rogers defined the helping relationship as "a relationship in which at least one of the parties has the intent of promoting the growth, development, maturity, improved functioning, improved coping with life of the other."[2] The characteristics that distinguish a helpful nurse-patient relationship from an unhelpful one are related primarily to the attitudes of the nurse and the perceptions of the patient.

Determining what is helpful and what is not depends to a great extent on who is perceiving the situation. In other words, a patient may not see a situation in the same way as his or her nurse. For example, a white nurse may see a black patient and two of her relatives arguing, with the patient obviously receiving much verbal abuse. The nurse also may perceive that the helpful thing to do is to intervene and stop the argument. On the other hand, the patient might prefer to take the verbal abuse than later face her relatives, who in all probability will make fun of her for having to be saved by a white person.

Certain values in a helping relationship must be observed by nurses if the relationship is to be productive in the long run. Doing a chore or making a decision for a patient may help in the short run, but it will not help the patient to become more self-directing in the future.

This final chapter does not attempt to provide a how-to-do-it approach with clearly outlined steps to follow. Lists are presented, but they are used primarily to summarize various thoughts. Helping relationships do not allow a rigid structure; therefore, this chapter presents a "be-it-yourself" approach, because health professionals need an attitude of being for others instead of doing for others. From this perspective, it is more important for the nurse to be *aware* rather than to be an expert. To be aware and to care about the world, values and life styles of patients are significant aspects of the helping relationship in which nurses try to promote positive intrapersonal, interpersonal, and intergroup relationships.

CHARACTERISTICS OF A HELPING RELATIONSHIP

Carl Rogers further stated that a helping relationship is one "in which one of the participants intends that there should come about, on one or both parties more appreciation of, more expression of, more functional use of the latent inner resources of the individual."[2] Relatedly, the job of the helper as seen by Alan Keith-Lucas is to provide "a medium, a situation, and an experience in which a choice is possible."[3] Ideally, through the helping relationship the fears that restrain patients can to some extent be resolved, and they can find the courage to make a commitment to a health plan and learn some of the practical skills necessary to make this decision a reality. Arthur W. Combs has stated that "the helper's basic beliefs and values rather than his grand schemes, methods, techniques, or years of training are the real determiners of whether or not the helper will be effective or ineffective."[4]

In a classic article entitled "The Characteristics of a Helping Relationship," Rogers asked a series of questions that he felt revealed characteristics of a helping relationship. If nurses can answer these questions affirmatively concerning their interactions with culturally different patients, it is likely that they will be or are helpful to all patients.

Can I be in some way which will be perceived by the other person as trustworthy, as dependable or consistent in some deep sense?[5]

This question is more than being rigidly consistent. It means being honest and congruent with our feelings so that we are a unified or integrated person.

Can I be expressive enough as a person that what I am will be communicated unambiguously?[5]

If we are unaware of our own feelings, a double message can be given that will confuse the situation and cause the relationship to be marred by the ambiguous communication.

Can I let myself experience positive attitudes toward this other person— attitudes of warmth, caring, liking, interest, respect?[5]

A professional attitude of aloofness is unhelpful; it creates a barrier or distance that protects scientific objectivity at the expense of establishing a helping relationship.

Can I receive him as he is? Can I communicate this attitude? Or can I only receive him conditionally, acceptant of some aspects of his feelings and silently or openly disapproving of other aspects?[6]

The nurse usually is threatened when she or he cannot accept certain aspects of the patient's beliefs or behavior. Clearly, the nurse must be able to accept those characteristics of the patient that she or he cannot accept in herself or himself.

Can I act with sufficient sensitivity in the relationship that my behavior will not be perceived as a threat?[7]

If the patient is as free as possible from external threats, he may be able to experience and deal with the internal feelings that he finds threatening.

Can I let myself enter fully into the world of his feelings and personal meanings and see these as he does? Can I step into his private world so completely that I lose all desire to evaluate or judge it?[8]

Evaluative comments are not conducive to personal growth, and therefore they should not be a part of a helping relationship. For example, positive evaluation is threatening because it serves notice that the patient is being evaluated and that a negative evaluation could be forthcoming. Self-evaluation leaves the responsibility with the patient, where it really belongs.

Rather than assisting a patient in making his own decisions, a nurse may impose her own opinions and solutions on the patient. Sometimes a nurse gives advice, moralizes, intellectualizes, and indirectly belittles the patient's feelings by failing to deal with them.[9]

Rogers listed four subtle attitudinal characteristics that are necessary for constructive personality change to occur. First, the nurse manifests empathic understanding of the patient. Second, the nurse manifests unconditional positive regard toward the patient. Third, the nurse is genuine or congruent, that is, her or his words match her or his feelings. Fourth, the nurse's responses match the patient's statements in the intensity of affective expression. These four conditions must be communicated to the patient. In an effort to conceptualize this process, Rogers formulated what he calls a process equation of a successful helping relationship: Genuineness plus empathy plus unconditional positive regard for the client equals successful therapy for the client (G + E + UPR = Success).[10]

The nurse can convey genuineness, empathy, and unconditional positive regard through four statements, including the feelings and actions that accompany them: "This is it," "I know that it must hurt," "I am here to help you if you want me and can use me," and "You don't have to face this alone."[11] These statements contain reality, empathy, and support or acceptance. It should be emphasized that the words of these statements are only one part of the communication process. As an old Indian once said about the treatment his people received from Anglos, "What you do speaks so loudly I cannot hear what you say!" To be effective, reality and empathy must be conveyed to the patient.

> Reality without empathy is harsh and unhelpful. Empathy about something that is not real is clearly meaningless and can only lead the client to what we have called non-choice. Reality and empathy together need support, both material and psychological, if decisions are to be carried out. Support in carrying out unreal plans is obviously a waste of time.[12]

Many studies on the nature of the helping relationship support the ideas of Rogers and Keith-Lucas. Various studies indicate three recurring themes as relevant to people who are considering entering nursing:

1. The nurse's ability to sensitively and accurately understand the patient in such a manner as to communicate deep understanding.
2. The nurse's ability to project nonpossessive warmth and acceptance of the patient.
3. The necessity for the nurse to be integrated, mature, and genuine.

Let us look at three characteristics of a successful helping relationship—genuineness, empathy, and acceptance—that seem so vital in the nurse-patient relationship.

Genuineness

Lowell wrote, "Sincerity is impossible unless it pervades the whole character." To be genuine in a nurse-patient relationship requires the nurse to be aware of her or his own inner feelings. If these inner feelings are consistent with the expressed behavior, it can be said that she or he is genuine and congruent. It is this quality of realness and honesty that allows the patient to keep a steady focus on reality.

To some nurses it may seem that reality is too brutal for the patient. Granted, the truth is not always painless; as an old saying goes, "The truth shall make ye free, but first it shall make ye miserable." It is also important to note that being open and honest is not a license to be brutal. A helpful, as opposed to a destructive, relationship is very much like the difference between a fatal dose and a therapeutic dose of a pain killer; it is only a matter of degree.

In the process of attempting to be transparently real, it is wise for nurses to evaluate their failures, their reasons for being less than honest. To protect patients from the truth about their health is to make a very serious judgment about them. It is to say that they are incapable of facing their real health problems. However, if the nurse provided only honesty in the relationship, it probably would not be very helpful to patients. The next component in the process, empathic understanding, is also needed.

Empathy

"First of all," he said, "if you can learn a simple trick, Scout, you'll get along a lot better with all kinds of folks. You never really understand a person until you consider things from his point of view—"
"Sir?"
"—until you climb into his skin and walk around in it."[13]

This passage from *To Kill a Mockingbird* accurately depicts the meaning of empathic understanding. It is literally an understanding of the emotions and feelings of another, not by the cognitive process but by a projection of one's personality into the personality of the other. It is a sort of vicarious experiencing of the feelings of the other to the degree that the nurse actually feels some of the pain the patient is suffering. Empathy requires the nurse to temporarily leave her or his own life space and to try to think, act, and feel as if the life space of the patient is her or his own. The Spanish writer, Una Muno, wrote, "Suffering is the life blood that runs through us all and binds us together."

The nurse communicates empathy when she listens and relates to the patient's complaints with understanding responses. If the nurse is pre-occupied with her own problems and feelings, her responses tend to be those of an efficient information-giver, a more comfortable role for the nurse but one which may cut off communication. Each of us needs the empathy of other people, and we are reassured when we feel that someone understands us. When positive emotions develop in the patient in response to the empathy of the nurse, they may provide the major motivating force in the patient.[14]

It is important that nurses maintain enough objectivity when they become empathic so that they can assist patients in overcoming health problems. Empathic understanding does no good unless it is communicated to the patient—to let him or her know that someone has a deep understanding of his or her predicament. This kind of understanding allows the patient to expand and clarify his or her own self-understanding. One way of communicating this kind of understanding is through active listening. Active listening is not mere tolerance; a nurse, for instance, has to really care and feel the emotions attached to the patient's words. Olga Roman Smiley and Charles W. Smiley cautioned:

Listen to the patient's tone of voice and note his manner of speaking, as well as his exact words. By listening, you are less apt to draw erroneous conclusions or cut off the patient so that meaningful material does not come out. Although silence appears to be an easy technique, it is hard to master. It can be used to give the patient time to organize his thoughts. It can be helpful to the nurse by preventing her from speaking too soon or jumping to conclusions. It can lead to empathy.[15]

The following three points express what listening with empathic understanding means:

1. Empathic listening means trying to see the situation the way the patient sees it.
2. Empathic listening means one must enter actively and imaginatively into the patient's situation and try to understand his or her life conditions.
3. Empathic listening does not mean maintaining a polite silence while we rehearse what we are going to say when we get a chance.

Once nurses are behaving genuinely and have empathic understanding toward the patient, the next step, which often occurs simultaneously, is acceptance.

Acceptance

It is worth repeating that nurses must be congruent or consistent in both their feelings and expressions of acceptance for patients. If nurses do not really accept patients yet attempt to express it, they will be giving a double message—acceptance and rejection. In such a case, the best that can happen is that patients will perceive these nurses to be phonies. The worst that can happen is that patient's self-esteem will be damaged. Double messages occur when feelings do not coincide with words.

A nurse's words may say, "I accept you and respect your feelings." But the nonverbal messages may be "I don't trust you," "Poor little insignificant you," "You are disgusting," and "You must be sick." Nonverbal messages that reflect more deeply held feelings are difficult to correct, because the owner does not have as much control over them as over words. Small children know this and are perceptive enough to sense these feelings. The words of Joe Louis to one of his boxing opponents illustrate this point: "You can run, but you can't hide from me."

The basic reasons for demonstrating acceptance are to build a relationship based on trust and openness, to establish a situation in which the patient is able to gain or maintain respect for self, and to develop an atmosphere through which the patient can come to respect others. The process involved in this aspect of the relationship is caring, and support is given through helpful feedback. Feedback is simply the expression of reactions to a behavior. In a sense, the patient will perceive the nurse's attitude of respect as an either/or proposition; either the nurse does or does not respect him or her. This may be an oversimplification, but if the patient perceives it in this manner, the consequences of that perception are real.

> As a health professional, the nurse assists patients to achieve optimum health states. She is responsible for doing something constructive with the behavioral feedback she receives from patients. For example, if a patient is angry and irritable, and translates these feelings into demanding behaviors, the nurse has two basic ways of responding: (1) She can avoid the patient, thus reinforcing his maladaptive behavior, or (2) the nurse can work with the patient to identify the source of his anxiety.[16]

To the extent that nurses can be themselves as persons, expressing their real selves, hopefully with empathic understanding for their patients, they will be helpful in promoting the health of their patients.

SOCIOCULTURAL CONDITIONS

This section deals briefly with the various views of human beings, the healthy nurse, social class and poverty, and social helping—a potpourri of sorts. In other words, it deals with the question asked by the little girl after being given a long list of information and data: "And what else?"

Various Views of Human Beings

Every human being has a totally unique inner nature. This inner self ("real self" according to Arthur Janov, "inner nature" according to Abraham H. Maslow) has characteristics that may be described in different ways. Maslow lists several ways of characterizing the inner self in *Psychology of Being:*

1. The inner self is biologically based. It is, in many ways, unchangeable or at least unchanging.

2. Each person's inner self is unique to him or her.

3. We may only discover the inner self; we cannot add to it or subtract from it.

4. The inner self is good or neutral—not bad.

5. If the inner self is allowed to develop, happiness is the result.

6. If the inner self is denied or suppressed, sickness develops.

7. Because the inner nature is not strong or overpowering, it may easily be suppressed by socialization.

8. Yet, even though denied, the inner self does not disappear. It merely persists underground forever pressing for self-actualization.[17]

Janov believes that the core of each person is the real self. The real self has real needs that must be met early in life to survive. Hunger, the need to be held, and the need to be loved are all real needs.[18] Obviously, if a child is not fed, he or she will die. This real need is universally recognized. The need to be held was not completely recognized until World War II, when the Naxis put infants into a room and only fed them. As a result of not being held, all the children died. The need to be loved is as universally recognized as it is misunderstood. The real self must be fed with real love—the unconditional love Eric Fromm talked about or the "ok-ness" Thomas A. Harris described. If an adult does not get real love, he or she will not die but will instead split with the real self to survive.

Several characteristics are frequently confused with the inner self. Some of these characteristics are entrenched in political philosophy, public education, religion, and superstition. Biblical phrases such as "spare the rod and spoil the child," for example, imply some basic instinct in humans toward evil. Superstition, added to religious phrases such as this, implies that the evilness must be beaten out of the person so that "the demon won't creep out." Hence, the inner self is often considered evil.

Certain defensive feelings, such as jealousy, hate, and hostility, are often thought to be inborn in human beings. According to A. S. Neill, this is not true. Neill worked with children in his Summerhill School and found that after psychological treatment, children could refrain from expressing feelings of hate, hostility, and jealousy. Because they had learned these feelings, they could learn to refrain from expressing them.[19]

Janov claims that primal patients do not express (or have) feelings of hate, hostility, or jealousy. According to Janov, anger may be real or unreal; fear may be real or unreal; guilt may be true guilt or socialized guilt. Hence, these feelings are not always inborn in the individual.

Defenses are not part of the patient's real self but are added for protection, which is not protection at all. Transactional analysts say that defenses are seen in games, manipulations, ulterior transactions, and similar endeavors undertaken by children and adults. We are not born manipulators; we are taught to be manipulators. Maslow believed some defenses are desirable. He further believed that frustration, deprivation, and punishment are ways to fulfill and feed our inner selves. Whether they are expressing the real or unreal self, a disproportionate number of nonwhite patients display jealousy, hate, and hostility. An equal number become manipulators to survive.

The environment's effect on the patient is filtered through each person's perceptual apparatus. Thus a black patient may in reality be living in a ghetto, but if she does perceive herself to be a ghetto dweller, that perception has more effect on her behavior than her environment. A nurse may be open, flexible, and democratic, but if a patient perceives her or him to be closed, rigid, and authoritarian, the consequences of that perception will stifle the nurse-patient interaction. Humanistic nursing takes a relativistic view of reality. It leaves the patient as the center of decision making and responsibility. If one holds to the behavioristic or Freudian views, the patient is not considered the initiator of his or her acts and thus is not responsible. The Freudian view of the helping relationship tends to make helping a manipulative relationship, with the patient being the object rather than the subject of the relationship.

Many basic needs affect the nurse-patient relationship. Maslow divided these basic needs into five major categories:

1. Physiological needs (food, water, and shelter).
2. Safety or security needs (free from physical and psychological attack).
3. The needs for love, affection, and belonging.
4. Esteem (self-concept) needs.
5. The need for self-actualization.

Until the first four needs are met, the fifth need, which is a rather abstract concept of potentiality and self-development, is virtually unseekable.

> If the needs of the indigent are to be met, health workers must understand how the culture of poverty influences the behavior of the poor, and how their own middle-class norms and values intrude and influence their value judgments and promote a negative response to health services by the poor. The poor are often stereotyped as lazy, sexually promiscuous, dirty, irresponsible, and uncaring. The person with the middle-class values of cleanliness, gratification deferment, and individual responsibility often views with contempt those with differing characteristics and those dependent on public assistance.[20]

In another vein, Donald Snygg lists three pertinent points for the nurse to be aware of. First, the basic goal of all individuals is for a feeling of increased worth, of greater personal value. (This goal is never completely reached.) Second, given one success, a degree of self-enhancement, human beings will always aspire to more success. Third, satisfaction of the need for greater personal value can be and is sought in a number of alternative ways.[21] Consumer goods and good health are of value to the patient only as they contribute to the feeling of positive self-worth.

Patient participation in the health plan is a goal often sought by nurses, but the authoritarian nature of their methods prevents most patients from being optimally involved in their rehabilitation. The key requirement for participation is freedom. In most health care settings, there are too many barriers in the path of patient freedom. Studies comparing the maze-learning ability of rats raised in a cage and periodically run through mazes with that of free-roaming rats conclude that the free-roaming rats outperform the caged rats in maze learning and more complex behavior. But rats are not people!

In hospitals that patients perceive as authoritarian, social dimensions become more than a boundary; they become barriers to openness. Patients become prisoners cut off from communicating with their jailers (nurses). Under these conditions, patients can easily become defensive, psychological cripples. In the following passage, Earl C. Kelley describes this process:

> Defenses are necessary, provided they do not become so impervious that they imprison that which they defend. It often happens that defenses are inadequate for the dangers of living. This happens most often to the very young, who have tender psychological selves and inadequate protection. In these cases, which are numerous, the self becomes damaged, and in serious cases crippled. These psychological cripples have to behave as cripples do, and their actions are at wide variance with what is "expected" of them in our culture. From this group society gets its criminals, its deviates, its so-called insane. The person is crippled by conditions over which he has little control, and then because he behaves in a crippled fashion we say he is delinquent, or "insane."
>
> This is not because we are inhuman, or devoid of human compassion. Our hearts go out to the physical cripple, and great deference is properly paid to him. If we could see the psychological cripple our blame, hostility, and rejection would be changed to love, and tender nurture. We would not expect him to step lively, and look out for himself. We would cease to subject him to the many forms of rejection which we have devised for those who do not conform.[22]

It should be obvious from the preceding discussion that both the nurse's and the patient's frames of reference are important in health care. The question now arises: What are the criteria for a socially and psychologically healthy nurse? One answer, of course, is that the healthy nurse is mature, which is what the next section is about.

The Healthy Nurse

William James once said, "An unlearned carpenter of my acquaintance once said in my hearing: 'There is very little difference between one man and another; but what little there is, is very important.' " We have already built a case for the assumption that the inner self is good and desirable. We may also assume that a healthy nurse is a person who *is* her or his inner self, and a healthy nurse who is her or his inner self is self-actualizing. Or stated another way, health is self-actualization. The healthy nurse is free to make choices. She or he is free to sift through alternatives and choose which alternative is best. She or he is free because of this awareness of alternatives.

All people have options. All people make choices every day. Yet, not all choices are made out of awareness. An example of a nurse making an unaware choice is losing control of her temper and blaming the patient for this loss, such as "You *made* me angry." An example of making a choice through awareness is expression of direct anger. If anger is turned inward, it becomes depression. If anger is turned outward with responsibility and directly at the source of anger, the result is anger with awareness.

> When a patient comes for ambulatory care, we, the caregivers, expect him to take an active part in making decisions and setting goals. But these expectations are not always realized and conflict results—conflict in what we want from the patient and in what the patient wants from us. The anger that a caregiver feels can be used as a signal to look at what is disturbing the patient.[23]

The healthy nurse is a self-regulated person. Self-regulation is learned early in life and continues to strengthen and develop as the nurse matures. Self-regulation means the right to live freely, without undue outside authority. The healthy nurse operates in the here and now. She or he is primarily concerned with the present, not the past. And to repeat for emphasis, the healthy nurse is aware of choices and accepts responsibility for her or his behavior.

The healthy nurse is a perceptive person. She or he does not see everything in dichotomous terms—good or bad, childish or mature, and so forth. She or he has insight into the behavior of patients yet does not exploit that insight. She or he uses insight to empathize with the suffering of her or his patients. On the same note, that insight gives the nurse the ability to vicariously identify with the pleasures of patients.

It is also important to note that nurses who accept patients perceive them positively and attempt to understand them to facilitate an improved health care climate.[23] Several studies have shown that if a nurse has a positive perception of the patient, that is, if she or he thinks the patient is a capable person, the patient responds favorably to treatment. It is extremely important that nurses by aware of their racial/ethnic beliefs and value systems. The following four aspects of a nurse's value system are important. First, a nurse is often unaware of her or his racial/ethnic beliefs until forced to look at them. Second, some of the nurse's values conflict with others. Third, the values a nurse espouses are often different from her or his actions. Fourth, some nursing values are impossible to realize because they are inconsistent with the facts of life. Gilbert C. Wrenn made five suggestions that can be considered values and principles of a basic humanistic nursing credo:

1. I shall strive to see the positive in the patient and praise it at least as often as I notice that which is to be corrected.

2. If I am to correct or criticize a patient's action, I must be sure that this is seen by him or her as a criticism of a specific behavior and not as criticism of himself or herself as a person.

3. I shall assume that each patient can see some reasonableness in his or her behavior, that there is meaning in it for him or her if not for me.

4. When I contribute to a patient's self-respect, I increase his or her positive feelings toward me and his or her respect for me.

5. To at least one patient, perhaps many, I am a person of significance, and he or she is affected vitally by my recognition of him or her and my good will toward him or her as a person.[24]

Social Class and Poverty

Nurses should be aware of some other ideas about helping. Specifically, most writers suggest that the following must occur before individuals will ask for help. First, they must recognize that something is wrong that they can do nothing about without help. Second, they must be willing to talk to someone about the problem. Third, they must give that person some right to tell them what to do. Finally, they must be willing to change in some way.

All of this is very threatening to the patient's equilibrium and self-concept. In hospitals this puts lower-class patients in a particularly difficult situation because of their relatively low self-esteem. To them, seeking help may be a degrading process.

> The feeling of powerlessness which characterizes the culture of poverty stems from poor people's dependency on organizations to meet their socioeconomic and health needs. Frequently, these agencies are impersonal, bureaucratic structures that decide how much financial assistance a family will receive for food and clothing, whether or not they will have a telephone, where they are to live, what they are to learn, and where they are to receive their health care.[25]

SOCIAL HELPING

Numerous studies have focused on the helping relationship with lower-class persons. August B. Hollingshead and Frederick C. Redlich observed that therapists have more positive feelings toward patients whose social class standings are comparable to their own.[29] It seems reasonable then that nurses also tend to have more positive feelings for patients of their own ethnic or socioeconomic class. George Banks, Bernard G. Berenson, and Robert R. Carkhuff found that helpers who are different from their clients in terms of race and social class have the greatest difficulty effecting constructive changes, whereas helpers who are similar to their clients in these respects have the greatest facility for doing so.[27]

It is important to note that ethnic minority group patients need more (or a different kind of) attention than other patients. Of course this is an overgeneralization, since each patient should be looked at individually to determine his or her needs. Even so, it is imperative that nurses be cognizant of barriers created by ethnic or social class differences. If Chicano patients are hesitant to trust an Anglo nurse, for example, it may be because they do not trust members of that particular ethnic group, or it may be because the nurse's nonverbal messages are "stay away." Rather than guess, it is better to ask patients what they think the difficulty may be. If this is done tactfully, this will get the issue out in the open with a minimum of defensiveness. It may be that the patients are not aware of their nontrusting behavior, or the nurse may have been projecting her or his own nontrusting attitude onto the patients. It is best to get and keep these feelings, perceptions, and thoughts out in the open so that trust can be built. This does not mean that the nurse-patient relationship is always nice and sweet.

Most nonwhite patients' problems are rooted in their social environments. Certainly family therapy is an alternative. Another alternative is social action designed to change health care organizations. One of the reasons why many nurses are continually frustrated is because the problems they are called on to solve are themselves the products of other institutional or community organizations. If nurses really want to be helpful, some of them will have to be active in community change. The most significant changes they can make, however, involve their own jobs.

Frequently a patient's rehabilitation depends not on his or her adjustment to a particular health facility but instead on being placed in another one. This kind of environmental changes is not without a theoretical foundation; it is modeled after milieu therapy, preventative and community or social psychiatry. We can take as our illustration the model of milieu therapy, in which the hospital environment serves as a therapeutic instrument, and patterns of human relationships are consciously attuned to the treatment or developmental needs of the residents. When this model is applied to nonwhite patients, it becomes clear that more often than not nonwhite patients do not get the institutional treatment they need, because community health resources are not attuned to their needs. There are at least seven steps nurses can and must take if all patients are to be aided and allowed to become fully functioning persons:

1. Regard each patient as a vital part of the health care process.
2. View all patients positively, because whatever diminishes a patient's self—humiliation, degradation, or failure—has no place in nursing.

3. Provide for individual differences.

4. Apply the criteria of self-actualization to every health care experience.

5. Learn how things are seen by their patients.

6. Allow rich opportunities for patients to explore themselves and their health care environment.

7. Help patients to become independent.

Since sensitivity to their own feelings is a prerequisite to effective helping, it may be beneficial for nurses to undergo some type of multicultural sensitivity training. Numerous studies show extensive evidence for the idea that nurses trained in such programs are more successful in helping Third World patients. If the research studies reviewed are correct in their assertion that helping can be accomplished only on the terms of the healthier person in the relationship, it becomes necessary to have some criteria for determining who is best able to assist culturally different patients. Nurses who have not gotten themselves together emotionally are not able to assist patients in getting themselves together.

Many studies have been conducted that indicate the importance of the interpersonal relations between the nurse and the patient. The implications of these studies should be self-evident. The nurse-patient relationship may be for better or worse, that is, the development of patients' health adjustment may be helped or retarded because of the type of relationship they have with nurses. When patients believe that nurses value and respect them, they are likely to value and respect themselves.

Three major assumptions about the universality of helping should be remembered. First, everyone at times has emotional problems that we experience as unpleasant and painful. Second, everyone seeks help for his or her personal problems. Third, everyone offers help to others who are experiencing emotional difficulties. When William Menninger was asked how many people suffer from emotional illness, he answered, "One out of one of us." The help we seek may come from a spouse, colleague, friend, or nurse. It is clear that a part of a patient's needs must be met in her or his relationship with the nurse.

SUMMARY

It has been proposed by several organizations that nursing education include skills needed to effectively work with culturally diverse patients. Nurse commitment to cultural pluralism is exemplified by those who demonstrate a willingness to both accept change and to change themselves. The role of the nurse in implementing ethnic and cultural pluralism includes the following dimensions of intergroup relations: identity consciousness, validation of differences, minority group advocacy, collaborative and cooperative strategies, conflict resolution, and risk taking.

Validation of differences suggests that nurses go beyond simply valuing cultural dissimilarities; they must take an active stance in protecting cultural differences.

Minority group advocacy requires "placing one's self in another's shoes; it means listening rather than telling. . . . Advocacy thinking should lead to a clarification of differences between persons, and to a recognition of when it is or is not possible to collaborate."[28]

Nurses can best serve themselves and their patients when they recognize and prepare for conflict situations. Conflict is inevitable in society. It can be a destructive force that breeds differences, hostility, and alienation, or it can become a creative force that encourages open and constructive problem solving.

Nurses should understand that social changes require risk taking. Risk nothing, or everything, and your commitment is questioned. Risking something specific in a thoughtful, calculated manner seems to be the best strategy for change. Black, Indian, and Latino nurse caucuses are excellent illustrations of group efforts to make the nursing profession more active in affirmative action and multicultural education.

It is hazardous enough to risk educational and employment opportunities or peer approval with one's eyes open. To do so in ignorance is to invite needless failure and pain. Ethnicity and poverty complicate nurse-patient interactions; however, they are neither irreversible assets nor liabilities. It is our hope that this book has added a measure of understanding about multicultural problems in nursing.

References

1. Robertson, H. R. 1969. Removing barriers to health care. *Nurs. Outlook* 17:45.

2. Rogers, C. R. 1958. The characteristics of a helping relationship. *Personnel Guid. J.* 37:6.

3. Keith-Lucas, A. 1972. *Giving and taking help.* Chapel Hill, N.C.: University of North Carolina Press, p. 46.

4. Combs, A. W. 1969. *Florida studies in the helping professions.* Gainesville, Fla.: University of Florida Press, p. 3.

5. Rogers, C. R. 1958. The characteristics of a helping relationship. *Personnel Guid. J.* 37:12.

6. Rogers, C. R. 1958. The characteristics of a helping relationship. *Personnel Guid. J.* 37:13-14.

7. Rogers, C. R. 1958. The characteristics of a helping relationship. *Personnel Guid. J.* 37:14.

8. Rogers, C. R. 1958. The characteristics of a helping relationship. *Personnel Guid. J.* 37:13.

9. Ramaekers, Sister M. J. 1979. Communication blocks revisited. *Am. J. Nurs.* 79:1080.

10. See Rogers, C. R. 1961. The process equation of psychotherapy. *Am. J. Psychotherapy* 15:27-45.

11. Keith-Lucas, A. 1972. *Giving and taking help.* Chapel Hill, N.C.: University of North Carolina Press, p. 70.

12. Keith-Lucas, A. 1972. *Giving and taking help.* Chapel Hill, N.C.: University of North Carolina Press, p. 88.

13. Lee, H. 1960. *To kill a mockingbird.* New York: Popular Library, p. 34.

14. Robertson, H. R. 1969. Removing barriers to health care. *Nurs. Outlook* 17:45.

15. Smiley, O. R.; and Smiley, C. W. 1974. Interviewing techniques for nurses. *Comm. Health* 6:102.

16. Seeger, P. A. 1977. Self-awareness and nursing. *J. Psychiatric Nurs.* 15:25.

17. Maslow, A. H. 1962. *Toward a psychology of being.* New York: D. Van Nostrand Co., pp. 3-5.

18. Janov, A. 1970. *The primal scream.* New York: Dell Publishing Co., Inc.

19. Neill, A. S. 1960. *Summerhill.* New York: Hart Publishing Co., Inc.

20. Robertson, H. R. 1969. Removing barriers to health care. *Nurs. Outlook* 17:44.

21. Snygg, D. 1971. The psychological basis of human values. In Avila, D. L.; Combs, A. W.; and Purkey, W. W., editors. *The helping relationship sourcebook.* Boston: Allyn & Bacon, Inc., p. 86.

22. Kelley, E. C. 1971. Another look at individualism. In Avila, D. L.; Combs, W.; and Purkey, W. W., editors. *The helping relationship sourcebook.* Boston: Allyn & Bacon, Inc., p. 315.

23. Gruber, K. A., and Schniewind, H. E., Jr. 1976. Letting anger work for you. *Am. J. Nurs.* 76:1450.

24. Wrenn, G. C. 1958. Psychology, religion and values for the counselor. *Personnel Guid. J.* 36:43.

25. Robertson, H. R. 1969. Removing barriers to health care. *Nurs. Outlook* 17:44.

26. Hollingshead, A. B.; and Redlich, F. C. 1958. *Social class and mental illness.* New York: John Wiley & Sons, Inc., p. 176.

27. Banks, G.; Berenson, B. G.; and Carkhuff, R. F. 1957. The effects of counselor race and training upon Negro clients in initial interviews. *J. Clin. Psychol.* 23:70-72.

28. Larson, R. C.; and Elliott, L. F. 1976. Planning and pluralism: Some dimensions of intergroup relations. *J. Negro Ed.* 45:95.

Part III Review

SUMMARY

We have only scratched the surface of methods for establishing rapport with culturally different patients. Concern for their status causes some Third World people to view every white person with deep suspicion. Chicanos, for example, are on their guard when around Anglos. The rise in nationalism among Third World people sometimes results in prejudice against whites. Extreme nationalistic sentiments result in the erroneous belief that only a health provider from a patient's own ethnic group is qualified to assist him or her.

The challenge to the health professional is to demonstrate that competence and empathy are not traits unique to members of a particular ethnic group. For example, competent, sensitive white nurses can, when judged by their deeds, be considered as black as any of the black patients assigned to their wards. Blackness is more than a condition of the skin: it is thinking and behaving in ways acceptable to black Americans. Black patients grudgingly admit that these nurses have "soul." Similarly, competent black nurses have been able to demonstrate to white patients that some black Americans have "culture."

The first step in establishing rapport with patients is to help them relax. To do so, caregivers must be relaxed. If they are worried about being physically or verbally attacked, nurses will not relax. Generally, patients are also anxious about their initial contact with health professionals. For most low-income patients, the presence of professionals produces feelings of great discomfort. Even their decision to withdraw involves anxiety. During these stressful periods, health plans or conversations related to them may only serve to panic patients. Nurses must learn to slow the pace and talk about less threatening subjects. A few minutes of informal conversation can often reduce stress.

Some culturally different patients approach nurses in ways that are outright defensive. Most individuals using defense mechanisms usually do not have faulty personalities. Instead, it is their home and health environments that are faulty. Protection of the ego is normal, and disproportionate use of defenses indicates a lack of security. Rationalizations, reaction formation, regression, and other defense behaviors are ways patients try to maintain their psychological balance. Patients who imagine that they are objects of a caregiver's rejection develop rigid, persistent, and chronic ego-protection devices. Continued feelings of rejection will result in behavior inappropriate to reality. An example is the Native American patient who imagined that all Anglo nurses disliked him. To protect himself, he withdrew from all voluntary contact with them. One concerned nurse asked him, "Why do you avoid me?" He answered, "Because you don't like me. You smile at all the white patients but you never smile at me." Issues that center on race or ethnic identity frequently cause patients and nurses to overreact.

Many nurses are disappointed when their patients respond to their efforts by being unfriendly. These nurses vindictively conclude that their patients are inferior people; they see patient faults that do not exist. There is a bit of irony in situations where historically rejected patients (low-income ethnic minorities) reject their rejectors (nurses). Unfortunately, few nurses appreciate this irony. When nurses discover that they are not very successful with Third World people or low-income people, they tend to avoid future assignments in inner-city and depressed rural area hospitals.

It is understandable and regrettable that student nurses who have not been adequately prepared to work with culturally different people develop negative attitudes about assignments to hospitals containing large numbers of such patients. Nurses who fear Third World people seek employment in white suburban communities with grossly exaggerated claims of "no problems."

Recommendations

With the preceding observations in mind, we make the following recommendations to individuals concerned with improving transcultural health care:

1. Determine which language the patient prefers to speak and, where possible, speak it or use an interpreter. If you do not speak the patient's native language(s), do not criticize them for speaking it among themselves and with their relatives. Admonishing patients to "speak only English here" is likely to alienate them.

2. Become familiar with local medical beliefs and practices. Clark recommends that "the use of ridicule should be avoided in all situations. ... For example, if a mother suggests that her child is suffering from 'fallen fontanelle,' a doctor or nurse might point out that Anglos call this disorder by another name—dehydration. Differences in ideas of etiology might simply be ignored. Conflict might be avoided by saying, 'Yes, I know about that disease, but it seems to me that this is something else.' "[1]

3. Prescribe meals containing food common in the patient's diet, such as Spanish rice, chili sauce, tortillas, and pinto beans for Chicanos. When in doubt about food preference, ask the patient. This strategy will avoid serving "hot" food when patients would prefer "cold" food and vice versa.

4. Allow relatives to visit as often as possible; however, it is not recommended that patients be spatially segregated by ethnic backgrounds in rooms, wards, and floors.

5. Avoid patronizing or condescending approaches to patients or their relatives. Treat people as you would like to be treated.

6. Never make fun of a patient's religious beliefs. Religious freedom is a constitutional and human right of all persons.

7. Take advantage of opportunities to learn about people in other cultures.

Questions for Further Study

1. When should health care providers insist on Western instead of traditional Third World treatment of sick persons?

2. What are the ethical issues inherent in imposing Anglo medical values and practices on non-Anglos?

3. What specifically should the health care provider know about ethnic food preferences?

4. How, if in any way, do ethnic group beliefs influence personality development?

5. What are the best ways to find out an ethnic group's traditional medical beliefs and practices?

6. How does religion affect the practice and transfer of medical practices?

References

1. Clark, M. 1970. *Health in the Mexican-American culture: A community study*. Berkeley: University of California Press, p. 226.

EXERCISES

Exercise 1: Challenge

At a party you become involved in an argument with a friend, who believes that health professionals should not become personally or emotionally involved with poor patients/clients. "We don't need any more bleeding heart liberals," he chides you. "Besides, they don't appreciate people who try to help them. They don't want to do anything except have a lot of illegitimate babies, live off welfare, and try to force our children to go to school with their illiterate brats."

1. How will you respond?
2. What erroneous assumptions is your friend making?
3. What if the assumptions are true?

Exercise 2: Transcultural Goals

Now that you have read this book, select two or three transcultural goals that are important to you. Focus on strategies for achieving these goals. Basically, the steps for achieving personal goals are:

1. Set realistic goals.
2. Analyze the factors that support or block your goal achievement.
3. Plan ways to lessen the effect of blocking forces and still maintain the supporting forces. (Set definite, realistic time limits.)
4. Experiment with new behavior and evaluate its effectiveness.

Factors That Support Your Goals

Factors in self:

Factors in others:

Factors in work/school situation:

Factors That Block Your Goals

Factors in self:

Factors in others:

Factors in work/school situation:

Exercise 3: Counseling Styles

It is important that health care providers understand and feel comfortable with their own unique counseling styles. The following questions may have more than one answer, but you are asked to circle the letter (a, b, c, or d) of the *one* response in each question that best reflects your point of view.

1. An effective practitioner:
   a.   Remains detached from her or his patients.
   b.   Is a member of a health care unit that performs special functions.
   c.   Is mainly a resource person for the patient.
   d.   Is really just an ordinary member of the medical team.
2. During a group counseling session, I would guide by:
   a.   Staying out of the discussion most of the time.
   b.   Using occasional interventions to focus the discussion on relevant issues.
   c.   Supporting ideas valued by leaders in the group.
   d.   Providing behind-the-scenes leadership.
3. I would invite patient discussion of my behavior to show:
   a.   That I am an expert in my field.
   b.   That I am a real person.
   c.   That he or she need not be afraid of me.
   d.   That it is safe to try out new behavior.
4. The most vivid example of communication behavior that shows Third World people that they are important is:
   a.   Not interrupting.
   b.   Talking very little.
   c.   Agreeing with a shy person.
   d.   Not giving negative feedback.
5. When patients express their feelings, I would:
   a.   Help them explore the causes of their feelings.
   b.   Keep uninvolved.
   c.   Try tactfully to indicate that feelings have no place in a health care discussion.
   d.   Encourage them to withhold personal feelings until they can meet with me in private.
6. If a patient becomes angry with me, I would:
   a.   Respond objectively to facilitate rehabilitation.
   b.   Reflect his or her feelings to help him or her better think them through.
   c.   Respond naturally to be myself.
   d.   Not respond.
7. My main goal in counseling low-income, poorly educated patients would be to encourage them to:
   a.   Do things and analyze them.
   b.   Explore basic motivations of human behavior.
   c.   Learn how to cope with health problems.
   d.   Visit a local folk healer for additional assistance.
8. It is most helpful to patients when the care provider:
   a.   Shares gossip and food.
   b.   Surprises them with unexpected visits.

    c.   Administers the health plan efficiently.

    d.   Learns local customs.

9. If a minority-group patient wants to take over the counseling function I would:

    a.   Clarify professional and patient roles.

    b.   Encourage him or her to assume leadership.

    c.   Help him or her to see how inadequate he or she would be.

    d.   Confer with a colleague before making a decision.

10. Which of the following is the most important characteristic of an effective health professional:

    a.   Ability to maintain consistent behavior.

    b.   Unusual skill in facilitating patient independence.

    c.   Ability to handle herself or himself with minimum strain in conflict situations.

    d.   Strict adherence to institutional regulations.

Note: Perhaps you would like to discuss your answers with a person whose behavior you believe best represents your profession. Keep in mind the counseling trilogy of congruence, empathy, and positive regard as benchmarks of effective counselors. To this list we could add commitment to individual growth and self-actualization. In many instances these characteristics conflict. Do your responses and that of other persons suggest that you highly value these characteristics? If not, what do you seem to value more?

Index